HOW TO
GET PREGNANT
WITH THE
NEW TECHNOLOGY

HOW TO GET PREGNANT WITH THE NEW TECHNOLOGY

A World-renowned Fertility Expert Tells You What Really Works, What Doesn't, and Why

SHERMAN J. SILBER, M.D.

Illustrations by William C. Andrea

WARNER BOOKS

A Time Warner Company

This book is not intended as a substitute for the medical advice of physicians. The reader should regularly consult a physician in matters relating to his/her health and particularly with respect to any symptoms that may require diagnosis or medical attention.

This book contains many references to actual cases the author has encountered over the years. However, names and other identifying characteristics have been changed to protect the privacy of those involved.

Warner Books, Inc., 666 Fifth Avenue, New York, NY 10103

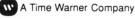 A Time Warner Company

Printed in the United States of America
First printing: January 1991
10 9 8 7 6 5 4 3 2 1

Library of Congress Cataloging-in-Publication Data
Silber, Sherman J.
    How to get pregnant with the new technology : a world-renowned
fertility expert tells you what really works, what doesn't, and why
/ Sherman J. Silber.
        p.   cm.
    Includes bibliographical references and index.
    ISBN 0-446-51498-5
    1. Human reproductive technology—Popular works.   I. Title.
RG133.5.S55   1991
616.6'9206—dc20   90-50279
                                                                    CIP

Book design by Giorgetta Bell McRee

To my faithful, hard-working staff, at my office and at St. Luke's Hospital in St. Louis. For over a decade they have acted as tireless workers, organized scientific and medical personnel, and as concerned, warm counselors to my patients. The many advances we have made would not have been possible without their exceptional dedication.

ACKNOWLEDGMENTS

I would like to thank my friend and colleague Dr. Robert Cohen, also of St. Louis, Missouri, and my colleagues from around the world (many of whom are mentioned in this book) who have shared their knowledge and new ideas so selflessly. It has been this international sharing of new advances that allows us today to help most infertile couples have a baby.

I would especially like to thank Dr. Ricardo Asch and his team at the University of California/Irvine for their collaboration and friendship over the years. Their creativity has helped greatly to popularize the new reproductive technology by dramatically improving pregnancy rates around the world, even in institutions that otherwise would not have ventured into this "brave new world."

CONTENTS

HOW TO GET PREGNANT WITH THE NEW TECHNOLOGY

PREFACE

The Infertility Epidemic

Twenty-five percent of couples in their thirties are infertile. Only 1 percent of teenagers are. There is a worldwide, emotionally wrenching epidemic of infertility, making it our nation's number one public health problem. Even in a country like India with severe *over*population, the most common reason for a visit to the doctor is infertility. From our teen years (when the last thing we really want is a child) to our mid-thirties when we finally feel emotionally and financially secure enough to start our family, there is a twenty-five fold decline in our ability to get pregnant.

If you are in your thirties, have been working hard establishing yourself, and are now just casually thumbing through this chapter at a local bookstore because you're thinking maybe in a few years you might like to start a family, you should realize that there is a 25 percent chance you will not be able to do so without medical intervention.

These startling figures came out of the National Center for Health Statistics in 1985 and were presented to the United States Congress through a panel assembled by the Congressional Office of Technology Assessment in 1988. I was one of five physicians on that Congressional Advisory Panel. We have all witnessed an explosive increase in couples desperately struggling to have a child but it wasn't until these statistics were formally assembled that we were stunned to find out just how staggering the problem is.

What accounts for this dramatic increase in infertility over the last twenty years? We could speculate about the increase in sexually transmitted diseases, environmental pollution, declining sperm count from absorption of toxic substances, and even the increased tension and anxiety of modern life. These may very well be contributing factors, but a major reason is simply that by the time the modern couple decides to have children, usually in their thirties, the human animal is just not as fertile as it was when younger.

Further analysis of these statistics, however, shows that age is not the only factor. In 1965, 18.4 percent of couples in their thirties were infertile, whereas in 1982, this figure had jumped to 24.6 percent. In younger, less infertile groups ages twenty to twenty-four, in 1965, only 3.6 percent were infertile; and in 1982, 10.5 percent were infertile. So we are no longer in a position of just *speculating* that there is an infertility problem which is on the rise. Hard, cold statistics show that nearly a quarter of the population that is trying to start a family cannot do so without medical help. A major contribution is the putting off of childbearing until later years, but this alone does not completely explain the increase in infertility because it is on the rise in younger people as well.

After this detailed report submitted to the U.S. Congress, what is the government doing about it? As one might expect, basically nothing. But there is help available. With dramatic new technology, virtually any couple (with a few exceptions) can have a child. But you are going to have to understand the myriad complexities of your own reproductive system in order to get the right help instead of the wrong help and also to figure out how to position yourself with your health insurance company in such a way as to get them to help bear the burden of the cost (as they should).

One of the views of the Congressional Advisory Panel that I was on (which consisted of lawyers, psychologists, sociologists, and religious leaders as well as doctors) was that society clearly benefited from this putting off of childbearing until the thirties. Both men and women are now able to obtain fuller educations, develop themselves in their careers, and contribute dramatically to the intellectual and economic prosperity of the modern world. This would not occur so readily if we were saddled with children as teenagers or in our early twenties. So if society is collectively making a decision to put off childbearing, it should be no one's position to advise couples condescendingly just to "hurry up" and have children when they're young. Luckily the new reproductive technology is a cost-effective solution for such couples, even though the insurance companies and government bureaucracy are often too dense to realize it.

THE NEW REPRODUCTIVE TECHNOLOGY

In *The New York Times Magazine* in December of 1989, a forty-one-year-old writer named Paulette conveyed her sense of loss at trying to have a child in her late thirties, not succeeding, and now finding herself a successful forty-one-year-old writer who sadly "will probably never have a baby." It wasn't until she reached age thirty-eight that she decided to stop using birth control pills and tried to get pregnant. She read a book called *Fertility Awareness* and hoped she could get pregnant "naturally" with just a little bit of help from knowing more about the timing of her cycle and the quality of her cervical mucus. It wasn't until she reached forty that she saw a local doctor who began "fertility testing," including mucus testing, hormone testing, and "two endometrial biopsies" (a tiny piece of the lining of the uterus is sampled to see if it is capable of sustaining a pregnancy).

She was then given a grand diagnosis of "luteal phase defect." This was a very popular diagnosis fifteen years ago, and many women were treated with progesterone supplementation in the second half of their cycle in an effort to "overcome" this problem. Later she was given an ovulatory stimulant pill, Clomid, because of the view that luteal phase defect is sometimes caused by a subtle "ovulation defect." She then went through a procedure called "intrauterine insemination" in which her husband's sperm was placed directly inside her uterus even though previous testing had shown that her cervical mucus was quite able to allow his sperm to penetrate on its own. These are simple, old methods of treatment that sometimes work and certainly make sense in a young woman trying to have a baby. But not for Paulette.

In fact, what Paulette went through is the conventional wisdom of trying to make a diagnosis and then using simple, non-invasive treatment appropriate to that diagnosis. The problem with this conventional wisdom is that, first, many of these "diagnoses" are just normal variants which have nothing to do with why the woman is not getting pregnant, and second, when time has almost run out, fiddling around for too long with the old-fashioned approaches may waste the few precious years you have left.

With the new in vitro fertilization (IVF) and GIFT technology, we can bypass all of the incredible hurdles that sperm and eggs have to go through (even in a fertile couple) in order to achieve a pregnancy. We simply have to admit our ignorance that we often really don't know why a couple isn't getting pregnant. The benefit of the new technology is that we can avoid being fooled and self-deceived as doctors into making artificial diagnoses (albeit well-meaning) trying to pinpoint the cause of the problem. With the new technology, we realize that it is an amazing ordeal for sperm and eggs to actually meet each other and, if they do fertilize, for the resulting embryo to manage to implant in the womb and become a successful pregnancy. In young couples, this happens more easily. But in older couples, despite the appearance of normalcy, it just doesn't happen so easily, and they may need all the help they can get in bypassing these hurdles.

I celebrated New Year's with our son's high school biology teacher (and swimming coach) and his thirty-nine-year-old wife, Pam, playing with their six-week-old baby, who never would have existed without the new technology of IVF and GIFT. She told me to make sure to tell everyone in this book how awful it is to go through the conventional series of "diagnostic" tests and ineffective treatments for years with one contradictory diagnosis after another and ineffective treatments. She had gone through seven years of this at the previous clinic she had used. She had two laparoscopic operations to remove tiny little implants of "endometriosis" and never got a satisfactory answer to her question of how her mother could have had five children despite huge implants of "endometriosis." When surgery didn't help, Pam was placed on progesterone, because they suddenly discovered "luteal phase defect," and finally Clomid. She had literally hundreds of pills and doctors' visits and tests.

Yet during a twenty-minute interview with them less than a year ago, I was able to tell her more accurately that I really didn't know why she wasn't getting pregnant. But her husband's sperm count was low (less than 20 million per cc), and she was in her late thirties. That was enough reason for them to be infertile, and I recommended *no more tests*. She was thrilled when I suggested we proceed right to the new technology with GIFT. I recommended no more hormone tests, X rays, laparoscopies, hamster tests, endometrial biopsies, basal body temperature charts, postcoital tests, etc. She was fed up with trying to figure out *why* she was infertile and getting nowhere. She conceived with the GIFT procedure, and now she and her husband have a healthy baby. She has no idea why she was infertile and neither do her original doctors who spent so much of her money on wild-goose chases.

MISLEADING DIAGNOSES OF THE CAUSE OF YOUR INFERTILITY

The Simple Unexplainable Effect of Age

Even in the best-conditioned athletes, age has a way of slowing us down, sometimes imperceptibly year by year, and it doesn't mean that there is any particular physical ailment or diagnosis to explain that slowdown. This is usually (though, of course, not always) the case in a couple who suddenly starts trying unsuccessfully to have babies in their mid-thirties.

In 1982, the French reported in the *The New England Journal of Medicine* on 2,193 supposedly "normal" women (whose husbands had no sperm whatsoever in their ejaculate) undergoing artificial insemination with fertile donor sperm. These were "normal" women and they were being inseminated with certainly normal sperm. There is no logical reason why they shouldn't all have gotten pregnant. Yet it was very clear that "normal" women under thirty had a high pregnancy rate, and "normal" women over thirty showed decreasing pregnancy rates the older they got. A more recent study from Ontario published in 1989 in *The Journal of Fertility and Sterility* looked at over 2,000 couples with "unexplained" infertility. The chances of getting pregnant with simple, conventional methods of treatment were directly related to how young the woman was. No other factor studied was significant except for age.

Just recently I saw a woman, typical of many others I see every month, who got pregnant very easily as a young teenager after her first sexual experience and gave the child up for adoption. Five years later, again she got pregnant quite easily with a single sexual experience and kept this baby as a single mother. She continued to have completely regular, normal periods for six more years, got married, and then used condoms for birth control for three years until she and her husband were certain that their marriage was a stable one. By the time they decided to try to have children, she was thirty-three years old, and her menstrual cycles by now had become irregular, varying from twenty-five to thirty-two days. All of her tests otherwise were normal, but now she couldn't get pregnant.

What happened to her subsequently is a terrifying story which exemplifies the pitfalls I am hoping to help you avoid with this book. She saw a doctor who diagnosed her as having "endometriosis" and "adhesions," despite the fact that her organs were quite normal. He performed major surgery on her to remove the endometriosis and release the adhesions. As long as insurance companies require a "pathological diagnosis" in order to get treatment paid for, and as long as major surgery results in no difficulty getting insurance payment (whereas in vitro fertilization requires major verbal acrobatics to get payment), women like her run a good chance of being mistreated in this fashion.

The "Endometriosis" Myth

The most common, overused "diagnosis" for infertility is "endometriosis." Endometriosis is a condition whereby some of the lining of the uterus has leaked back into the abdominal cavity and has implanted in little tiny nodules either in the abdominal wall, on the outside of the fallopian tube, or possibly in the ovary. When doctors perform a "laparoscopy" as part of an infertility investigation to see if the woman has a normal uterus, tubes, and ovaries, most of the time the examination is normal. Nonetheless the diagnosis of "endometriosis" is frequently put on the operative note just because the insurance company is much happier to pay for laparoscopy when they see a "pathological" diagnosis. The euphemism used to avoid the guilt of outright deception is to call it "minimal lesion" endometriosis. Doctors are often so anxious to find a diagnosis to determine the "cause" of infertility (not to mention the desire for patients to get insurance reimbursement) that many couples walk out of their long series of expensive infertility tests thinking incorrectly that they now know why they haven't gotten pregnant. This might be harmless if it weren't for the fact that it may lead to unnecessary or improper treatment.

The "Male Factor" Myth and "Varicocele"

There are there many popular "diagnoses" which may lead to inappropriate surgery that gets an infertile couple no closer to getting pregnant. The doctor may obtain a sperm count on the husband, find that it is "low" (below 40 million per cc), and not be aware of the fact that patients with low sperm counts often have little difficulty getting their wives pregnant. The husband may then be put on all kinds of totally ineffective drug treatments such as Clomid, Pergonal, HCG, testosterone, or, worst of all, be given that common diagnosis of "varicocele."

A varicocele is a varicose vein of the testicle (usually on the left side) that is present in 15 percent of all males on the planet. It is just a common, normal anatomic variant, but it has been blamed for close to 40 percent of "male infertility." In many of these cases of "male infertility" there is really nothing infertile about the man's sperm anyway, but even so the varicocele has little to do with it. A careful study of 651 infertile couples with varicocele was published in the *British Medical Journal* by the Australians in 1985 demonstrating absolutely no difference in pregnancy rate among couples whose husbands had the varicocele operated on versus those who did not have the varicocele operated on. Similar studies have been repeated in Belgium and in Sweden. Fifteen percent of the men who come to the office for a vasectomy because they already have had all the children they wanted are found to have a varicocele on physical examination, and in my experience that is the same incidence of varicocele in infertile couples. It has been argued that 40 percent of infertile men have varicoceles, and it is implied that the varicocele is the cause of the infertility. But many of these so-called "minimal lesion" varicoceles are really not varicoceles at all by the common definition and are no different from what is found in a normal, fertile population.

But what happens to these couples once the diagnosis of varicocele is made in the man? Typically, the men get operated on, sometimes on one side, sometimes on both sides, and then they wait six months to see if the sperm count improves. Since sperm counts, like the weather, vary from month to month around a mean average value, it only makes sense that if you get one sperm count before this unnecessary surgery and one sperm count after this unnecessary surgery, at least half of the men will appear to have some improvement. But this is an illusion created simply by the variability, the up and down of sperm counts, and the failure to make note of those whose sperm counts have gone down after varicocelectomy.

We see many men who were sent by their wives' gynecologists to a local urologist, who then makes a diagnosis of varicocele (even though there is none). He tells them the sperm count is too low, puts the man through surgery, and then claims some kind of improvement in sperm count. Meanwhile, the wife has wasted a year without treatment. The wife, her husband, and her gynecologist have all been under the illusion that they knew what the problem was, and that the "problem" was being corrected.

Sometimes the diagnosis of "poor cervical mucus" leads a woman to being placed on cough medicine in an effort to loosen up the mucus. Sometimes the diagnosis of "autommunity," i.e., that the wife is in some way allergic or immune to her husband's sperm, leads to the couple's being told to use condoms for a year in order to lower her "antibody levels." Sometimes the diagnosis of "low sperm count" which doesn't improve despite a wide variety of different therapies leads the couple to try artificial insemination with "donor" sperm, and the woman still doesn't get pregnant because the "low sperm count" really wasn't the cause of the problem in the first place.

In fact, the ability of the sperm to fertilize has very little to do with the sperm count but rather with a combination of not too fully understood factors, including quality of sperm motion, structure of the sperm, and, quite shockingly, the quality of the wife's eggs. Very poor sperm can often fertilize excellent eggs, whereas the best-quality sperm may be required to fertilize an egg from a relatively infertile woman. The most interesting example of this comes from cases of artificial insemination with donor sperm.

In couples whose husbands have absolutely zero sperm in the ejaculate, the use of donor sperm for artificial insemination results in a high pregnancy rate. For couples in whom the sperm count is low (i.e., there are some sperm present), the use of donor sperm results in a much lower pregnancy rate. Thus, we are often fooled into thinking the low sperm count was the cause of the infertility, when, in truth, in many, many cases it is not a cause of infertility. Only when the sperm count in the husband is zero is it clear that the cause of the infertility is bad sperm. Thus, infertility is in most cases a problem of "the couple," and cannot easily be attributed specifically just to the husband or just to the wife.

THE NEW TECHNOLOGY (IVF AND GIFT) BYPASSES EVERYTHING THAT CAN GO WRONG NO MATTER WHAT THE SO-CALLED "DIAGNOSIS" IS

The new technology of in vitro fertilization (IVF) and GIFT takes into account all of these problems and solves the quandary of our frequent ignorance of why couples are not getting pregnant. If the cause of the problem really is "low sperm count," the new technology allows sperm to be placed right next to the egg where they do not have to go through the incredible ordeal of transport up through the vagina, then the uterus, and finally the fallopian tube, a journey which results in only 10,000 out of the original

100 million sperm making it. If the cause of the problem is poor ovulation on the part of the woman, the hormonal stimulation of the ovaries and the removal of eggs from the ovaries removes the obligation for ovulation. If the problem is poor cervical mucus blocking the entrance of sperm into the womb, the new technology bypasses that problem. If the problem is "endometriosis" (a highly questionable but very popular viewpoint), again the new technology bypasses the theoretically unfavorable environment for fertilization that endometriosis supposedly creates in the woman's pelvis. If the problem is poor pickup of the egg by the fallopian tube from the surface of the ovary (a tricky feat in which the fallopian tube has to "reach over" and grab the egg by twisting back on itself), IVF and GIFT once again bypass this event.

Almost anything that can go wrong in the arduous process which sperm and eggs normally have to go through is bypassed and made easy by the new technology. In a sense, we are "introducing" the sperm directly to the egg in an ideal environment in which they can truly get to know each other and making things much easier for them to get along. The fact is that no matter what the diagnosis (except that of completely blocked fallopian tubes or terribly low sperm count), the GIFT technique will result in a pregnancy rate of 45 percent for each treatment cycle attempted despite many, many years of prior infertility and despite what the diagnosis is, whether correctly or incorrectly having been made.

Change in Thinking Now from the Early 1980s

My first book, *How to Get Pregnant*, emphasized simpler treatments for infertility in the 1980s. It also explained as much as we knew at that time about the details of just exactly how difficult it is for the sperm and egg to meet and result in a successful pregnancy. I have received hundreds of thousands of happy responses from people who have read that book, and the methodology described in much of that book is still valid (particularly the chapters on the function of the male and the function of the female). But now, years later, there is a whole new technology that has vastly simplified the problem and, indeed, for many couples may well be the most cost-effective, quickest, and least painful way of solving their infertility problem. In the early 1980s, in vitro fertilization remained a last-resort, new-horizon-type approach available only to those unusual couples in whom other treatments simply wouldn't work. It was much more expensive than any of the other available fertility treatments, and the pregnancy rates were estimated to be 2 percent or less. But now it is different.

In vitro fertilization techniques, and particularly modifications of in vitro fertilization such as GIFT, are yielding pregnancy rates as high as 45 percent per attempt, are being performed without the need for surgery, and are being done on an outpatient basis or on a one-day hospital stay. These high pregnancy rates are being achieved despite the fact that the infertility problems we see today are worse. First, couples are waiting until their late thirties to try to have children. Second, many infertile couples are getting pregnant using the simpler, conventional methods described in my earlier book, and that leaves large numbers of "more difficult" cases remaining for whom the conventional techniques didn't work.

We know now that it is a waste of time for the man to have a varicocelectomy operation, or for the woman to go on a half year of Danocrine therapy to shrink up her endometriosis. We know the treatment of the husband with Clomid or routine doses of Pergonal and various other drugs will do nothing to increase his sperm count (see Chapter 5.) In other words, after going through the 1980s, *we now know better what really works and what doesn't work.*

We understand more fully, by virtue of the in vitro fertilization experience, just how people do and don't get pregnant, and we can bust some of the old myths. We can save the woman unnecessary surgery for "minimal lesion endometriosis." We can actually see the follicle developing in the ovary with a simple ultrasound test and know exactly when she ovulates by when the follicle disappears or reduces in size, and we can avoid the emotional drain of literally years of fruitless testing and slingshot-style therapy. Paulette does not have to waste her few valuable remaining years of potential fertility by just testing her mucus and wondering whether she's having sex at the right time. Tammy, who got pregnant easily as a teenager and now in her late thirties is happily married and wants a child, does not have to go through unnecessary surgery for endometriosis. Furthermore, her husband doesn't have to go for years on Clomid to try to increase a low sperm count that really isn't too low.

Very often, by the time a couple has gone through years and years of wasted, inappropriate infertility treatments, they're just too worn out or their funds are absolutely exhausted, and they can't even consider the new technology of GIFT or IVF, which would have been so much more likely to have helped them. Cynthia is a thirty-two-year-old woman treated for infertility for ten years with Clomid, artificial insemination, several laparoscopies, two varicocelectomies on the husband, and several operations to lyse adhesions despite the fact that in truth the cause of her infertility all these years had been completely idiopathic (that means we just don't know). Yet now that she would have a 45 percent chance for pregnancy per treatment attempt with GIFT, she is just too tired, frustrated, and emotionally depressed to go any further.

ACHIEVING PREGNANCY WITH CONVENTIONAL METHODS VERSUS THE NEW TECHNOLOGY

It is important not to be overly negative about the conventional treatments that have certainly helped thousands of couples. So do not misinterpret the focus of what I am saying. Shortly after my first book came out, I heard from a lady who wanted to thank me for my simple solution to her problem. I had seen her and her husband almost a year earlier after being told that his sperm count was too low. She reminded me that I had taken one look at her oily skin, her history of acne, the hair on her toes, and told her she probably had an elevated male hormone level affecting the quality of her ovulation. She was writing to thank me and to let me know that despite several years of being told nothing could be done for her because of the husband's low sperm count, she got pregnant just two months after she was started on Clomid.

That same day I also heard from a lady whose husband was about to undergo a varicocelectomy operation because his sperm count was "so low." But she got pregnant before he had a chance to have his surgery. When they rechecked his sperm count, it was very high (over 50 million), despite his never receiving any treatment. She got pregnant after simply timing their intercourse to her ovulation day in the cycle. There was one couple who had been infertile for many years in whom the wife ovulated perfectly on day fourteen of every twenty-eight day cycle like clockwork. In fact, it was because her ovulatory cycle was so perfect and so regular; she always ovulated on Tuesday or Wednesday, and her husband, who is a traveling, workaholic businessman, was only in town on the weekends. So for all these years, they were infertile and never got pregnant simply because they were having sex only on the weekends. With her absolutely regular, predictable cycles, she always ovulated during the middle of the week. A simple rescheduling of their intercourse resulted in her getting pregnant rather quickly without any high technology.

One lady begged me to review her case even though she and her husband couldn't travel to our clinic in St. Louis. At that time, we were estimating the quality and time of ovulation from basal body temperature charts (rather than ultrasound and simple LH urine testing, which is available today). Her basal body temperature charts clearly showed poor ovulation, but her doctor had insisted on not treating her because he felt the husband's sperm count was too low. In fact, the local urologist had put the husband on the male hormone testosterone, which would only make his muscles bigger but would certainly lower rather than raise his sperm count. After her husband discontinued taking these steroids and she went on Clomid, she promptly became pregnant and I still receive a Christmas card every year from her despite the fact that we never met. There are countless, similar stories which tell why we should not completely throw out the old methods of fertility treatment.

THE INFERTILITY PROBLEMS WE TREAT TODAY
ARE WORSE THAN THOSE IN THE EARLY 1980s

The problem of infertility in our modern society is getting worse, and the simpler methods don't work for everyone. They should be discontinued after they have been shown not to be effective for a couple, and the newer technology used before too much time, energy, emotion, and money have been wasted on old-fashioned approaches.

It is years since I originally wrote *How to Get Pregnant* and first made the public at large aware of this rising epidemic of infertility. Since then, the problem has gotten much worse, but the solutions have gotten better. With refinements in the new technology of in vitro fertilization, GIFT, and microsurgery, the most seemingly insoluble cases of infertility can be solved and most people can get pregnant. In addition, simple infertility problems can be solved more quickly. However, you are not likely to be able to benefit from this new technology unless you learn how it works.

CHAPTER 1

How Does the New Technology Work?

SOLVING SEEMINGLY IMPOSSIBLE INFERTILITY PROBLEMS WITH THE NEW TECHNOLOGY

In the mid-1980s I saw a lovely woman who had undergone surgery by a well-meaning gynecologist for severe pelvic adhesions (scarring) caused by previous infections. (Nowadays if I were to see a woman with such severe adhesions in the pelvis, I wouldn't even attempt to try to solve her problem surgically, but would go straight to in vitro fertilization (IVF), a relatively simple, outpatient procedure.

At the time, the surgeon who explored her felt that her only option would be an effort to free up the adhesions so that the fallopian tubes and ovaries could be mobile and thus able to pick up the eggs in the proper fashion rather than be prevented from functioning by the solid scar tissue encasing them. Unfortunately, the doctor performing the surgery got into some problems with bleeding that were beyond his ability to handle and the only way he could solve the dilemma was by removing the woman's uterus (she was only twenty-five years of age). The doctor who removed her uterus did not feel the sense of tragedy he should have, because he was not aware that this lady could have gotten pregnant with in vitro fertilization without ever attempting the hopeless operation to open her completely cemented-down tubes and ovaries. If he had only known that all this lady needed was a uterus in order to get pregnant with the new technology, he might have avoided this foolhardy operation, sent her to a proper in vitro fertilization (IVF) program, and she could have had her baby. Now she could not even get pregnant with IVF.

Surrogate Pregnancy

Miraculously, four years later, I called this lady back to tell her what seemed absolutely incredible, that she could have a baby after all *even without her uterus*. She had to find a close friend who would be willing to carry her baby for nine months and then return her baby to her. Her own eggs and her husband's sperm would be used to get her friend pregnant using IVF or GIFT. Then, nine months later, her friend would give her baby back to her.

This is not the same as the infamous "surrogate motherhood" cases that have appeared in the media. "Surrogate motherhood" involves no medical technology whatsoever and is a procedure of highly questionable ethics. With the "surrogate motherhood" case you may have popularly read about involving "Baby M," a volunteer is artifically inseminated with sperm from a couple's husband and then paid to carry a baby who is genetically the surrogate's (not the infertile wife's). Nine months later the surrogate is required to give this baby (which is hers) up for adoption to the couple.

What I am referring to is something entirely different. A friend would simply voluntarily carry the genetic baby of the woman who has no uterus. Her friend, who would be paid nothing other than normal medical expenses, would then return the baby to her infertile friend who simply did not have a uterus.

Egg Donation

Couples who wait too long can even get pregnant after menopause. The only problem is it will require the donation of an egg either from an anonymous donor or from a good friend who has not yet gone through menopause herself. Most women go through menopause between the ages of forty-five and fifty-five but about 5 percent will go through their menopause well before the age of forty, so that at the young age of twenty-seven, for example, their childbearing days are just about over.

What about Paulette (to whom I referred in the Preface), who wrote the stirring article in *The New York Times Magazine*? Her biological clock is ticking and she's going to run out of fertilizable eggs fairly soon. That does not mean the end of her chance to get pregnant. A proper lining of the womb (endometrium) can easily be created by giving her the right hormones in the proper sequence to simulate a normal cycle, and put her husband's sperm along with one or more eggs from a good friend (or anonymous donor if she so prefers) into her fallopian tube at exactly the right time of her artificially induced cycle, and quite amazingly, she can get pregnant and carry and deliver a normal baby, virtually at any age!

Speaking of getting pregnant at an older age, a case was reported in 1989 of a grandmother giving birth to her own grandchildren using her daughter's eggs and her son-in-law's sperm. This procedure was necessitated because her daughter had no uterus. The grandmother was forty-eight years old, and her daughter was twenty-five. Their cycles were synchronized with hormones quite easily (as will be described in later chapters), and her daughter's eggs with her daughter's husband's sperm were used to create three embryos in a culture dish. All three embryos were then placed in the uterus (womb) of the grandmother-to-be and she got pregnant with triplets. Thus, in one delivery the grandmother gave birth to her own three grandchildren.

Perhaps the most amazing thing about these examples of apparently impossible infertility problems being solved with the new technology is just how simple it is. We're not talking about a procedure that requires difficult or expensive methodology.

Congenital Absence of Sperm Ducts

However, there are some seemingly impossible cases that do require very tricky technology and micromanipulative skill. One example is men who are born with completely absent sperm ducts. For almost twenty years, I had been bombarded by couples from all over the world for a solution to the problem of the male being born with completely absent sperm ducts. This is a particularly frustrating condition because the man's testicles are making perfectly normal sperm, but the sperm just can't get out and there are no ducts available to connect microsurgically. These cases had previously been completely hopeless (unless the couple was willing to opt for artificial insemination with donor sperm). Now, however, we have an extremely delicate method for microsurgically extracting sperm from right near the testicle, and getting the wife pregnant with it. This sperm normally should be unable to fertilize because they have not gone through the normal pathways which in most of us are necessary for the sperm to mature and develop the ability to fertilize. However, now it is possible to mature those sperm in vitro, i.e., in a culture dish, and then use them to fertilize the wife's eggs.

Advances like this seem to come when you least expect them. Several years ago, I had just finished telling my friend Dr. Richard Amelar (a fertility expert in New York) that a couple he had known for many years with congenital absence of the vas (and with whom he had become very close) should just give up because I didn't think the efforts in solving their problem were going anywhere. On that same day I had sent letters off to two similar patients in Colorado and Missouri, who had been repeatedly bugging me about why there couldn't be a "simple" solution to their problem. I told them that the complex requirements for maturation of sperm are beyond our understanding and that simply extracting them from near the testicle would not be of any benefit in getting the wife pregnant.

That same day, I flew out to California to begin what turned out to be a very fruitful collaboration with Dr. Ricardo Asch, who had originally developed the GIFT modification of the in vitro fertilization (IVF) procedure. With these three patients (who were only a small number of the thousands with whom I had corresponded over the previous years) freshly in mind, Dr. Asch and I pondered how we might be able to use the in vitro technology to approach this problem. We had not only to work out our scientific laboratory protocols, but also had to figure out how we could time the cycles of these patients' wives so that they could all be ready for the procedure around the same time when, by prior arrangement, our schedules would permit me and Dr. Asch to work together (since he was in California and I was in St. Louis). The result of that discussion was the methodology, very complex and indeed expensive, that has yielded full-term pregnancy with healthy, live babies in 25 percent of these otherwise hopeless cases. Dr. Amelar's good friends, and the couples from Colorado and from Missouri, were among our earliest such pregnancies. The new technology has "taught" us more about fertilization and getting pregnant than we ever dreamed of understanding years ago.

When we aspirated the sperm right out of the opening of the testicle of Dr. Amelar's friend, what we found initially was fairly dismal. Only about 10 percent of those sperm were mature enough to swim at all and they could barely make it forward at the slowest possible speed. These sperm looked like they were hobbling around on crutches because they were so poorly matured, they simply had had no sperm ductwork whatsoever in which to develop. We pushed the wife with hormones as far as we could to get as many eggs as possible out of her ovaries and, indeed, obtained twenty-six mature, good-looking, fertilizable eggs. Only two out of those twenty-six eggs were fertilized, obviously by a few lucky sperm that had to struggle their hardest under the best laboratory conditions to get in. That lady delivered a healthy little baby boy in the summer of 1989.

Another such case was a Boston policeman on whom we had tried the procedure once already and didn't get a single egg from his wife to fertilize. But this couple was persistent and wanted to try one more time. I didn't know why they tried again because I gave them very little hope. Yet this time, his wife's eggs did fertilize; she delivered healthy twin girls, and she even has a few embryos "frozen" for when they decide they want to try for a third child. Another one of these miracle patients is a professor of law, who has now become a good skiing buddy of mine and has helped me work through the legal and ethical implications of all these new techniques to make certain that we do nothing that would be unethical, unfair, or illegal. Because this technology is developing so swiftly, we haven't the slightest fear that the recently born children of these patients will have any difficulty having children themselves.

Micromanipulation: Fertilization "by Brute Force"

Another new development for otherwise impossible cases which requires great technical expertise is what scientists call "micro-manipulation," but what perhaps the layman might understand better simply as "fertilization of the egg by brute force." The way this works is that some men have sperm that are normal genetically but simply cannot move. They are motionless, non-motile sperm and, therefore, incapable of penetrating the egg on their own. This, too, is an extremely frustrating condition because these otherwise normal sperm are simply incapable of getting into the egg either because of no motility or very poor motility. With ultramicromanipulative instruments that can be attached to special microscopes, the wife's egg can actually be held secure with a microholding pipette (scientific word for eye-dropper), and another micropipette can be used to literally inject a sperm through the hard outer shell of the egg (what is called the "zona pellucida") so that this otherwise "dead" sperm is now able to fertilize the egg. Another variation of this "micromani-pulation," or "fertilization by brute force," is where a small hole or opening is drilled or dissected in the outer shell of the egg so that an extremely weakly motile sperm is able to find its way through this opening without having to exert much energy. (The sperm isn't injected directly into the egg, as that could injure it.)

Can you imagine the dexterity involved in this type of ma-nipulation? The sperm head is no more than 4 to 6 microns in diameter (that's approximately $\frac{1}{4,000}$ of an inch), and the size of an egg is approximately 100 microns in diameter ($\frac{1}{200}$ of an inch). Thus, "fertilization by brute force" is indeed a highly delicate procedure. To be quite frank, we are not certain yet whether this micromanipulation will pay off with increased pregnancy rates, but it is an area of research presently holding great hope. We have found for more than a decade that, in this field, one ought to be skeptical of any skepticism about future develop-ments.

TREATING COMMON INFERTILITY WITH THE NEW TECHNOLOGY

There was a tremendous furor of early skepticism and outright criticism of the new technology in the early 1980s. Dr. Ruth Hubbard, a Harvard University biology professor, warned the American Association for the Advancement of Science, "As a woman, a feminist, and a biologist, it is not worth opening a hornet's nest of reproductive technology for the privilege of having one's child." She continued, "How can we claim to know that the many chemical and mechanical manipulations of eggs, sperms, and embryos that take place during in vitro fertilization and implantation are harmless?" She was also concerned that in vitro fertilization required extremely costly and prolonged experimentation with highly skilled professionals and expensive equipment, "distorting our health priorities and funneling scarce resources into a questionable effort." She urged a complete halt to in vitro fertilization in the United States, and she was not alone.

Early Difficulties with In Vitro Fertilization (IVF)

Our government ordered a complete freeze on any support for medical research on the subject in the United States. In England, the originators of the procedure, Dr. Patrick Steptoe and Dr. Robert Edwards, had to perform their research and their first procedure in a sleepy little cottage because they could not get any government support or approval. In the United States, it took several years before the first private in vitro fertilization program was able to get through the legal, emotional, and religious barriers to be overcome in Norfolk, Virginia. The Department of Health, Education and Welfare (HEW) in the United States received petitions with 30,000 signatures protesting any federal funding for in vitro fertilization work, and so our government completely shunned any research support.

Interestingly, an advisory board commissioned by the Department of Health, Education and Welfare to study the ethical aspects of the procedure reported that this technology, which originated in England, should be employed in medical institutions in this country, and the same advisory board concluded that government financing for such research was "ethically acceptable." Nonetheless, the Department of Health, Education and Welfare of the United States never allowed any funding for this procedure and, as often happens best in this country, the technology developed quite well on its own on a private basis funded simply by patients who wanted to give the procedure a try. The enormous growth in this technology to the point where we know so much more about fertilization now (resulting in simpler and cheaper methods of helping hundreds of thousands of couples get pregnant who otherwise couldn't) came strictly from laissez-faire private enterprise research and development without any government plan and without any overall supervisory direction from any organization. In the first half of the 1980s, most of the new developments in the field represented technology imported from England, France, and Australia.

By 1982, four years after the birth of the first test-tube baby by Steptoe and Edwards in England, one hundred more babies had been born throughout the world through in vitro fertilization. The procedure has become so popular and ubiquitous that the original clinic started by Steptoe and Edwards by 1990 had been responsible for well over 1,000 healthy babies, and throughout the world every year thousands more healthy test-tube babies are being born.

Still it was a very experimental, very expensive, and highly unsuccessful procedure at this critical time in the early 1980s. That was when Professor Ed Wallach wrote a prophetic editorial in the journal *Fertility and Sterility* predicting almost all of the advances in the future that would make in vitro fertilization simpler, more cost-effective, and have a pregnancy rate high enough to merit its serious use on a large scale. He outlined future research in stimulating the ovaries to get more eggs, determining when to give the ovulatory triggering hormone HCG, monitoring the growing follicle with ultrasound, retrieving the eggs without surgery simply by ultrasound-guided needle aspiration, placement of multiple embryos instead of a single embryo to increase the pregnancy rate, and even freezing of extra embryos. He argued persuasively that if we are going to worry about the ethics of in vitro fertilization, there are a lot of things we do in medicine that ought to cause us to worry a great deal more. What Dr. Wallach's editorial did not predict was the development of GIFT.

GIFT (Gamete Intra Fallopian Transfer) Popularized the New Reproductive Technology

The idea of the GIFT procedure is so enticingly simple that all of us in the field just scratch our heads and say to ourselves, "Why didn't I think of that?" But we didn't, Dr. Ricardo Asch did, and that's why he deserves so much credit. In 1985, when he first suggested GIFT, the success rates with in vitro fertilization (IVF) were still so low that it was considered an absolute last-resort alternative and an exotic procedure performed only by a few centers with very low pregnancy rates. GIFT changed all that within a period of only a few years. Instead of taking the egg from the woman and the sperm from the husband and fertilizing the egg in a culture dish (in vitro) in an incubator over a forty-eight hour period, he simply held the eggs and sperm in culture long enough to prepare for loading them into a small little catheter and placed them directly into the woman's fallopian tube where fertilization normally takes place naturally.

"GIFT" is simply an acronym for G—Gamete, I—Intra, F—Fallopian, T—Transfer, which means transferring the sperms and the eggs (the "gametes") into the woman's fallopian tube. Instead of waiting forty-eight hours for the fertilization process to take place in an incubator, that step is bypassed. Sperm and eggs are simply placed directly into the fallopian tube and allowed to fertilize naturally. Then, at the right time, they travel on their own to the uterus as would occur in a normal fertile woman.

This simple idea literally tripled the pregnancy rates of standard in vitro fertilization (IVF), and set the stage for its massive popularization. You can't really have a program that does only GIFT without doing in vitro fertilization (IVF), nor should you have a program that only does in vitro fertilization and does not offer GIFT. They each have their separate places in the new technology for different types of patients. But the vast majority of infertile women will have the highest chance of pregnancy (reproduceable among many clinics around the world) with GIFT, assuming the wife has normal fallopian tubes. If, however, the fallopian tubes are diseased, then putting sperm or eggs into these diseased fallopian tubes is an error, and standard in vitro fertilization (IVF) must be resorted to. The advantage of GIFT is a very high pregnancy rate and a very minor surgical procedure, whereas the advantage of in vitro fertilization (IVF), despite a lower pregnancy rate, is that it can be used in any patient whether she has normal fallopian tubes or not, and it requires absolutely no surgery at all.

So Where Do We Go for Help?

So we come back to the original question, "How do you decide where to go?" When our U.S. Congressional Advisory Panel met during the years of 1987 and 1988, we amassed figures which showed that of 150 in vitro fertilization (IVF) clinics in the U.S., half of them had never achieved a pregnancy at all. Furthermore, of those that achieved pregnancies, the success rate varied from extremely low (less than 5 percent) to unrealistically high (greater than 30 percent). Evaluating the quality of the clinic and the chances of getting pregnant from that clinic was an extremely muddled mess at that time. In 1984, it was reported at the World Congress in Helsinki, Finland, that of over 10,000 women entering (IVF) cycles, there were only 600 live births, for a success rate of only 6 percent. In the United States in 1987, out of a total of 12,000 women undergoing (IVF) cycles, there were a little over 1,000 live births for an overall success rate of about 9 percent. Such a low success rate would hardly be encouraging to a couple.

It was for this reason that the congressional bureaucrats who reported on the discussions of our advisory panel promulgated the publicity that the success rate with this new technology is too low and the cost too high to consider it anything other than a last resort and that more resources should be spent on the "conventional" therapy for infertility. The bureaucrats also failed to accept the recommendation of the advisory panel that infertility was a medical condition or an illness, which would give strong weight to forcing insurance companies to pay for infertility treatment without the need to come up with a specific and usually erroneous pathological diagnosis.

The fact is that if you choose your in vitro fertilization program carefully, you have a chance of pregnancy and live birth of over 20 percent, and if your fallopian tubes are healthy (which is usually the case), you can undergo GIFT with the prospect of over 40 percent of having a pregnancy each cycle you attempt. Furthermore, we now have very good evidence that if you continue to go through multiple attempts, your chances remain just as good with each succeeding attempt at in vitro fertilization or GIFT for at least up to the seventh try. Thus, like flipping coins, your odds are very good that eventually you'll get pregnant with this technology. But you must choose the right doctor and the right program. This is a free enterprise, laissez-faire system, and it is very clear to most of the experts in this area that no government "regulation" is going to help you.

Even if "honest reporting" of results were mandated by all clinics with their books open to review by auditors (a regulation that I would certainly support), this would still not give you a simple answer of where to go, for the following reason: Some clinics might have a bad pregnancy rate simply because they restrict their attention to the most difficult cases with the longest duration of prior infertility, the greatest amount of scarring, the oldest women in their mid-forties, or couples in whom the sperm quality is miserable. If the clinic had the kind of expertise that encouraged these most difficult cases to be in preponderance at their doorstep, they could easily have a lower pregnancy rate than a clinic which takes on more routine cases.

That's one of the reasons why you must study this book and become a knowledgeable patient. It will help you choose the right doctor or the right clinic. It'll make you savvy about how to get this paid for by your insurance company. It will give you the depth of understanding which you need in order to go through the many preliminary steps which are part of every IVF or GIFT cycle.

CONCLUSIONS

This book will review the basic *How to Get Pregnant* principles from 1980, but will debunk some of the terrible myths of conventional treatment, like endometriosis, varicocele, treatment of men with low sperm counts, among others. This book will encourage resorting earlier to in vitro fertilization (IVF) or GIFT technology as a way of getting more infertile couples pregnant more cheaply and quickly and with less pain. But understand that a couple shouldn't undergo this treatment without a full understanding of how it works. Otherwise there are too many steps and it's too intimidating.

This technology is certainly more cost-effective than so many of the treatments that insurance companies routinely pay for, but a couple is still going to need the savvy to figure out how to get the insurance company to pay for this procedure. The insurance company needs to understand that it will save rather than cost more money. This book will explain the differences between in vitro fertilization and GIFT with its variations, why such high pregnancy rates can be obtained, and what kind of clinics are able to obtain these pregnancy rates. Additionally you will learn how to watch carefully and pick the right place by interviewing the doctors and the nurses who are directly involved, so you can evaluate their results realistically.

A "list" of "specialists" or "clinics" is never going to be reliable. I can assure you that anyone and everyone who says that they are "fertility specialists" gets on such a list. There is no list of recommended doctors or clinics that any author will publish which will be reliable for you. In an effort to maintain neutrality and avoid libel suits, organizations such as The American Fertility Society, the American Medical Association, RESOLVE (a lay organization of infertile couples), county medical societies, and various books and manuals can never do a frank job of discerning and deciding which clinic is the one that is right *for you* or is most likely to give a successful result. For the energy, the time, and the money that must be put into this effort, you must make a good choice. For that, you must understand the new technology.

CHAPTER 2

Why Are Humans So Infertile?

HUMANS WERE NEVER REPRODUCTIVELY VERY EFFICIENT

In all other animals except for the human, the desire for sex is timed to correspond exactly to that moment when the female is about to ovulate. The human inclination to have sex at any time during the month or year is peculiarly human, separates us completely from the rest of the animal kingdom, and is reproductively extremely inefficient. In all species, there is only a very brief period of time, a matter of days during each month, that intercourse is likely to lead to pregnancy. The timing of sex is very important if a species is to have a very high fertility rate.

A period of fourteen days is required for a follicle to develop in the ovary from day one of menstruation until that egg is sufficiently matured so that it is ready for ovulation. After ovulation, there is another fourteen-day period after the egg is fertilized (assuming sex has occurred at the right time), when the embryo grows and then implants in the uterus, or "womb." If intercourse occurs at some time other than those few days around the time of ovulation, it is very unlikely to lead to a pregnancy.

Animals go through what is an "estrous" cycle, or "heat,"

whereas humans go through a menstrual cycle. In the normal cycle of any animal, as the follicle (or follicles) destined to ovulate begin to grow and prepare the egg for maturation and ultimately fertilization, that follicle (the little blister within which the egg is located) is producing tremendous quantities of the female hormone estrogen from its "granulosa" cells. This high production of estrogen during the developing of the follicle takes place in the first half of the cycle, beginning in the human on the first day of menstruation. In all animals except for humans, this increasing estrogen level caused by the developed follicle getting ready to ovulate the egg, chemically triggers the female to desire sex. When this happens, any farmer or animal trainer knows the animal is "going into heat." Whether it's a cow, moose, pig, or a rat, the female assumes a peculiarly hunched body position, getting ready for sex. Only that time in the cycle will she allow a male to get near her. It is the extremely high level of estrogen that occurs just prior to ovulation (because the follicle is now finally ready to be ovulated) that triggers the sexual desire in all *other* animals. When animals have sex, it has been designed by nature to occur only at the time when it is likely to result in fertilization and a baby.

It is different for humans, who go through what is called a "menstrual" cycle and have the same high increase in estrogen level occurring just prior to ovulation because of the production of estrogen from the enlarging follicle as animals do. This high surge of estrogen occurs right around mid-cycle just prior to ovulation. The difference between humans and all other animals, however, is that we do not feel any "heat." In humans, the female is just as apt to accept the male in a sexual act at any time during the month, and unless she is one of those rare women who are extremely tuned into what her body is doing, she will have no idea whether she is having sex at a time of the month that is likely to lead to pregnancy or not.

Sexual desire in the human is much more complex and is not driven by the female hormone estrogen. In fact, in the human female, sexual drive comes from the male hormone testosterone, the same hormone that is constantly turning on sexual drive in the male. This is unique in the animal kingdom and is specifically a human phenomenon. Of course, the female level of male hormone is about one-tenth the male level, explaining the lower chemical sexual drive in the female than in the male. The small amount of testosterone which the female makes is, however, quite adequate for her to become willing and interested in being a sexual partner. The amount of testosterone in the circulation is fairly constant in the male from day to day and from year to year. This is true in the female also, although there is an ever so slight increase in testosterone just around the time of ovulation. Thus, we bear a slight resemblance to our animal friends in the sense that in the human, "female-initiated" sex, is more common around the time of ovulation than any other time. But this effect can only be noticed in a small way in large population studies. Usually husbands and wives have sex fairly randomly through the month, whereas animals only have sex on a few very specific days when the female's estrogen level triggers her interest just prior to ovulation.

WHY IS SEX IN THE HUMAN SO REPRODUCTIVELY INEFFICIENT?

Many sociological studies have demonstrated that for the average happily married couple with no psychological problems, and a life not too cluttered by excessive workaholic pressures, sex occurs on an average of two to three times per week. Under this circumstance, sex is likely to occur not only at times when it won't lead to pregnancy, but it is also likely to occur at a time when it will. But what if you have a very busy schedule and a hectic, crowded life with both partners working, a tremendous amount of stress, and a sexual frequency that is more erratic than just a steady two to three times per week? If that is the case and you don't know when you are ovulating, you might be having sex at the wrong time. In humans, sex occurs simply because it is an enjoyable expression of human feeling.

Why should human beings be different and what is the benefit to us of having this totally random interest in sex unrelated to whether or not it is likely to lead to a baby? It may be related to our family system. The survival of our intelligent form of life as humans depends upon a well-developed family system and an educational program designed to teach our truly helpless young (born without any instincts of how to hunt or survive) how to gain the knowledge necessary to survive in the world, and this allows the creativity to achieve with each new generation a new and better world.

Humans are the only animals that make love facing each other. Throughout the animal kingdom, the female squats in her position of "heat" and the male "mounts" on top of her facing her rear end. They never get to look at each other. Only in the human race does intercourse become the equivalent of "making love." Only in the human race is there the direct facing of one another, indicating that some kind of communication is occurring other than just a chemically triggered desire for orgasm.

Furthermore, only in the human race is there a sexual interest between the male and the female that persists on a regular basis. This reproductive pattern promotes the development of love, permanent mating, and a family system. And it is because of this pattern that human beings are so infertile when compared to the rest of the animal kingdom.

SEASONAL TIMING OF SEX IN ANIMALS

Although the cow breeds once a month, most animals breed only at a particular time of the year in which getting pregnant is likely to lead to the birth of the baby in the spring months (when it is most likely to survive through a warm summer while growing and preparing for its first winter). For example, the moose (or any other antlered deer species) has tiny testicles during mid-winter and spring, no horns, and certainly no interest in sex. It's a good thing, because if he were to impregnate a cow moose at that time, she would wind up delivering in the late fall and the baby moose would most assuredly die. But after June, when the days are getting shorter, the decreasing daylight stimulates a little gland in his brain called the "pineal" to release a hormone called "melatonin," which in the human has very little effect but in most all other animals regulates the season of breeding.

As the days get shorter, the moose's testicles gradually begin to get bigger, and he begins to produce sperm and the male hormone testosterone. (In every animal, testosterone is chemically the same male hormone as produced by humans.) As the moose produces testosterone during the late summer and early fall months, he begins to grow antlers or horns very much the way human males develop a beard, pubic hair, or hair under the arms under the influence of male hormone. In fact, the expression "horny" comes from the fact that as the moose develops higher testosterone levels and gets a charged-up interest in having sex, he is also growing his horns. In the fall season, the moose's testicles reach the maximum size, producing huge amounts of sperm and male hormone, and his horns have reached their maximum dimensions, preparing him for the bitter fights he will have with other males in preparation for the "rutting" season, when he will finally mate with a nearby female moose. His sexual desire for this female moose is purely chemically mediated and in no way relates to any type of evaluation of each other's personalities. When the mating season is over, his testicles again begin to shrink, he stops making testosterone and sperm, and he leaves the female moose to go back on his private wanderings.

Bears have a similar mating pattern except that the mating season is reversed. Whereas the moose's testicles get bigger beginning in late summer and early autumn as the days get shorter, the bear's testicles begin to increase in size in late winter as the days get longer. In fact, it is the increase in the growth of the bear's testicles and the increased production of testosterone that wakes him up out of hibernation. If a bear were castrated while he was in hibernation, he would never awaken. Testosterone wakes him up, gets him out of the den in spring, and when it reaches its maximum level, he, too, mates purely under chemical urges that he doesn't understand and shortly thereafter leaves the female to carry on the job of rearing the young completely on her own.

THE NECESSITY OF A FAMILY SYSTEM IN HUMANS AND, THEREFORE, INFERTILITY

We know that the human mind today is not any different organically than it was 40,000 years ago with the first emergence of Cro-Magnon man. Yet 40,000 years ago, they were busy learning more efficient methods of hunting and producing primitive art on the walls of caves. Now that same exact brain is being used to send men into space and to probe the very mysteries of DNA and the genes that produce life. How can that same primitive brain be responsible for our incredible civilization? The reason is the immense flexibility and capacity for learning that is unique to humans compared to other animals, who are simply born with all the instincts necessary for survival and successful behavior. Instead, humans are born with an enormously educable brain. For this to work required a family system and a relatively small number of offspring per parent so that the lessons learned in each generation could be passed on from parent to child. This could never have occurred if we were just having sex with each other triggered by increased estrogen or testosterone levels timed specifically to when it was likely to lead to having a baby.

Reproductive Inadequacy of the Human Male

But it is not just the inadequate timing of human intercourse that leads to our relative infertility compared to other animals. It is simply an embarrassing fact that human sperm production is very low compared to sperm production in any other animal. Most male animals produce about 25 million sperm per day per gram of testicular tissue. Humans produce only 4 million sperm per day per gram of testicular tissue. In other words, on a per weight basis, comparing humans to any animals, large or small, humans produce one-sixth the amount of sperm of all other animals (with the exceptions only of the gorilla, the orangutan, and the goose). Compared to all other animals the human male is a reproductive disaster.

The average bull ejaculate contains about 10 billion sperm, whereas the average fertile man's ejaculate would contain no more than 100 to 300 million sperm. Imagine that the average bull produces in a single ejaculate thirty to one hundred times more sperm than the average human, despite the fact that the actual volume of ejaculate coming from the bull is no more than that of the human. The bull's sperm are moving at literally three times the speed of the human sperm, in a perfectly straight line, and there are virtually none that are abnormal, weak, or deformed-looking. The human ejaculate is lucky to have 60 percent of the sperm moving at all, most of them move rather slowly compared to that of the bull, and easily 40 percent of the sperm have abnormal structures with atypical head shapes and unpurposeful circular motion instead of linear progression. The average fertile man's sperm just looks terribly sick when you compare it to that of a bull.

Another example of superior animal fertility is the pig which ejaculates an entire pint of sperm when he has sex with the sow; the completion of the orgasm requires a full half hour. In addition, the pig has little screwlike grooves on the end of its penis which correspond to similar grooves in the female pig's cervix. Thus, the male pig literally "screws" his penis into the cervix of the female so that during this entire half hour in which a pint of sperm is delivered directly into the uterus, there is no way for any leakage or waste to occur. The amount of sperm in a single pig ejaculate is about four hundred times the amount of sperm in a single human ejaculate, and none of it is lost.

Spiders have sperm so perfect that when the male spider inseminates the female, although the sperm number may be relatively few, each one is a "jewel" and results in fertilization. In the human only about .001 percent of the sperm ejaculated has any chance of ever getting near the egg, and only a small fraction of the sperm in a human ejaculate is really any good.

If you were to look at the microarchitecture ("histology") of the human testes compared to that of any other animal, you would see a striking difference; their testicular microarchitecture is perfectly structured with an orderly wave of sperm production beginning from the earliest immature forms (called spermatogonia) proceeding in a perfectly sequential wave through many steps toward the final product of mature sperm. At any given point along what is called the "seminiferous tubule" of the testicle, you see a perfectly organized progression of sperm production. However, the arrangement seen in human testicle biopsy, even in a "normal" man, is a chaotic mess.

In almost all animals, there is a "wave of spermatogenesis" which allows one to follow the production and maturation of various stages of sperm production from beginning to end in a perfectly logical, sequential fashion, and the end result is an enormous number of literally perfect sperm. But in the human, anywhere in the seminiferous tubule is a chaotic "mosaic" arrangement of a helter-skelter variation in the different stages of spermatogenesis organized in a completely random fashion.

Thus, even the "normal" man who does not represent a case of "male infertility" has very low sperm production, a high percentage of abnormal sperm in every ejaculate, and a completely abnormal and disorganized testicular architecture compared to the rest of the animal kingdom.

WHY IS HUMAN SPERM COUNT SO POOR?

Many people have worried that the human sperm count is declining and there have been numerous popular newspaper articles complaining that industrial pollution and chemical toxins surrounding us are the cause, thus precipitating the infertility crisis we presently face. But a cold analysis of the data available does not substantiate this hysterical fear. Mean sperm counts from fifty years ago are not significantly different in the United States than they are today. Fear that the sperm count was declining was precipitated simply by the realization that 10 percent of "fertile" men coming in for a vasectomy have sperm counts in a "very low range," i.e., below 10 million per cc.

On the other hand, it is true that our sperm count has been declining. However, it has not been declining over the last fifty years, but rather over the last hundreds of thousands of years *because of our monogamous mating pattern and family system.*

Is the Environment Causing Our Sperm Count to Go Down?

Before explaining how our family system (which has been responsible for the greatness of human life) has caused this gradual erosion of male fertility, we should discuss the concerns of environmentally conscious researchers who fear, quite justifiably, that modern life can have a very negative impact on reproduction.

The first example to document this fear came from a personal observation of Dr. Robert Schoysman, who has for decades run a major artificial donor insemination program in Brussels, Belgium. Sperm donors were usually medical or law students, and many of them had offered several specimens over a period of several years. Occasionally someone who had been a very fertile sperm donor would suddenly turn up with consistently low counts that had to be rejected for use in the donor insemination program. This finding puzzled Dr. Schoysman. When he looked into the matter, he found that it was almost always in times of great emotional stress, like final exams and term papers that were due around the time, that the donor's sperm count declined.

In a similar vein, Dr. Michael Jondet in Paris told me several years ago that, whereas in the past he would have to reject about 30 percent of volunteers for sperm donation because the count was not high enough, at present he has to reject approximately 70 percent of potential donors. He had no explanation for this striking change but said he had to wonder whether the stress of modern life for students was having some as of yet scientifically undefined impact on the sperm count.

Dr. James Overstreet, from the University of California at Davis, one of the world's major authorities on sperm fertilizing ability, tells of a single anecdotal experience from his sperm bank in Sacramento. There was a student who had been a very fertile donor and whom he had known for several years who suddenly turned up one day with a sperm count that had gone virtually to zero. He assumed there was some kind of laboratory error and had another collection performed and, indeed, found once again that the count was close to zero. He then had a personal interview with this student to try to figure out if there was anything different he was eating or in his behavior that might explain this strange and sudden loss of fertility in an otherwise normal sperm donor. Dr. Overstreet found out that this student's life had just completely fallen apart in the last several months; his personal problems were so extreme that he virtually broke down in front of him.

A single anecdote doesn't prove anything, but stories like these cause even the most sophisticated scientist to wonder whether in some way stress might have some impact on lowering sperm production in some men.

Again, before the potentially dangerous effect of environmental contamination on sperm production is completely discounted, let's look at what happened to the Chinese between the 1920s and the early 1930s in the small village of Wang Cun in the Jiangsu Province when, for a period of ten years, not a single child was born and nobody could understand why. The village was panic-stricken and threatened with extinction. They tried praying to Buddha and moved their ancestors' tombs to "luckier" sites. Some of the villagers married previously fertile widows from other villages (who had given birth to children in other places), but they all became strangely barren when they moved to Wang Cun. Then, suddenly, in the mid-1930s, "the curse was lifted," and women began to get pregnant again. It was not understood until many years later that the cause of this sudden sterility of an entire village was because of a change in the method of cooking, switching from soybean oil to a cheaper, crude cottonseed oil. When the price of soybean oil went down again in the mid-1930s, the villagers switched back to soybean oil away from crude cottonseed oil, and fertility returned.

We now know that cottonseed oil does not necessarily cause infertility if it has been prepared first by heating. But if the cottonseed oil has been prepared by a cold press process without preheating, a chemical in the cottonseed oil, now called gossypol, suddenly and dramatically stops men from producing sperm. (This is the basis of modern Chinese research on a male birth control pill.)

Thus, although it is clear from large-scale population studies that overall the human sperm count has not suddenly declined in the last fifty years (but rather over several tens of thousands of years), nonetheless we should be aware there may be environmental and emotional factors that can cause fluctuation in sperm count in ways that we don't yet understand.

Monogamy and Lack of Sperm Competition

But the major reason that the human male is so reproductively inadequate, even the most of fertile of human males, lies in our monogamous mating system and family life, and the inherent lack of "sperm competition." This is a fascinating dilemma that we are forever locked into, and it deserves a detailed explanation, not only because we will understand ourselves and our infertility better, but because it will explain why all of the so-called medical treatments for raising sperm count that urologists prescribe without any scientific basis don't—and can't possibly ever—work. It will explain why we have to resort to the new technology to get wives pregnant when the husband's sperm counts are inadequate, rather than waste time with most futile hormonal stimulation approaches, which can't possibly have any impact on their sperm production; their poor sperm production is genetically determined by tens and hundreds of thousands of years of mating history.

"Oligospermia," or a low sperm count, is part of being human in the fullest sense. In family system and mating patterns humans are closest to the gorilla; we are quite different from chimps or smaller monkeys. The ferocious-looking gorilla, who weighs five hundred pounds, has a very tiny penis and very small testicles. On the other hand, the chimpanzee, which weighs only one hundred pounds, has an enormous pair of testicles, huge compared to that of a human. Why should chimps, who are also great apes and intelligent like the gorilla, have such a tremendous sperm count and be so extremely fertile, when gorillas are probably one of the only other animals on the planet whose sperm production is as poor as that of humans?

Chimps are very promiscuous. They travel in troops of thirty to forty and all of the males copulate with any female who goes into "heat." There is not a single male who does not copulate with any female who has reached her time of ovulation. They have a troop system but not truly a family system. Gorillas, on the other hand, are virtually monogamous (one male has sex with one female or sometimes with two females, to whom he remains emotionally attached). When the gorilla's female mate goes into heat, he can be certain there is no other male gorilla who will go near her or have sex with her. They have a truly faithful family system.

If only one male copulates with a given female, there will be no competition from the sperm of any other male, and if she does get pregnant, she will have done so from whatever few sperm that male happens to have. On the other hand, if several males were to copulate with a given female, she is most likely to get pregnant from the male who had the best and highest sperm count. Therefore, in a promiscuous mating pattern the male offspring of the female is most likely to come from sperm of the male having the highest sperm count. In a monogamous mating system, as in the gorilla or the human, since there is no competition among sperm from different males for fertilizing the egg, the female is more likely to give birth to a male offspring whose father had a relatively low sperm count.

Evolution of Male Infertility

When we stop to think that it only takes one sperm to fertilize an egg, very often we may ask why we need so many sperm if only a few are necessary for a male to impregnate his mate. Well, one reason for those millions and millions of sperm is not just to increase the female's chance of getting pregnant but to make it less likely that another male who copulates with her will get her pregnant. In monogamous animals, such as the human or the gorilla, males with very poor sperm counts are more likely to have offspring but their male offspring are more likely to also have poor sperm counts when they grow up. If only one male copulates with a given female, there will be no competition with sperm from any other male and she is likely to get pregnant with whatever sperm he has. But if several males copulate with a given female, she is more likely to get pregnant from the male with the best sperm count.

Why can't we humans make sperm well? Why is male infertility the most common and difficult problem that infertility specialists have to deal with? The answer is that oligospermia, or poor sperm production, is an inherited part of being human.

Anywhere you look in the animal kingdom, you can describe very accurately the mating system simply by looking at the weight and size of the testicles. The more promiscuous the mating system, the larger the testicles. The more monogamous the mating system, the smaller the testicles and the lower the sperm count. This relationship is obvious when you compare turkey testicles, for example, to goose testicles. The goose is one of the few other animals that has a faithful, monogamous family system in which one male mates with one female for life in what appears to be a lasting, loving relationship. Turkeys, and other ground fowl, on the other hand, have sex quite indiscriminately with any female that is around. The goose's testicles are extraordinarily small and tiny and even difficult to find, whereas turkeys and roosters have respectable, large testicles. Throughout the animal kingdom, monogamous animals with loving, lasting relationships with a single partner are likely to be poor sperm producers. The species does not become extinct because the female retains her fertility. If other problems don't intervene, such as age or disease, she is able to get pregnant with a very small number of sperm.

Human populations with a strictly monogamous lifestyle are much more likely to have low sperm counts and small testicles than those with a more promiscuous lifestyle. One famous study performed in the 1980s in Hong Kong on autopsied men compared the testicular size of Chinese males from Hong Kong to that of Caucasian males from the same city. Chinese males had testicle sizes averaging one half that of Caucasian males, showing that many thousands of years of completely monogamous lifestyle resulted in lower sperm counts than in populations where there has been a break from strict monogamy.

OUR WORLDWIDE INFERTILITY EPIDEMIC

Infertility is a global problem. It is not just something that has recently cropped up in the United States. In Russia, China, the Near East, and certainly in Europe and South America, the story is the same. Amongst Catholics where large families are traditional, most would choose in vitro fertilization (IVF) or GIFT (despite the negative views of the papacy) if it were necessary for them to have a baby. Orthodox Jews view having children and populating the earth as the first commandment of the Bible and will use all the human resources at their disposal to fulfill that first commandment. The dedication of Muslims to solving their infertility problems is extraordinary and can best be exemplified by the following account.

A patient, who had just arrived in St. Louis for a complicated microsurgical operation to reconnect his blocked sperm duct-work, told me through a translator from the St. Louis Islamic Center that he was sitting at an oasis in the Middle East pondering his misery at not being able to have a child when along came a Bedouin on a camel. The Bedouin sat down beside him and they chatted. He explained that doctors in Riyadh, Saudi Arabia, as well as specialists he had visited in Cairo told him that he has "epididymal blockage," which means blockage of the very delicate microscopic sperm ducts, and although he was making sperm, the sperm could not get out. They told him the surgery for this was very complex and they gave him a low prognosis for success. He didn't know what to do because life seemed so meaningless if he could not have a child.

The Bedouin then stared off at the sky with a prophetic gesture and said, "Go to St. Louis." In the middle of the desert, this religious Muslim asked, "Where is St. Louis?" As it turns out, the Bedouin was related to a patient from Saudi Arabia, on whom I had operated successfully for a similar condition several years earlier. The story had spread very quickly throughout Saudi Arabia that his sperm count was now normal and his wife has had several children. Needless to say, this patient, on the advice of a Bedouin he had never seen before in his life, flew from the Arabian desert to St. Louis, in order to have microsurgery to correct his sterility. Such is the dedication of people to have a child despite seemingly implacable odds.

In China, where one quarter of the world's entire population resides (1.2 billion people), infertility is the most vexing problem of "upwardly mobile" couples who put off childbearing (as the government has told them to) and then find they can't have children. For that reason, China called its first World Congress on Infertility in October of 1988. Although the facilities are meager and primitive, there is no shortage of patients for in vitro fertilization and GIFT.

In India, the country with one of the world's most difficult overpopulation problems, threatening its economy and way of life, making it seem almost impossible to pull out of poverty because of the enormous population overgrowth, a major disaster in almost 20 percent of households is the inability to have children. Smallpox, which is unheard of today, was a scourge of

India thirty or forty years ago, and every male child who survived it wound up with epididymal obstruction, i.e., blockage of the sperm ducts, which could only be treated with very sophisticated, modern microsurgery such as that developed in St. Louis. Whenever a couple from Saudi Arabia, India, or Pakistan arrives, and the husband has a couple of small scars on his nose, I know that he had smallpox as a child and I know why they are seeing me.

HUMAN DESTINY AND INFERTILITY

If we look at the most remote areas of the world, where humans live today the same as they did 40,000 years ago, we begin to understand better why infertility isn't really a curse, but rather an intrinsic part of being human, and in fact how it has insured our survival. The !Kung tribesmen (commonly referred to as the African Bushmen) live in the Kalahari Desert much the same as they did 40,000 years ago. The !Kung have an average of only four children per family and get pregnant only about once every five years, the only human tribe whose birth pattern is the same as that of the gorilla. Yet they use no modern birth control, and in fact live the most basic, primitive existence on the face of the earth. They represent mankind at his raw earliest. They have no agriculture and so the food supply is at best unpredictable. They live strictly by hunting and gathering. They own virtually nothing and they are chronically undernourished. They are very small people and speak in a strange clicking sound that makes it very difficult to find translators. If they had more children, they surely could not feed them.

The !Kung breast-feed their children exclusively for four or five years (indeed this is necessary because there is so little food available that it must all be given to the adults, with nothing left over). The child has to derive his or her nutrition strictly from the mother's breast. This constant suckling, without any relief bottles or heaping teaspoonfuls of baby food, completely suppresses ovulation in the female until such time as the child is about four years old and truly able to get around and eat the same food as the adults. The family system is secure, and their immense intelligence is unquestioned by any anthropologists who have ever been with them. In a sense they represent the beginning of our human ascent, which would not have been possible if our ancestors were turning out litters of children.

So when orangutans and gorillas (like geese) developed family mating systems and reduced fertility, in a sense it was a step toward humanity of which the !Kung tribesmen of the Kalahari Desert are the earliest examples. Trillions and trillions of little baby ants and baby bees are born every year but instinct governs their function completely. There is not a lot that a baby ant or bee has to learn. Human babies are born with a mind that is an open book. It is their early experiences and the education afforded by their family in a society that can devote its resources to the education of limited numbers that has resulted in the fullest expression of our humanity.

SEXUALLY TRANSMITTED DISEASES

Probably 10 percent of human infertility is caused by tubal obstruction, and that is usually, although not always, caused by infectious diseases transmitted sexually. One-third of African men are sterile because of epididymal obstruction caused by sexually transmitted disease, an absolutely incredible figure. The infertility caused by sexually transmitted disease requires the most complex medical treatment. Very delicate microsurgery is needed to bypass obstruction either in the male or the female. Furthermore, in the female, the lining of the fallopian tubes is often so badly damaged by a disease that surgery alone is not adequate and in vitro fertilization may be necessary.

The diseases of gonorrhea and syphilis, which are the most popularly known sexually transmitted diseases, actually arose in the Renaissance around the 1400s. The French, of course, blamed it on the English and called it the "English Pox," and the English, naturally, blamed it on the French, calling it the "French Pox." The fact is that gonorrhea and syphilis were rampant everywhere in Renaissance Europe and these diseases were strictly a result of the increasing promiscuity associated with the liberalization of values during that time. We noticed the same phenomenon in the United States and Europe in the 1960s. The tremendous increase in infertility among women between the ages of twenty to twenty-four who normally would be undergoing no age-related decline in fertility is caused by the increase in sexually transmitted disease.

It is not that a promiscuous sexual pattern will always lead to sexually transmitted disease in a particular culture. For example, well before the arrival of the white man, Eskimos had a very promiscuous-style sex life. A husband would offer his wife to a guest for a night and he would be terribly insulted by a refusal. In the original Eskimo culture, if a young girl were to get pregnant (which was frequently the case) prior to a marriage being arranged, it would be no problem because she would just give the child to someone else in the community who wanted it. The extended family would take care of the child; the promiscuous sex life was perfectly well accepted. It was with the arrival of white explorers and the germs that they carried that the introduction of sexually transmitted diseases occurred.

It is not the promiscuous mating pattern of certain groups but rather the change from a monogamous mating pattern to a promiscuous one which causes a rampant increase in sexually transmitted disease, most of which leads to sterility and some of which leads to death. This, for example, is why AIDS eventually had to develop. Anyone who has studied the medical history of the Renaissance could have predicted in the 1960s that some terrible disease, most likely generated by a very "weak" organism which would be only capable of contagiously spreading through intimate contact, would have to develop. If the organism (or germ) were strong enough to be transmitted through casual contact, it would be rampant in the population. Chicken pox, for example, is one of the most contagious of all diseases and few grow up without getting it. Human immunity to it is very strong because we have had hundreds of thousands of years of experience with it and it is very easily transmitted from one person to the next. But sexually transmitted diseases are usually relatively uncontagious organisms that would never get anywhere if it weren't for the variety of intimate contacts allowed by an increasing promiscuity in the mating pattern of the society.

Ironically, when our sexual patterns change toward mating approaches that should lead to greater numbers of children as in the rest of the animal world, it just results in the spread of diseases which make the infertility problem even worse.

IS IN VITRO FERTILIZATION ETHICAL, AND SHOULD SOCIETY PAY FOR IT?

Professor Donald Coffey from Johns Hopkins University, who is one of the great DNA biochemists and philosophers in this country, has pointed out that if you look at everything in the world from the smallest molecule to the largest star, we humans are the average-size thing in the universe. Fifty percent of things in the universe are larger than us and 50 percent are smaller. Dr. Coffey points out that the chances of this happening, as well as just the mere chance that the molecule of DNA could ever just form on its own by accident and thereby direct the formation of life by accident, are almost infinitely low. He argues that there is a "human destiny" and that the design of DNA was to create enough flexibility within our development to find that human destiny and make it occur on our own. Right now there exists a terrible problem with infertility. There are those who would reject the new technology as being "unnatural," and possibly, therefore, unethical. These people are afraid of the future.

Every advance has its danger and we can't hold back now. Charles Lindbergh, flying his little airplane without a window across the Atlantic Ocean to Paris, never dreamed of 747s; he simply couldn't have imagined them. The greatest aviator in history could not foresee the future that he was unlocking with that solo flight. Four hundred thousand years ago, man discovered fire; 100,000 years ago, we began to bury our dead; and 40,000 years ago was the beginning of art. Should we have been afraid of fire? There are those who are afraid of art and free speech. But, as Dr. Coffey points out, "Every pessimist in the history of the world has been proven to be wrong."

There was no one in North America, not even Indians, 40,000 years ago. There was no complex civilization here 400 years ago. Our society is an anachronism in human life. We don't want to be "natural"; if we wanted to be "natural," we would still have typhoid, bubonic plague, polio, and enjoy the prospect of getting old. We who want to have children don't like infertility either.

The normal facets of our biology are causing 25 percent of us to be infertile. Those who are infertile do not want to stifle the creativity of our human mind because of the irrational fear of pessimists who, as we know, have in the past been proven to be wrong. The new infertility technology of IVF, GIFT, and microsurgery is the creative human solution to the problem of infertility that is part of our human condition.

CHAPTER 3

How You Get Pregnant Normally

Getting pregnant is not an easy task. The arduous journey which sperm must make through the female genitals to reach the egg, as well as the simultaneous adventure of the egg getting matured by hormones in the first half of the cycle in order to become genetically ready for fertilization, erupting from the ovary, getting grabbed by the fallopian tube, fertilized, and then hustled along into the womb at exactly the right moment to implant, constitutes an incredible odyssey fraught with excitement and peril every step of the way. Failure of the sperm or egg to make an important connection anywhere along this complicated itinerary will prevent pregnancy from occurring.

A BRIEF INTRODUCTION TO THE VAGINA, UTERUS, TUBES, AND OVARIES

The vagina is an elastic canal, about four to five inches long. At the end of this canal, in the deepest recess of the vagina, is a structure called the "cervix," which is the entrance to the womb, or "uterus." The uterus is a hard, muscular, pear-shaped structure with a narrow, triangular cavity inside, so small that it would barely hold a teaspoonful of fluid (see Figures 1 and 2). Yet this is where the fertilized egg must implant itself and grow during the next nine months into a full-size baby. The uterus has a remarkable capacity to expand so as to allow room for this growing baby, pushing aside and squashing all the other organs of the mother's abdomen. At the end of the nine months, its muscles contract during labor to squeeze the baby out into the world.

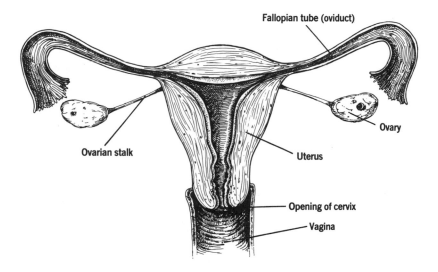

Figure 1. The female reproductive organs.

Far back in the corner of the uterus on each side is a microscopic canal that leads into the fallopian tubes, through which the sperm must squeeze their way in order to reach the egg, and in the opposite direction through which the fertilized egg must pass in order to reach the uterus. These microscopic canals leading from the uterus into the fallopian tubes are only about one-seventieth of an inch in diameter (the size of a pinpoint).

The fallopian tubes are four inches long and hang freely in the abdomen. They widen at the end into a large, flowerlike opening called the "fimbria" near the ovaries, but they are not directly connected to the ovaries.

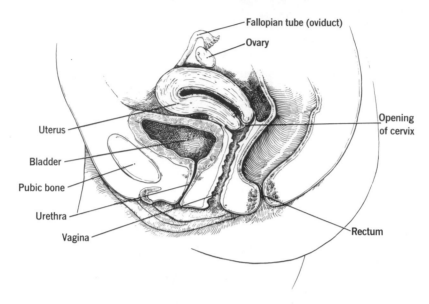

Figure 2. The female reproductive organs (side view).

The ovaries are the organs that make the female's eggs and sex hormones. They lie outside of the uterus and fallopian tubes. When an egg is extruded every month from the surface of one of the ovaries, it is released freely into the abdominal cavity rather than directly into the tube. The open end of the tube, the fimbria, then comes to life like an octopus tentacle when ovulation occurs and actively grasps the egg after its volcano-like eruption from the surface of the ovary. The end of the tube thus reaches out for the egg and actively swallows it, nourishes it before and during fertilization for three days, and then transports it ultimately into the uterus (see Figure 3).

Unlike the testicle, which is continually churning out billions of new sperm, the ovary never produces any new eggs. When a woman is born, she has within her ovaries all of the eggs she will ever have. No new eggs are formed. While the male seems wastefully to produce billions of sperm every week, the female simply matures one of her existing eggs for ovulation each month. (She eventually runs out of this limited supply, and her ovaries

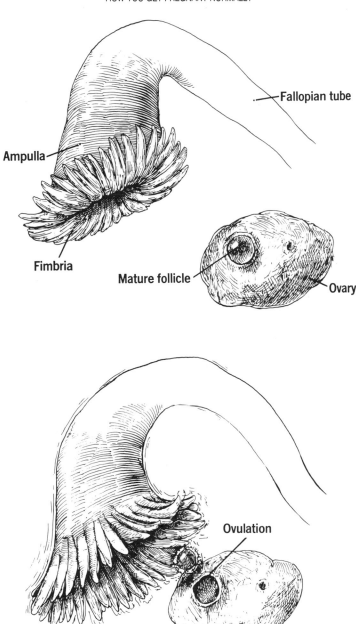

Figure 3. Ovulation

shrivel up at the time of her menopause, usually sometime between ages forty-five and fifty-five.) The ovaries mature and release only about 400 such eggs during the course of a woman's lifetime. Generally, the most fertilizable eggs are released earlier in life. Thus with advancing years, though a woman may still be able to get pregnant, she is much less fertile than she was in her youth.

The fact that the woman's eggs have already been manufactured and merely need to be extruded properly (whereas the male's sperm must be continually manufactured by an inexorable assembly-line process) makes it much easier to increase the fertility of a woman than a man. When a woman's internal clockwork goes wrong and she ovulates improperly or not at all, usually it is not difficult to improve her fertility with hormone or drug therapy. The eggs are already there, and only require a little bit of guidance. Hormonal manipulations to enhance the woman's fertility are much more likely to be successful than hormonal manipulations of the man, which are generally worthless.

HOW DOES THE EGG REACH THE TUBE?

The journey of the egg, or "ovum," through the tube and finally into the uterus after fertilization is extraordinarily hazardous. The woman's tube is not simply a passive channel through which the egg is transferred; many events must work in precise synchrony in order for successful pregnancy to occur. It is when these events get fouled up that GIFT or IVF procedures help to bypass the difficulties.

The egg must first be picked up from the surface of the ovary at the time of ovulation and transported by the fimbria into the wide area of the tube called the "ampulla." Fertilization takes place here, only halfway toward the womb, by sperm coming up from the uterus. The fertilized egg is prevented from leaving this portion of the tube for several days by a tightening of the narrow region of the tube called the "isthmus" nearer the uterus. Once fertilized, the egg must first be nourished for several days in the ampulla of the tube before it can be allowed to pass into the uterus.

The fertilized egg, or embryo, cannot be allowed to pass into the womb until it is two or three days old. If it is transferred into the uterus too soon, it will not be ready to implant, and it will die. If the transfer of the egg into the uterus is delayed too long, a "tubal," or "ectopic," pregnancy will occur (i.e., the fertilized egg implants in the tube rather than the womb). This eventually destroys the tube and requires surgery. Because the journey of the egg from the ovary to the site of fertilization, its nourishment in the tube, and the precise synchrony of the continuation of its journey into the womb is so intricate, problems with this egg and embryo transport process are frequently responsible for female infertility.

There are, on the surface of the fimbria, microscopic hairs called "cilia," which constantly beat in a direction toward the uterus at a fantastically rapid speed and create a kind of conveyor-belt effect for moving the egg along the tube toward the uterus. When the egg is grasped by the fimbria it is ushered along until it finally disappears into the tube. While it appears almost as though a mysterious force field is in operation, it is the beating of the microscopic cilia that lure the egg into the tube within a matter of minutes.

The cilia work this magic by digging into the sticky gel, called the "cumulus oophorus," that surrounds the egg and moving it along by transporting this whole sticky, goocy mass, rather than by specifically moving the tiny egg. The egg itself is invisible to the naked eye, but the gel which surrounds it is easily visible. If this sticky substance were not present, and the egg were just placed bare upon the surface of the fimbria, the beating of the cilia would never move the egg along. The cilia are only able to dig in and transport the egg with this sticky, gooey material encasing it.

Because the ovary hangs freely in the abdominal cavity, it would seem remarkable that the egg ever gets into the tube. It would appear that the egg would just fall off the ovary and be lost. A foul-up in this egg pickup process may be responsible for many cases of infertility for which we have no explanation. With the GIFT procedure (see pages 269–75) most of these women can now eventually get pregnant.

The process of grasping the egg and moving it into the interior of the tube requires only about fifteen to twenty seconds. Once the egg is safely within the tube, it is transported within five minutes toward, but not into, the narrower region of the tube located two-thirds of the way toward the uterus. Here, the egg must wait for a successful sperm coming from the opposite direction to challenge its way into the egg's tough outer membrane, the "zona pellucida," score a direct hit, and thereby establish pregnancy. While the egg is held in this location by the tight resistance of the narrow region of the tube, the much tinier sperm nonetheless must struggle through this area of resistance in order to arrive from the opposite direction.

The fertilized egg is then retained in the tube while it goes through the very earliest stages of development. Once the egg has been allowed to develop in the tube for two or three days, the "isthmus" suddenly opens up and the early embryo passes quickly into the uterus.

HOW DO SPERM REACH THE EGG?

If the egg is not penetrated by sperm soon after ovulation, it becomes overripe and dies. After the egg is released from the ovary, it is only capable of fertilization for about twelve, or possibly at most twenty-four hours. The likelihood of intercourse in the human taking place during such a specific twelve-hour interval in any month is rather slight. So nature must provide some mechanism for providing a continuous flow of healthy sperm to the site of fertilization. That way, if intercourse is perhaps one or two days off the twelve-hour limit, some sperm can still arrive at the site of fertilization at the right time. For this reason, complicated barriers to sperm transport are necessary, providing a steady, continuous flow of a small number of sperm into the site of fertilization instead of a sudden, brief flooding with sperm only to then disappear before the egg is available.

The success of test-tube fertilization demonstrates that, if eggs can be recovered at precisely the right time, they can be fertilized in the laboratory with only a small number of sperm. Then the complicated mechanism provided by nature to allow a slow, continuing flow of a small number of sperm at a time is not necessary, and the large numbers of sperm normally required for fertilization through intercourse are not needed.

Ejaculation into the Vagina

Most of the spermatozoa in the ejaculate are contained in the very first portion of fluid which squirts out of the penis and enters the vagina. The remaining squirts usually contain very little sperm. Thus at the first moment of ejaculation, the female's "cervix" (the opening leading into her uterus) is bathed by a high concentration of sperm. Within just a few minutes after ejaculation (see Figure 4), sperm begin to invade a very thick fluid (called "cervical mucus") which is pouring out of the opening to the uterus, called the cervix. The sperm must be able to invade the cervix via the cervical mucus by virtue of their own swimming ability. Nothing about the sexual act will help those sperm get into the cervix. They simply have to swim into the mucus on their own, and this requires a great deal of coordinated, cooperative activity on their part.

Ejaculation is a very tense moment for the sperm, as the vagina

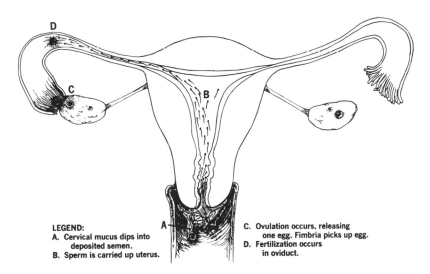

LEGEND:
A. Cervical mucus dips into deposited semen.
B. Sperm is carried up uterus.
C. Ovulation occurs, releasing one egg. Fimbria picks up egg.
D. Fertilization occurs in oviduct.

Figure 4. Sperm invading cervical mucus from vagina.

presents a very harsh, acid environment which would normally immobilize them quickly. The alkalinity of the semen (the fluid which contains the sperm), as well as the alkalinity of the cervical mucus, allows the sperm to survive in this difficult vaginal environment. Any acidity at all quickly kills sperm.

Yet even the semen is a potentially dangerous milieu for the sperm; any sperm that remain in the semen for over two hours are likely to deteriorate. In order to survive long enough to get to the egg and fertilize it, the sperm must gain rapid access to the cervical mucus. Any sperm that have not penetrated the cervical mucus within a half hour after orgasm will not be able to do so later on, because by then they will have lost their ability to swim into the more friendly environment of the cervix. The invasion must take place promptly; any sperm left behind will never be able to catch up.

Sperm Invasion

The deposition of semen in close proximity to the cervix thus undoubtedly aids the sperm in their rapid invasion of the cervix. Spermatozoa can be seen invading the cervical mucus within seconds after ejaculation, but most will not make it. Of some 200 million sperm deposited into the vagina near the cervix, only 100,000 ever get into the womb. Thus over 99.9 percent of the sperm never have a chance of getting beyond the vagina.

Once the sperm enter the canal of the cervix, they are capable of fertilizing the egg for as long as forty-eight hours. They may actually live for up to six days, but they seem capable of fertilization for only two days after intercourse. Since the egg is only fertilizable for twelve hours after ovulation, it is important to have a continuing flow of sperm across the tube so that whenever the egg reaches the area, there will be sperm available. In this sense the canal of the cervix can be looked upon as a receptacle through which platoons of spermatozoa migrate and in which some are detained in order to ensure a continuous supply of smaller numbers, over a more prolonged period of time, to the deeper recesses of the female where fertilization takes place.

Of course, these delaying mechanisms can do more harm than good in infertile couples if events do not allow the invasion of sperm to be mounted successfully. (That is where GIFT or IVF solve the problem by bypassing all these barriers.)

To understand how this invasion of sperm gets launched effectively, we must first understand that remarkable liquid which covers the opening of the womb, the cervical mucus. The cervical mucus presents a very effective barrier to bacteria and thus protects the womb against infection. It is a selective filter which favors normally active sperm, and excludes other objects (including poor-quality sperm) from access. But it doesn't even permit access to normal sperm except during a specific period at mid-cycle, when ovulation is imminent and fertilization is possible. Cervical mucus resembles a thick, clear liquid which can be poured from one container into another. However, in a technical sense it is not a liquid. As it is being poured, it can actually be cut with a scissors; thus, although it seems to behave as a thick liquid, it also has the characteristics of a very pliable, transparent plastic.

Cervical mucus is absent or very scanty during most of the monthly cycle, gradually becoming more abundant around the middle of the cycle, when ovulation is about to occur. Just prior to ovulation it becomes almost optically clear, although it is translucent at other times. At the moment when fertilization is possible, near the time of ovulation, the mucus can be stretched out into a very thin strand; but at other times in the cycle it is more sticky, and instead of stretching, it will break. All of these changes in the cervical mucus which occur around the time prior to ovulation are designed to help sperm gain access to the uterus. The more liquidlike character, the greater transparency, and the greater stretchability (called "spinnbarkheit") are all characteristics which favor the successful invasion of an army of sperm. When the mucus is sticky and thick, not as abundant, and translucent rather than transparent, it is difficult if not impossible for any sperm to gain access.

Microscopically, the cervical mucus consists of a dense mesh which, during most of the monthly cycle, represents a solid barrier to invasion. Just prior to ovulation, under the effect of the female hormone estrogen, the amount of mucus production rises ten-fold and the water content of the mucus increases. The otherwise impenetrable, dense mesh opens up, and allows a successful invasion of sperm.

When semen first reaches the cervical mucus after ejaculation, a clear barrier line can be seen separating the two different fluids. Semen does not "mix" at all with cervical mucus. Soon, however, "phalanges" of sperm begin to penetrate into the mucus, forming branching structures which invade into it. Observing the sperm's penetration of the cervical mucus under the microscope is an exciting event. Sperm at first seem to bounce against the cervical mucus without any evidence that they will ever be able to gain access. Their movements while in the ejaculate are haphazard, and not specifically aimed toward the mucus. However, within a matter of minutes one or two spermatozoa begin to make an indentation in the line separating the cervical mucus from the ejaculate. Once one sperm has been able to initiate the penetration of the mucus, other sperm then quickly follow at that same point of entry. Sperm then continue to invade the cervical mucus at that point much like a single-file line of army ants. Only one or two spermatozoa can pass at a time through this line of entrance.

Once initial penetration has occurred, more sperm are able to continue easily across this beachhead into the cervix. They swim in a straightforward direction along parallel rows of the invisible microscopic molecular structure of the mucus. Sperm which can move only in a curved path, or wiggle in place, are incapable of taking part in this invasion of the cervix, and are left behind in the vagina to die. Once this beachhead in the cervical mucus has been established, sperm can reach the fallopian tubes in about thirty minutes.

Pregnancy would not be likely if *all the sperm* got into the fallopian tubes at one time, because they would soon pass on into the abdominal cavity, and not be available to fertilize the egg except during a very brief, lucky interval. If they were not lucky enough to pass through the fallopian tube at exactly the moment of ovulation (or within twelve hours of ovulation), they would be long gone by the time the egg arrived. Thus nature had to invent some mechanism for allowing a continuous entry to the site of fertilization by a smaller number of sperm. To accomplish this the cervix and the cervical mucus act as a reservoir from which, over a period of time, spermatozoa are slowly released into the uterus and up to the fallopian tubes over a period of several days. But the problem is that only several thousand out of the 200 million sperm that started in the vagina ever get into the fallopian tubes where they can meet the egg.

Capacitation of Sperm

During the course of their odyssey toward the site of fertilization, the sperm undergo a process call "capacitation," which is not fully understood. It used to be thought that unless sperm reside for a certain period of time outside the male reproductive tract and in the specific fluids of the female reproductive tract, for some unknown reason they are not capable of fertilization even though in every other respect they look normal. It was thought that this process of capacitation could only occur in the specific fluids of the female reproductive tract while the sperm migrate on their journey toward the egg. However, test-tube in vitro fertilization has demonstrated that capacitation of sperm (once considered one of the greatest problems in successfully achieving test-tube babies) can occur in relatively simple nonspecific fluids available in any laboratory.

All that is necessary to start the capacitation process going is to remove the sperm from the semen by "washing" it (see pages 234–43). Removing the sperm from semen and placing them in any laboratory "culture media" fluid results in a dramatic tripling of their swimming velocity, so that even though they are mere human sperm, they begin to swim more like the sperm of more respectable animals like horses or bulls. Thus sperm seem to have a natural tendency toward developing capacitation for fertilization on their own and simply require a period of several hours outside of semen. In nature this happens when they leave the semen and enter the cervical mucus. However, the old concept that this can only happen to sperm while they are journeying through the female tract has finally been discarded.

OVULATION

All of the eggs a woman ever releases were actually made years earlier, while she was still in her mother's womb. In men, sperm production continues every day for his entire postpubertal life by the hundreds of millions, but a woman starts her life with only a few hundred thousand eggs, and that is all she will ever have. After she reaches the age of menstruation, each month one of her eggs develops sufficient maturity to be released and offered to the tubes for fertilization. Only about four hundred such eggs will be released during her lifetime. During each of these menstrual months, for every egg which is successfully developed and extruded, there are about 1,000 that try to develop but instead lose out and die. Thus, each month from 1,000 eggs one is selected that will mature to the point where it can be extruded and fertilized. Each month, the ovulated egg may come from either of the two ovaries; it is a matter of chance which ovary will successfully mature a follicle during a given cycle. Somewhere between her mid-forties and fifties, she will run out of these eggs, and go through the menopause.

The process whereby a matured egg is extruded from the ovary is called ovulation. Since many women who seem unable to have children owe their problems to a disturbance in ovulation, and since part of in vitro fertilization (IVF) or GIFT is stimulating the ovaries to prepare many, many eggs for fertilization, we should understand how this repeatable, monthly series of changes leading to ovulation occurs naturally in the ovary. Then later we will unravel the hormonal events of the menstrual cycle which regulate the clocklike orderliness of this event.

All of the hormonal events taking place during the month between menstrual periods are directed at preparing the egg to be genetically ready for fertilization, and preparing the uterus (womb) and the cervix for the moment of ovulation, so that the sperm and the egg have the best opportunity for joining up to form an embryo, which then can implant in a properly prepared uterus and thus result in successful pregnancy.

Formation of the Follicle

From the time of sexual maturity on, about 1,000 undeveloped eggs, or "oocytes," each month leave their prolonged resting phase and start to mature. This initiation of development is a continuous process, in marked contrast to ovulation, which occurs only once a month. Once the egg starts to develop, it proceeds inexorably, and no longer has the choice of returning to being quiescent. It either wins the race to ovulate, or it must degenerate and die.

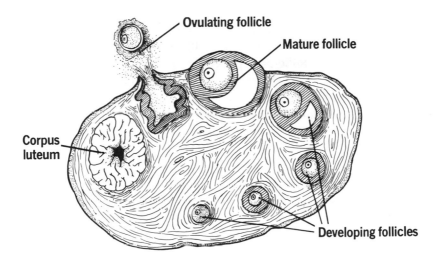

Figure 5. Formation of the follicle, and ovulation and transformation of the ovulated follicle into the corpus luteum.

The most striking feature of the egg's development is the growth of its surrounding fluid-filled compartment, called the "follicle" (see Figure 5). The growth of this follicle is stimulated by the hormone FSH (follicle-stimulating hormone) produced by the pituitary gland in the early phase of the monthly cycle. The time required for the egg to develop the proper follicle necessary for ovulation is about fourteen days. Although the follicle-stimulating hormone (FSH) stimulates all of the developing eggs during the month to form follicles, one of the eggs always gets a head start over the others, and once it obtains that lead it never relinquishes it. The other eggs developing that month then degenerate. *However, if huge doses of FSH were to be given to the woman at the beginning of the cycle, far in excess of what her pituitary would normally secrete, she would develop many follicles instead of just one.*

The follicle is a spherical, bubblelike structure which bulges up from the surface of the ovary, and which contains the egg. The egg (which is only ½₀₀ of an inch in diameter) is surrounded and protected by a mass of sticky, gelatinous fluid called the "cumulus oophorus" and hangs on a stalk to the follicle wall. However, most of the fluid in the follicle is clear yellow, and the follicle itself is fairly large (four-fifths of an inch in diameter). Occasionally two follicles successfully reach maturity, and they are both ovulated. In that circumstance the woman may have fraternal, or nonidentical, twins. Indeed, some of the drugs used to stimulate ovulation in women who would not otherwise ovulate may work better than expected, and, as mentioned, cause the development of more than one follicle. Therefore, multiple births are more common in women who require medical treatment to help them ovulate.

Two or three days prior to mid-cycle, when the follicle has reached its maximum size (usually, two centimeters, or four-fifths of an inch), it produces an enormous amount of the hormone "estrogen." This increased level of estrogen prior to ovulation stimulates the cervix to make more (and clearer) cervical mucus in order to allow sperm invasion. This dramatic increase in estrogen production by the follicle then stimulates the pituitary gland to release another hormone, different from FSH, called "LH" (luteinizing hormone). The sudden release of LH is what triggers ovulation. The increase in estrogen indicates to the pituitary that the follicle is ripe, and this beautifully times the release of the LH hormone. Ovulation then occurs normally thirty to fifty hours after the beginning of this "LH surge."

Release of the Egg

Under the influence of the mid-cycle LH surge, the wall of the follicle weakens and deteriorates, and a specific site on its surface ruptures. The bulging follicle is then extruded from the surface of the ovary through this ruptured area (see Figure 5). Observed under a microscope, ovulation appears similar to the eruption of a volcano. Occasionally women actually feel several hours of discomfort in their lower abdomen during ovulation; this discomfort is called "Mittelschmerz." In women who require hormone treatment to stimulate ovulation, so many follicles may grow so large that when ovulation occurs it causes strong cramps and (rarely nowadays) they may even become sick enough to require several days of rest in the hospital (see hormone treatment, pages 251–57). However, this sort of complication is not very likely with modern dosage monitoring. It is mentioned only to underscore what a dramatic intra-abdominal event ovulation is.

Production of Progesterone

The ruptured, empty follicle then undergoes another dramatic change, called "luteinization." Prior to ovulation, the follicle had produced only estrogen. After ovulation, it produces the other female hormone, "progesterone." Before ovulation occurred, it was impossible for the follicle to make progesterone. Thus the production of progesterone "implies" that ovulation has occurred. In the old days, the production of progesterone used to be the basis for all our clinical methods of evaluating ovulation. The production of progesterone by the transformed follicle after ovulation is the key to successful implantation of the embryo in the womb during the second two weeks of the cycle.

The rupture of the follicle at ovulation transforms it into a completely different endocrine gland, which manufactures this different female hormone, progesterone, which has an entirely separate purpose than estrogen. The new structure that forms monthly from the ruptured follicle is called the "corpus luteum." This is Latin for "yellow body" and simply signifies that the follicle turns yellow as it changes its identity. As soon as the corpus luteum (which has formed in the ruptured follicle) begins to produce progesterone, the cervical mucus (which had become maximally receptive to sperm invasion just prior to ovulation) is suddenly caused to become sticky and totally impermeable to the invasion of sperm. In addition, progesterone causes the entrance of the cervix to close dramatically, even though just prior to ovulation it had been gaping in readiness for the entry of sperm. Although estrogen in the first half of the cycle stimulates the buildup of a thick, hard layer of tissue called the "endometrium" to line the uterus prior to ovulation, this lining does not become receptive to the fertilized egg until after ovulation, when the secretion of progesterone causes it to soften. If the uterine lining is not "softened" after ovulation (i.e., transformed from "proliferative" to "secretory") by progesterone, implantation of the embryo cannot occur.

The corpus luteum manufactures this progesterone over a very limited time. If no pregnancy develops, the corpus luteum ceases to produce progesterone by ten to fourteen days after ovulation. With this cessation of progesterone production by the ovary, the soft lining that was built up in the womb to prepare for the nourishment of the fertilized egg is shed and the woman menstruates. The drop in progesterone (and estrogen) production by the ovary during menstruation then stimulates a new increase in FSH (follicle-stimulating hormone). A new follicle then develops, estrogen production resumes, and the cycle begins again.

The presence of progesterone only *implies* that ovulation has probably occurred; ovulation may not have actually taken place. The hormone LH may stimulate the transformation of a follicle into a corpus luteum even though a proper egg may not have been released or picked up by the fallopian tube. In the past the only methods we used to have for determining whether or not a woman ovulated (and indeed for pinpointing the time of her ovulation) were indirect and based solely on the assumption that when progesterone is produced by the ovary, ovulation must have occurred. Now we can peer right into the follicle with ultrasound, and in addition measure every hormone related to egg maturation and ovulation quickly and simply.

HORMONES THAT CONTROL OVULATION AND THE MENSTRUAL CYCLE

The cycle which animals go through are called "estrous" cycles. No animals except for man and the apes have "menstrual" cycles. In a "menstrual" cycle the buildup of the lining of the womb is so lush, and the drop in hormone level supporting that lining is so abrupt, that at the end of the cycle the lining actually sheds and the woman bleeds for four to five days in what is commonly known as her "period." In all other animals, however, this shedding does not occur, and the thick lining of the womb merely returns to the thinned-out condition which marks the beginning of the next cycle.

Since most women are unaware of when they ovulate, we must try to understand the events in the menstrual cycle more fully than do animals, who simply "do it" at the right time automatically. We will arbitrarily call the first day of the menstrual cycle "day one," which is the day that bleeding commences. Menstruation normally takes place over about four to five days. Thus the fourth day of bleeding would be the fourth day of the menstrual cycle. Bleeding usually ceases by day four or five and in most cases resumes after day twenty-eight of the cycle. Although the first day of menstruation represents a shedding of the lining of the uterus (womb) from the previous month's cycle, it is actually the *beginning* day one of the next cycle.

On the first day of menstruation the pituitary hormone FSH is already stimulating development of a follicle that will take precedence over all other follicles trying to get started for that next month (see Figures 6 and 7). Interestingly, FSH which in females causes the follicle to develop, is the exact same hormone which in males helps to stimulate sperm production. As the follicle is stimulated by FSH from the pituitary to develop over the next ten to fourteen days, it produces increasing amounts of the female hormone estrogen, *but no progesterone*. Estrogen produced by the ovarian follicle then, in turn, inhibits further pituitary production of FSH, so that the FSH level begins to drop prior to ovulation. Keep in mind that there is always a "feedback" mechanism whereby the very estrogen which FSH

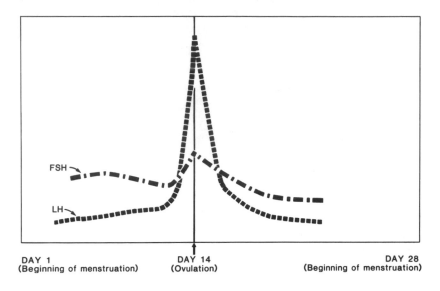

Figure 6. Hormone changes associated with normal ovulation.

causes to be produced by the ovary inhibits the pituitary from making more FSH. This is so-called "negative feedback."

By day twelve to day fourteen of the menstrual cycle, the follicle is usually quite ripe and appears on the surface of the ovary as a fluid-filled bubble ready to burst. In the meantime, the estrogen which has been produced by the follicle during this first half of the cycle is stimulating the uterus to prepare a thick lining to receive the fertilized egg. This first half of the cycle is called "proliferative." This thick, "proliferative" uterine lining is not ready to receive the egg until it is "softened" in the second half of the cycle by progesterone.

Estrogen in the first half of the cycle has also caused the cervix to produce enormous quantities of optically clear mucus, allowing the greatest receptivity to sperm penetration. It also causes the entrance to the cervix, which is generally closed, to open between day nine and day fourteen, and it is almost gaping with an abundant outflow of clear mucus just prior to ovulation. Estrogen has thus prepared the way for sperm entrance.

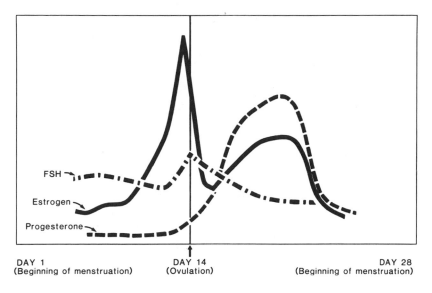

DAY 1
(Beginning of menstruation)

DAY 14
(Ovulation)

DAY 28
(Beginning of menstruation)

Figure 7. Hormone changes associated with normal ovulation.

The final effect of estrogen (in high quantities) is to trigger the release of a different "LH" pituitary hormone or "lutenizing hormone." The triggering of LH release by increasing levels of estrogen is called "positive feedback." This enormous surge of LH from the pituitary is what causes the follicle to burst, and the ovulation occurs about thirty to fifty hours later. Actually LH does a lot more to the egg (*to make it fertilizable*) than just cause ovulation (release of the egg from the ovary). (See pages 71–73.)

After ovulation, as mentioned, the ruptured follicle forms the yellow "corpus luteum" which produces "progesterone." Over the next ten to fourteen days progesterone makes the lining of the uterus soft, delicate, and spongy, so that it can adequately nourish the fertilized egg, which cannot implant unless this change in the lining occurs. Progesterone also causes the cervical mucus to dry up and the cervix to close. This second half of the cycle is called the "secretory" phase and is under the domination of progesterone. It is sometimes also called the "luteal" phase because progesterone is produced by the corpus luteum. If the egg is not fertilized, the corpus luteum has a very specific limited lifetime of ten to fourteen days. At the end of that time, if the woman is not pregnant, the ovary stops producing progesterone, the uterine lining can no longer support itself, and it sheds on what becomes day one of the next menstrual cycle, when she starts to bleed.

As we shall see later, almost all women have the machinery necessary to produce the right hormones and a proper egg, and yet may not be fertile simply because the precise synchrony of events required to regulate the system is misfiring. It is as if a fine automobile were missing its spark plugs and points. Maturation of the follicle with its production of estrogen under the influence of FSH, the stimulation of LH release by this production of estrogen, the induction of ovulation by LH release, and the subsequent transformation of the follicle into a corpus luteum which produces progesterone must occur in a precise and orderly fashion. The mere production of estrogen and progesterone, and the release of FSH and LH, are not sufficient. Fortunately, in most cases of "misfiring," the proper synchrony can easily be restored.

HOW THE PRIMITIVE REGION OF THE BRAIN CALLED THE "HYPOTHALAMUS" CONTROLS THE MENSTRUAL CYCLE

The entire cycle of follicle development, ovulation, and menstruation depends upon the precisely timed release of FSH and LH from the pituitary gland. In the male, FSH and LH released from the pituitary gland stimulate the production of sperm and the male hormone "testosterone." In the female, FSH and LH are necessary for the ovaries to function. In the male, FSH and LH production is constant and, therefore, sperm and hormone production is constant. In the female, there is a delicately synchronized increase in FSH at the beginning of the cycle to promote follicle growth, an LH surge at mid-cycle to promote ovulation, and then a gradual drop in pituitary hormones which causes a drop in estrogen and progesterone production by the ovary, menstruation, and then in turn a sudden increase in FSH to begin a new cycle.

We know that release of FSH and LH in the pituitary is controlled by a hormone called GNRH (gonadotropin releasing hormone) released by the brain. A primitive region of the brain called the "hypothalamus" sits right at the base of the brain and above the pituitary gland. The hypothalamus causes the pituitary to release FSH and LH by sending the hormone GNRH directly to it from the brain. It used to be thought that in some way the male and the female brains were different (and indeed they are in most other animals), because in the male the brain supposedly directed a constant production of FSH and LH, whereas in the female the brain seemed to direct a cyclical production of FSH and LH. We now know that this area of the brain in humans functions identically in the male and female, and that rather it is only the ovarian response that directs all of the cyclical production of FSH and LH in the female quite differently from the male.

This new discovery was made by the pioneering work of Dr. Ernst Knobil, then from the University of Pittsburgh, and now located in Houston, Texas. By releasing GNRH, the primitive region of the brain is simply permissive in allowing the pituitary to stimulate the ovary in the female and the testicle in the male. The brain secretes small pulses which last only a minute or so of the hormone GNRH about every ninety minutes just like a clock in both men and women. Puberty begins when the brain starts secreting this hormone at ninety-minute intervals without letup. It is the constant, never-ending release of GNRH that causes the pituitary gland to start secreting FSH and LH, bringing on puberty to boys and menstruation to girls.

We know that in men with deficient sperm or testosterone production, the FSH and LH levels are higher because the pituitary is "overworking" in an effort to stimulate whatever testicular tissue remains. The same phenomenon occurs in women. We know that when the ovary runs out of eggs, and women can no longer produce estrogen (thereby going into menopause), the FSH and LH levels from the woman's pituitary go sky-high in an effort to stimulate what little ovarian tissue may still be remaining. Thus there is a "negative feedback" mechanism whereby the production of estrogen from the ovary inhibits the release of FSH from the pituitary, and a decreased number of eggs available in an aging ovary leads to an increase in FSH and LH release from the pituitary. We used to think that this feedback inhibition worked by decreasing the brain's release of GNRH. We now know that is not true.

Something very strange happens at mid-cycle in the woman compared to the man when the increasing levels of estrogen which normally serve to inhibit the release of FSH and LH (negative feedback) suddenly cause a reverse effect, and the high levels of estrogen now cause instead a "postive feedback." The exact opposite of inhibition takes place, and the surge in estrogen at mid-cycle causes the pituitary to suddenly release a huge amount of LH along with some extra FSH, and this stimulates ovulation. Because this "positive feedback" is not found in the male, we had always assumed that, in this sense, the male brain was quite different from the female brain and that only the female had this unusual positive feedback response resulting in the mid-cycle surge of LH. The cyclic pattern of hormone production in the female, which is quite different from the constant pattern of hormone production in the male, was thought to be due to a difference in the female brain's release of GNRH. Knobil's experiment proved beyond a shadow of a doubt that in truth the male and the female brain are quite the same. If the hypothalamus were destroyed (as he did in monkeys), there would be no further GNRH secretion, the pituitary would then subsequently cease to make FSH and LH, and either the ovaries or testicles, depending upon whether it is a female or a male, would shrivel up and completely stop functioning. On the other hand, if small doses of GNRH were injected once every ninety minutes in these monkeys, the males would once again continue to produce sperm and testosterone on a steady basis, and the females would once again begin their normal pattern of cyclic ovulation and menstruation. GNRH released from the brain simply allows it all to happen, but really doesn't direct anything.

CLINICAL IMPORTANCE OF GNRH RELEASE FROM THE BRAIN FOR IVF (IN VITRO FERTILIZATION) AND GIFT

Why am I spending so much time talking about this fascinating phenomenon of the relationship of the primitive region of the brain to the pituitary, the ovaries, and the testicles? The reason is that it bears very heavily on how we can obtain the most fertilizable possible eggs from the female for in vitro fertilization (IVF) and GIFT procedures. When the ovaries are stimulated to make more eggs by administering FSH (a necessary step in the in vitro fertilization process), the tremendous increase in estrogen production over a normal level can cause an *early increase in LH secretion* which may result in premature ovulation with complete loss of the eggs or, at best, can hurt the fertilizability and subsequent pregnancy rate of the eggs obtained. This problem was demonstrated by Steptoe and Edwards in reviewing their first 1,000 babies from in vitro fertilization, and since 1988 has become a standard concern in the stimulation of follicle development for IVF. In order to prevent this *premature LH increase* while at the same time stimulating ovulation in the woman, we needed to have a better understanding of GNRH, the hormone from the brain that allows the pituitary to release FSH and LH.

If GNRH were *released constantly rather than at pulsatile intervals of ninety minutes*, a peculiar reverse phenomenon takes place. The pituitary, rather than being stimulated to release FSH and LH, would become completely paralyzed after two to five days and would no longer secrete any FSH or LH at all until the constant release of GNRH is stopped and regular pulsatile ninety-minute secretion is resumed. Thus, we can completely turn off the pituitary whenever we want to by simply giving a constant dose of GNRH. It's as though the pituitary needs a ninety-minute rest before each new GNRH stimulus in order to function properly. If the pituitary doesn't get this ninety-minute rest, it behaves just as though there were no GNRH at all. This process is called "down regulation."

GNRH is chemically a very simple hormone called a "polypeptide" that can be easily synthesized by drug companies. When a small modification is made in the structure of the GNRH (again, an easy thing to do), we have what is called a "GNRH agonist" which, if injected just one time a day, stays around in the bloodstream at a constant level rather than being immediately destroyed within minutes as the brain's normal GNRH would be. Thus, by giving an injection of "GNRH agonist" simply once a day, you are creating the same effect as infusing a constant level of GNRH all day long and giving the pituitary no "rest." There are several "GNRH agonists" on the market, "Lupron" (leuprolide) being the popular one in the United States, and "Buserelin" being the popular one in Europe. Using Lupron along with our stimulation cycle, we completely turn off the pituitary and prevent it from interfering with the proper development of the large number of eggs necessary for IVF and GIFT procedures because *we no longer have to worry about a premature LH surge* (see Figure 8).

FERTILIZATION OF THE EGG IN THE FALLOPIAN TUBE

The goal toward which all of these processes lead is fertilization of the egg by the sperm. This is a beautiful and moving event to observe under the microscope, and only in the last decade have scientists come to understand fertilization well enough to duplicate it in a test tube and thereby produce a normal baby.

Fertilization of the egg occurs in the fallopian tube ampulla. But because sexual intercourse usually does not coincide with the moment of ovulation in the human, our eggs may very well have to wait in vain for the arrival of spermatozoa. The egg is capable of being fertilized only for a brief period of about twelve hours after ovulation. If it has to wait too long for sperm to arrive, all the effort that went into preparing the egg during the previous two weeks will have been wasted.

The number of sperm which actually reach the site of fertilization is terribly small when one considers the enormous numbers that are deposited in the vagina. The likelihood of fertilization is related to the number of sperm present because

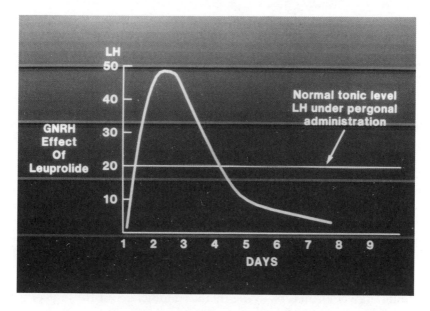

Figure 8. Graph showing an initial increase in pituitary secretion of LH during the first four days of Lupron (leuprolide) treatment and after that the decline to zero secretion level.

the actual contact of a sperm with the egg is governed mostly by chance. However, large numbers are not necessary when the sperm and egg are placed right near each other. That is why in vitro fertilization and GIFT procedures are so useful in couples with male infertility.

HOW IS THE EGG PREPARED FOR FERTILIZATION DURING THE FOLLICULAR PHASE OF THE CYCLE UNDER FSH STIMULATION?

Successful fertilization and getting pregnant depends on what happens to the egg from the very beginning of day one of the menstrual cycle under the stimulation of FSH until it is ready for ovulation. Incredible genetic cellular changes take place beginning each month with the elevation of FSH at the start of the woman's menstruation. It may simply appear that as the follicular half of the woman's cycle develops, all that is happening is that FSH is stimulating one or more follicles to develop in the ovary. In truth, some very complex cellular events are taking place in the egg during this monthly development and growth of the follicle. Furthermore, the release of LH stimulated by the estrogen surge at mid-cycle does much more than just cause ovulation. It sets up another critical genetic preparation of the egg without which fertilization would be impossible.

Thus far only a superficial description of what happens during a menstrual cycle has been given: 1) follicular growth and estrogen production in the first half, 2) ovulation at mid-cycle, hopefully with fertilization, and then 3) preparation of the uterine lining for embryo implantation in the second half of the cycle allowed by the production of progesterone from the corpus luteum, newly formed from the ovulated follicle. But these events are only the outward signs of a very complex genetic preparation for fertilization.

"REDUCTION DIVISION" ("MEIOSIS") OF THE EGG'S CHROMOSOMES

Every cell in the body has forty-six chromosomes consisting of twenty-three pairs, which carry all of our genes. However the sperm and the egg at the moment of fertilization must have only twenty-three single chomosomes, not forty-six, so that when the sperm and the egg unite, it results in a fertilized egg with the normal number of forty-six chromosomes.

When sperm leave the testicle, they have only twenty-three chromosomes. Sperm precursors in the testicle have forty-six chromosomes like every other cell in our body. But in the process of sperm production, the chromosomes are reduced by a process called "meiosis" to half the normal number.

The eggs have forty-six chromosomes until the very moment the sperm penetrates an egg and initiates fertilization. Fertilization cannot possibly occur unless the egg's forty-six chromosomes can be reduced to twenty-three. The moment the sperm penetrates the egg, half of its chromosomes must be extruded. Then two half sets of chromosomes, one from the male, and one from the female, merge into a new individual with the normal number of forty-six chromosomes. Without the hormonal stimulation of FSH causing follicle development, followed by the release of LH at mid-cycle, the eggs would not be genetically prepared for this complex event of "meiosis" to occur.

The miracle of this separation of chromosomes is the most complicated event in the whole reproductive process, and it determines the genetic makeup of the child. This event, when the chromosomes separate, results in the genetic variability of the offspring. It is the moment when the penetrating sperm triggers the egg to start the second "reduction division" of meiosis, the moment when, out of a billion possibilities, the DNA of one individual, specific person is created.

At the time of a woman's birth, all of her eggs are fixed in the beginning phase of the first "meiotic division." The remaining stages of the "meiotic division" will not begin again until years later when her egg is finally stimulated by FSH to form a follicle at the beginning of one of her menstrual cycles. Then the LH surge at mid-cycle causes the egg to resume "meiosis." This resumption of meiosis triggered by LH would not occur without the prior preparation caused over the preceding two weeks by FSH and follicular growth.

DEVELOPMENT OF THE EGG DURING GROWTH OF THE FOLLICLE

At the beginning of the cycle, from day one of menstruation, increased FSH production from the pituitary stimulates rapid growth in the egg. The egg will grow during this early follicular phase from a tiny 20 microns to its normal mature size of 140 microns (from $\frac{1}{1,000}$ of an inch to approximately $\frac{1}{200}$ of an inch in diameter). At this time also, the very tough outer membrane, like the shell of a chicken egg, the "zona pellucida," forms around the enlarging egg. This occurs before one can even see a follicle forming on ultrasound. Next the follicle expands to form a fluid-filled cavity around the egg.

When the follicle forms, many compact layers of "granulosa" cells begin to surround the now enlarged egg, and the outer sheath of these granulosa cells produces the hormone estrogen. Recent work by Dr. Neil First, from the University of Wisconsin, has shown that even a brief deprivation of estrogen to the maturing egg during this stage will result in the egg's immediate death. If FSH stimulation were to suddenly cease or be reduced dramatically, estrogen production by the granulosa cells would decline and the egg would die.

The egg remains embedded on one side of the follicle in a mound called the "cumulos oophorus." The cells around the egg remain compact until the very latter part of this second stage of the follicular phase. When the egg is finally ready for LH to trigger the important genetic events that will allow fertilization after ovulation, these cells spread out in a radial pattern, giving a sunburstlike appearance that is called the "corona radiata." If this widely disbursed sunburstlike appearance of cumulus cells surrounding the zona pellucida of the egg is present, physicians performing in vitro fertilization know that the egg is adequately "mature" for fertilization to occur. It is the most easily observable sign that the egg has gone through enough FSH stimulation to be ready for the genetic events of "meiosis" which will ultimately lead to the possibility of fertilization.

It is quite astounding that there is little difference in the maximum diameter of the egg of almost any species even though the size of the follicle containing the egg is generally related to the size of the animal. Thus, eggs of a whale could easily pass through the oviduct of the smallest mammal, like a rat, even though the whale's follicle containing that small egg could easily be as large as a whole rabbit. The increasing size of the follicle has nothing to do with any increase in the size of the egg, but merely is an indication that the egg is being properly prepared for what it has to do when it receives the surge of LH at mid-cycle.

RESUMPTION OF MEIOSIS AFTER THE LH SURGE

LH *begins* the resumption of meiosis (reduction division to half the normal number of chromosomes), but the penetration of the egg by a sperm is what causes the *completion* of that process. After the LH surge, the *first* meiotic division occurs, but this division does not reduce the number of chromosomes. This is an equal division in which forty-six chromosomes are still left within the egg nucleus.

The "first polar body" is a small, little divided nucleus that is pinched off from the main body of the egg, which tells you that first meiotic division has occurred under the influence of LH, meaning that the egg is now prepared to undergo the all-important second meiotic division. It is thus prepared for the entrance of a sperm.

The time required for the LH surge to cause the extrusion of the "first polar body" is about ten to twelve hours. This is what tells us the egg is ready to be fertilized. This is always completed well before ovulation, and it must be completed before eggs are obtained for in vitro fertilization.

PENETRATION OF THE EGG BY A SPERM

For a sperm to enter and fertilize the egg, it must dig its way through several layers of protecting shields that surround the egg. All of these outside walls protecting the inner confines of the egg represent an impressive barrier to sperm penetration, and a sperm cannot dig its way through these protective membranes without the aid of chemicals released from its warhead, the "acrosome" (see Figure 9). The acrosome surrounds the front portion of the sperm, much like a battering ram. Chemicals released by the acrosome first dissolve the jellylike "cumulus oophorus," enabling the sperm to pass through it and reach the tougher inner membrane, the zona pellucida. This very tough membrane represents perhaps the most formidable obstacle to sperm. To penetrate this barrier, the sperm cannot just haphazardly liberate chemicals, or the egg might be damaged. The

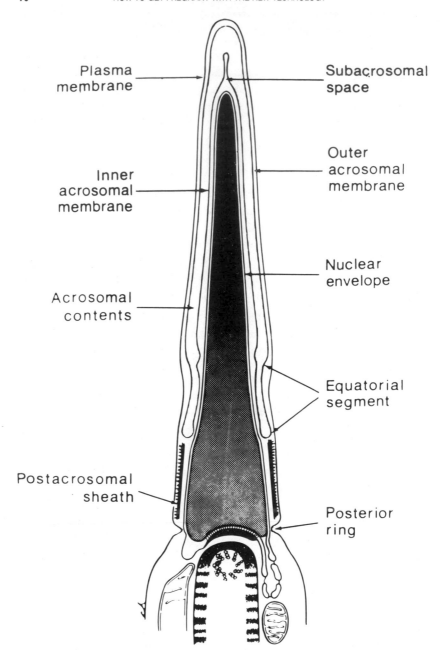

Plasma membrane

Subacrosomal space

Inner acrosomal membrane

Outer acrosomal membrane

Nuclear envelope

Acrosomal contents

Equatorial segment

Postacrosomal sheath

Posterior ring

Figure 9. Diagram of the sperm head with its outer acrosome battering ram before releasing its contents.

attacking chemicals must remain closely bound to the surface of the sperm and thereby cut an extraordinarily narrow slit into the membrane.

In order for the sperm to make its way through the sturdy zona pellucida, a process called the "acrosome reaction" is necessary. The acrosome "warhead" is attached around the front two-thirds of the sperm head, in a position much like an arrowpoint. Its contents are tightly contained because the leakage of "acrosin" at the wrong time prematurely would make it impossible for the sperm head to drill its way through the zona pellucida when it finally makes contact. During the "acrosome reaction," the inner and outer acrosomal membranes form holes which allow the release of acrosome particles that are actually deposited along the tunnel created in the zona pellucida by the penetrating sperm. When the sperm makes contact with the zona pellucida, in some marvelously mysterious way, this stimulates the acrosome to undergo its reaction and to release the acrosin, which helps the sperm head drill its way through the zona pellucida.

Once a lucky sperm makes contact with the zona pellucida (which is purely a random event), it takes a minimum of fifteen minutes before penetration can begin. Some sperm can be seen struggling to penetrate for as long as an hour before they make their initial penetration. If penetration hasn't occurred within an hour, however, something is wrong and the egg will probably not fertilize. Sperm enter the zona at an angle almost exactly perpendicular to the surface of the egg and appear to develop a channel within the zona as they move forward. Despite the important "drilling" effect achieved by the release of acrosin from the outer acrosomal membrane of the sperm head, it is very clear that without the vigorous, hyperactive beating of the sperm tail providing strong mechanical propulsive force, the sperm still would not be able to get in.

Once penetration of the zona has begun, it requires an average of twenty minutes for the sperm to get completely through; and once the sperm has gotten through, it immediately dashes around the "perivitelline space" (the narrow space between the egg membrane and the zona pellucida) and in less than a second plunges directly into the egg membrane itself. Very soon after the sperm head becomes embedded in the egg, its tightly packed

DNA begins to decondense (spread out a little), and the genetic material of the male now within the egg becomes the "male pronucleus."

COMPLETION OF MEIOSIS AND UNION OF THE MALE AND FEMALE GENES

When the first sperm has successfully invaded the "zona pellucida" of the egg, a remarkable event takes place. The membrane inside the "zona" which surrounds the egg fuses with the membrane of the sperm, and the sperm and the egg become one. The egg literally swallows the sperm as these two microscopic entities initiate the development of a new human being. Also at this moment the membranes surrounding the egg become transformed into a rigid barrier so impenetrable that other sperm, despite all the chemicals in their acrosomes, cannot possibly enter. Many sperm can be seen attempting to enter the egg in competition with the one that made it first, but their efforts are totally in vain. Once the egg has been successfully penetrated by a single sperm, it shuts its walls so tightly that none of the followers can possibly get through. This protects the fertilized egg from the entrance of the extra chromosomes (called "polyploidy") which would cause a genetically impossible fetus, and miscarriage. Penetration of the egg membrane by the sperm head also sets in motion the "second meiotic division" of the egg with the release of the second polar body. It is this "second meiotic division" that reduces the number of chromosomes to half so that sperm and egg genes can unite.

When the sperm head enters the egg its chromosomes are tightly and densely packed. As this "haploid" number of male chromosomes begin to unravel and loosen up in the egg, the sperm head no longer appears to be a sperm but rather becomes the "male pronucleus," which is sort of like half of the nucleus of an egg which has not yet completed its fertilization process. At this same time, the female nucleus, which is sitting on the opposite side of the egg near its membrane, is triggered in some way to undergo its second meiotic division within about twenty to thirty minutes after sperm penetration of the egg. This second

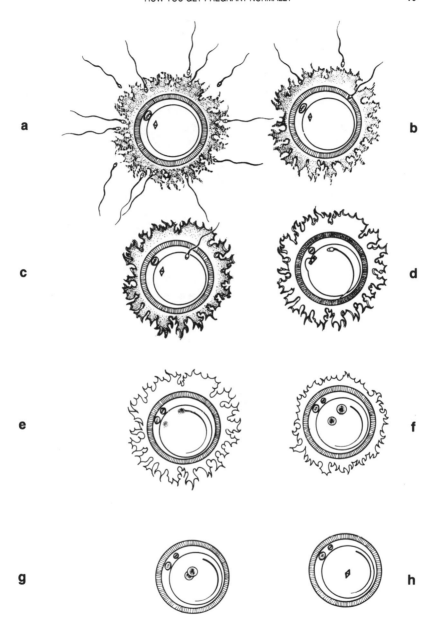

Figure 10. Diagram of the events of fertilization triggered by the entrance of the first sperm.

meiotic division causes extrusion of the second polar body outside of the egg and a reduction of the number of chromosomes of the female nucleus from forty-six to twenty-three, i.e., the "haploid" number which is required before fertilization can occur. Within eleven to eighteen hours the male and female pronuclei sitting on opposite sides of the egg appear extremely prominent and get ready to converge (see Figure 10).

This is truly an amazing event. The two pronuclei slowly and majestically move toward the center of the egg and join into one nucleus, which now has forty-six chromosomes and represents an entirely new human being. This process of the merging of the male and the female pronucleus is called "syngamy." After syngamy the fertilized egg is ready to divide. Division of the fertilized egg is called "cleavage."

EARLY DEVELOPMENT OF THE FERTILIZED EGG

Over the next three days the fertilized egg first divides into two, then four, then eight cells. The fertilized egg, or embryo, does not pass into the uterus for implantation until it is two or three days old. Thus all of us have spent the first few days of embryonic life in our mother's fallopian tube before being allowed into the womb. If the embryo is transferred into the uterus too soon, it will not be ready to implant and will die.

The first cleavage into two cells occurs sometime before thirty-eight hours after fertilization. The second cleavage (four cells) begins sometime between thirty-eight and forty-six hours after fertilization. The third cleavage (eight cells) begins between fifty-one and sixty-two hours after fertilization. If any one of those cells were to be removed, the remaining ones would still continue to develop into a normal baby. That is, each cell is still "totipotential" and could on its own develop into a completely normal human being. Each one of these early cells formed by the first three or four divisions of the fertilized egg is called a "blastomere"; each on its own would have the ability to form a completely intact individual.

Finally, by the third or fourth day, the embryo has 100 to 160 cells and is called a "morula." These cells have now "compacted" and no longer have totipotential individuality. It's at this stage that the embryo is passed from the fallopian tube into the uterus. By the fifth or sixth day after fertilization there are so many cells all still packed into the same hard, tough zona pellucida that individual cells can no longer be recognized. At this stage the pre-embryo is called a "blastocyst." On the sixth or seventh day after fertilization this "blastocyst" thins out a spot in the otherwise hardened shell of the zona pellucida and actually "hatches" just like a chicken hatches from its shell in an incubator. The blastocyst pushes its way out of this thinned-out crack in the zona pellucida and prepares for implantation (by the seventh day) into the wall of the uterus, or "womb."

Up until now the zona has protected the embryo. But now the embryo is ready for its most treacherous and frightening moment when the blastocyst hatches from its zona and has to attach to the endometrial lining of the womb. This is when the greatest risk of pregnancy failure occurs. If the blastocyst attaches successfully to the endometrium, then, and only then, can it be called a pregnancy. Then and only then can we call it a conception.

The woman has not conceived, and life has not begun, simply because of syngamy of the "male" and "female" pronuclei with cleavage of a fertilized egg. Such a fertilized egg could be allowed to live in culture media, finally cease to grow and develop, and just degenerate if it does not successfully attach to the endometrium and become a pregnancy. The mere fact that an egg has been fertilized does not mean that a pregnancy has been achieved.

PREGNANCY TESTING

If a pregnancy has been achieved the embryo begins to secrete the hormone HCG (human chorionic gonadotropin), and this HCG stimulates the ovary to continue to produce progesterone and estrogen, which is necessary for the maintenance of the lining of the womb. Without continued production of progesterone, the pregnancy could not survive. After about seven days, when the pregnancy is first established in the uterus, is when the embryo first begins to make HCG, which keeps forcing the ovary to make progesterone and thus prevents menstruation. After three months, the fetus, or rather the fetal placenta, makes its own progesterone, and the ovaries are no longer needed for production of any hormones at all. After nine months, the baby is ready to be pushed out of the uterus by the mother during labor.

The presence of HCG signifies an established pregnancy and thus is the basis for almost all of the routine pregnancy tests. When the doctor samples the patient's urine or blood and checks for pregnancy, he or she really is checking for the presence of HCG. If it is present, then the pregnancy test is positive. Since previous methods of analyzing this hormone were not very sensitive, the diagnosis of pregnancy could not be made with certainly until about four weeks after a missed period. However, with modern methods, pregnancy can be diagnosed with a simple test that the woman can perform herself in her home (or by the lab) within fourteen days of egg fertilization, or before she has even "missed her period."

CHAPTER 4

Figuring Out What's Wrong

Now that you know all of the intricate details about how pregnancy is supposed to take place naturally, with no painful testing or agonizing waiting, you'll want to know what tests your physician or clinic will be performing in order to find out what exactly is wrong with you or your husband, and why this incredibly complex series of events required for you to get pregnant is not happening correctly. As you may have already surmised, despite all of the testing that's available, you may never really find out why you're not getting pregnant. Since getting pregnant is such an incredibly complex process for the body to achieve, the real question is how does anybody ever get pregnant at all?

When I first wrote *How to Get Pregnant* in 1979, we all thought, perhaps smugly, that we had diagnostic tools for discovering the cause of infertility in over 90 percent of couples. In fact, we felt justified in that smugness by virtue of the fact that many couples got pregnant with the conventional treatments we had available at that time, which were applied according to the "diagnosis" of their problem. But it took a very long time for many of those couples to get pregnant. Many of them who were older ran out of time while waiting to get pregnant, many gave up treatment after years because of the emotional and economic cost of years of testing and treatment, and many simply did not get pregnant with the inadequate methods that were available at that time.

Those inadequate methods of treatment were based upon the misconception (pardon the double meaning) that a specific problem in the couple had been pinpointed and that solving that specific problem should result in the woman's getting pregnant. This was merely an illusion fueled by the general view in medicine: first you make a diagnosis, and then you apply a specific treatment. The fact is that the process of human reproduction is so incredibly fragile that a myriad of things can go wrong, and yet diagnostic testing will only reveal the most obvious and gross abnormalities.

That is why, despite government outrage at the so-called expense of the new technology, and in spite of media warnings that "simpler" methods of treatment would be more "cost-effective," and in defiance of the tangled worries of professional ethicists who, behind their ivory-tower desks, worry that we are "tampering with life," in vitro fertilization and GIFT programs are growing with extraordinary speed and have waiting lists too long to handle. The reason is that even after physicians and scientists "figure out what's wrong," there is a good chance they will be wrong, and the best hope for your getting pregnant (if simple, conventional methods of treatment don't work) is to bypass all the obstacles to fertilization that the body naturally presents and literally go around every aspect of the complex process described in Chapter 3.

In this chapter, I will outline some of the diagnostic testing you may go through, excluding tests on the husband's sperm (which will be covered in the next chapters). You should realize, however, that in the majority of women even if these tests come up with a "diagnosis," in most cases it does not in any way represent a definitive reason why you're not getting pregnant. Therefore, if the treatment of a specific diagnosis does not result in pregnancy, you should not delay for too long. If you're in your mid- to late thirties, you should go right to the new technology, which bypasses not just one problem but all of the problems that can crop up in this complex reproductive process. Ironically, the cost of these new reproductive technologies like in vitro fertilization (IVF) and GIFT is actually less expensive than many of the older, conventional methods of treatment.

I'll never forget years ago seeing a couple who were requesting a vasectomy; they had three children, were now in their mid-thirties, and did not want to have any more. Although the man had a quite normal semen analysis, I had never seen a more clearly infertile-looking woman in my life. She was overweight, her menstrual history was quite irregular, incompatible with any kind of regular ovulation, and she had oily skin with facial hair indicative of very high testosterone levels and severe hormonal imbalance. I was so fascinated by this couple that, despite the fact that they were coming in for a vasectomy (which I willingly performed), I did a complete infertility evaluation on them just as though they had come in complaining that they had not been able to get pregnant.

Daily hormone evaluations of the woman showed lack of ovulation, elevated male hormone levels, and no progesterone production. Whenever I saw her she had lots of clear cervical mucus but showed no sign of ovulation. Then suddenly one month she ovulated, as measured by an increased progesterone level and a drying up of her cervical mucus. This was clearly an "infertile" woman by any of our sophisticated hormonal testing, but she had three children and had only come to see me because her husband wanted a vasectomy. They had a very regular sex life, and I have to assume that their three children were the result of the few times in her whole life that she ovulated. But when she did ovulate there were always sperm continually moving up from her cervical mucus to the fallopian tube so that on her lucky day of ovulation, the sperm were ready. The majority of couples who are clearly infertile pass all our tests with flying colors, and yet this woman who had three children could not.

TESTS ON THE FEMALE

Going through expensive and sometimes painful tests without a clear understanding of what they are to accomplish is an intimidating experience which a woman may sometimes be afraid to question. This should not be the case. The purpose of this section is to explain what tests are actually needed. A large number do not give any information that helps in treatment, and many are expensive and uncomfortable. However, the testing should be simple and not overly expensive. Let's look at some of these tests and see what they really do and do not tell us.

History and Physical

Irregular Periods and Oily Skin

An abnormal menstrual history is a hint that there are problems. The clues to a woman's infertility may appear years before she has any interest in having children. When a girl's periods first begin, a stage in life known as "menarche," they are naturally very irregular. However, by age fifteen or sixteen they should have stabilized so that they come about every twenty-eight days, are of four to five days' duration, and tend to be a bit heavier the first or second day, tapering off to just a little spotting on the last day. There is a precise hormonal clockwork which regulates the development of the follicle, secretion of estrogen, buildup of a "thick" lining in the uterus prior to ovulation, the pouring out of large quantities of clear cervical mucus, the LH surge which induces ovulation, and the conversion to a "soft" lining in the uterus after ovulation when the ruptured follicle starts making progesterone. If this intricately synchronized clockwork of hormonal events is out of tune, the periods may be irregular. In a fertile woman, the normal buildup of a firm, thick lining in the womb, followed by a lush softening of that lining in the second half of the month, leads to an even and neat flow of menstrual blood. The uterus has a fresh start with each new cycle. However, if there is no ovulation, the lining of the uterus builds up unevenly, and bleeding can occur irregularly.

When the number of days between menstrual periods varies too greatly, this is a sign of error somewhere in the clockwork that regulates proper buildup of the lining of the womb and may be associated either with lack of ovulation, "poor" ovulation, or some deviation from the normal pattern of hormonal regulation. Certainly women with irregular periods can ovulate and get pregnant, but if they are ovulating, they may be ovulating late, or they are not ovulating each month. Some women may ovulate only twice a year and have very mixed-up periods in between. If the husband has a very high sperm count, the woman may very well get pregnant the one time she does ovulate.

When you examine the menstrual cycles of women who are very fertile (i.e., who got pregnant very, very easily), most of them (though not all) are like clockwork. They have the perfect, idealized twenty-eight-day cycles, with ovulation right in the middle on day fourteen. The perfect regularity of their menstrual cycles is a rough indication that all is right with their hormonal events, which as you have learned, are critical for normal fertilization to occur.

It used to be that the only way of knowing clinically that a woman has ovulated was if she produced progesterone in the second half of her cycle. Progesterone softens up the lining of the uterus so that a more complete and clean shedding of it will occur at the end of her cycle. When ovulation has not occurred, and progesterone has not been produced, the lining of the womb is somewhat tougher and flakes off in bits and pieces. Periods may not be heavy until several months' worth of this inadequately shed lining has built up. Irregular periods indicate a step-by-step peeling off of the lining rather than a heavy shedding of its entire thickness, and indicate hormonal and ovulatory irregularity.

Extremely painful periods have been thought to be a sign of a condition called "endometriosis" in which some of the tissue lining the inside of the womb is located in areas outside the womb. Thus when the lining of the womb begins to shed, supposedly similar shedding occurs outside the womb and causes pain. But "endometriosis" is one of the most overdiagnosed conditions on earth. Actually it is probably not a cause of infertility in most cases but rather a result of it. I have done tubal ligations on many "fertile" women and seen endometriosis in their pelvises. Of course, large lesions of endometriosis can cause infertility, and my negative comments will stir the wrath of those who make a living operating on *tiny* lumps of endometriosis that cause no harm.

But the major myth to be shattered here is not the treatment of endometriosis but rather that painful periods *do not* mean "endometriosis." They just mean painful periods, and they are not usually an indication of endometriosis, or any other specific infertility problem.

Using birth control pills will generally make irregular periods regular, because they artifically control the buildup and shedding of the lining of the womb. However, with the pill a much thinner lining develops and therefore the periods are much lighter. The woman who has had uncomfortable periods frequently is thus relieved of all of her menstrual discomfort when she goes on the pill.

Some women feel several hours of pain called "Mittelschmerz" at the time of ovulation. This is a sharp, crampy sensation felt on one side or the other, depending on which ovary is extruding the egg. For reasons we don't understand, most women do not feel this pain. Those who do feel this pain can tell exactly when they are ovulating.

Most women who do not ovulate regularly have a slightly increased amount of male hormone. It is not clear whether the increased production of male hormone is causing them not to ovulate, or whether their inability to ovulate is upsetting their hormonal clockwork to the point where too much male hormone is being produced. Regardless, there is frequently a definite increase in male hormone output in women who are not ovulating regularly. For this reason it is important to check for subtle signs of increased male hormone production. A small amount of hair on the breast, a slightly denser than usual amount of hair in the midline of the lower abdomen, a small amount of fuzzy hair around the anus, or even hair on the great toe are all signs of slightly elevated male hormone production.

Another sign of excess male hormone, which often turns up in the late teens (the significance of which is not realized until ten or fifteen years later when a woman is unable to get pregnant), is acne. Very frequently acne which persists beyond the mid-teens in a girl is a sign of elevated male-hormone production associated with lack of ovulation. Oily skin has similar connotations. Thus menstrual irregularity, abnormal body hair distribution, oily skin, and acne can be clues to an ovulatory disturbance.

Too Fat or Too Thin

The most obvious abnormality that may be a clue to the infertility problem is if a woman is either too fat or too thin. This may sound surprising but there is actually a fascinating hormonal explanation for the association of overweight and extreme underweight with infertility. The fat cells in your body absorb and slowly release the female hormone estrogen. Therefore, if a woman is obese, she has a lot of estrogen stored in her body that is slowly and gradually released constantly in a noncyclical fashion from places other than her ovaries. At the time of menstruation (day one of the cycle) she will not get as rapid and as high an increase in FSH production from her pituitary gland, because the estrogen constantly coming out of her fat cells is actually suppressing her pituitary gland. Without that early burst of FSH from the pituitary, the ovarian follicle gets a slow start and all of the hormonal events leading up to preparing the egg's chromosomes for ovulation and fertilization can be out of synch.

I had a very pleasant patient who happened to be 130 pounds overweight and had been infertile all of her married life. She had been through all of the testing performed at several fertility clinics and was now requesting that we perform GIFT on her since no other cause of infertility had been determined. I explained to her that we could not consider treating her with a procedure that involved even "minor" surgery unless she were to lose a hundred pounds and, thereby, become a safer operative candidate. I recommended her to several weight-loss programs which have had good results with the problem of massive obesity, told her to return after she had lost the weight, and then we would evaluate whether GIFT would be an appropriate procedure for her. She called one year later to tell me that after losing this significant amount of weight, her periods had become more regular, and she was now pregnant.

Being fat and having all this storage of estrogen not only can hurt fertility but can also increase the risk of getting cancer of the uterus later in life, for the same reason. It is well known by physicians that overweight women have a much higher risk of developing this cancer than women of normal weight. The reason for this increased risk of cancer of the uterus is that these women have an excess of continued estrogen release from their fat cells unopposed by any cyclic ovulatory production of progesterone. Thus, they continue to build up the hard, thick uterine lining that is typical of the first two weeks of the menstrual cycle. This can cause cancer of the uterus after menopause.

Ironically, there is one health *benefit* caused by obesity related to excess estrogen levels. As you may already know from popular articles, after menopause, if women do not receive estrogen hormone replacement, their bones thin out severely and they develop a condition called "osteoporosis." Without estrogen secretion in the female (testosterone in the male), calcium is gradually leached out of the bones and they become extremely weak and brittle. This leads to the classic "dowager's hump" seen in women in their sixties and seventies who have not been on estrogen replacement, and to the frequent incidence of broken hips that occurs much more commonly in postmenopausal women than in men (who never really go through a hormonal menopause). Women who are fat have a much lower risk of this osteoporosis because their fat cells continue to release estrogen even after menopause.

Excessive skinniness is also associated with infertility in the woman, but the reasons are a little more difficult to understand, and merely suggesting that a woman gain a few pounds is not necessarily the right approach. You'll remember from the previous chapter that the primitive region of the brain called the "hypothalamus" releases brief pulses of the hormone GNRH at ninety-minute intervals throughout postpubertal life. These ninety-minute pulsatile releases of GNRH are what permit the pituitary gland to secrete the FSH and LH, which in turn regulate the ovarian menstrual cycle.

There is a condition called "anorexia nervosa" in which strong emotional problems interfere with the functioning of the "hypothalamus," and the pulsatile release of GNRH does not occur. This "anorexia" is also associated with an inappropriately decreased appetite. The appetite center of the brain is very close to that same area in the hypothalamus which releases the GNRH. Thus, in some extremely skinny women, there is an inadequate pulsatile release of GNRH from the hypothalamus resulting in inadequate secretion of FSH and LH, and a poor menstrual cycle.

But the association of extreme skinniness and infertility is not that clearly understood. Many athletes and long-distance runners, who have hardly any body fat, also have scanty periods, are infertile, and yet seem to show no emotional disturbance related to decreased appetite. Therefore, some doctors still feel that perhaps just adding a little bit to the percent of body fat would help regulate the hormonal balance in these women.

AM I OVULATING?

Basal Body Temperatures (BBT)

The least expensive method of determining ovulation is to keep a daily basal body temperature chart, although this test is becoming unpopular now that simple home ovulation test kits (LH dipstick) for urine are available. The "basal body" temperature (BBT) is taken immediately upon waking up in the morning, before getting out of bed or having any activity whatsoever. Before ovulation, this temperature will always be about one-half to one degree Fahrenheit lower than after ovulation. The production of progesterone (which can only occur after ovulation) is what raises the body's basal temperature, and it is thus the progesterone production that we are measuring. Charts for recording these monthly temperatures are available at almost any pharmacy, or from your doctor (see Graph 1).

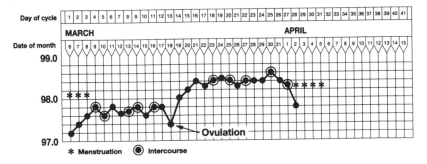

Graph 1. Normal Basal Body Temperature (BBT)

It seems easy to do, but there are pitfalls and incredible aggravation associated with this inexpensive way of determining your ovulation. If the temperatures are not taken first thing in the morning, *before you even move to get out of bed*, they may give a falsely elevated reading and be difficult to interpret. Every evening before going to bed you must place the thermometer by your nightstand within easy reach. If you forget to do this, you will have to get out of bed in the morning to get your thermometer. Even this slight degree of activity can raise your temperature above the basal level and make that day's temperature reading worthless. Upon awaking in the morning you simply grasp the thermometer before doing anything else, put it under the tongue for three minutes, and lie still.

Another problem is that it tends to become a daily nuisance, constantly reminding you about your problem and weighing heavily on you emotionally. I can't tell you how many women have called to tell me they finally got pregnant after just getting disgusted with their thermometer and throwing it out the window or into the fireplace.

A third problem is that although it gives a picture of progesterone production, it is only an indirect one and usually must be verified with direct assays of blood progesterone levels, since the temperature can be affected by such things as colds, flu viruses, keeping late hours, or even having a poor night's sleep. Remember: The basal body temperature refers to the body temperature after a night of normal, restful sleep. The body temperature normally reaches its lowest levels after all mental and muscular activity has ceased for several hours. That is why the best time to record this basal temperature is just upon awakening. Your temperature during the rest of the day is affected by your daily activities and will not be an accurate reflection of whether you are making progesterone.

The basal body temperature of a very highly fertile women usually follows a very characteristic pattern during each menstrual cycle. A low temperature range spans the first fourteen days beginning from the first day of menstruation. This low range is generally in the area of 97.2°F to 97.6°F. Around day fourteen there is a sudden increase in the temperature (up to one degree) which is maintained daily until menstruation begins and the

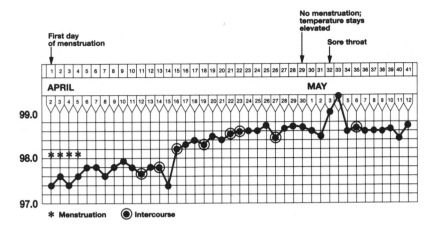

Graph 2. BBT—Pregnancy

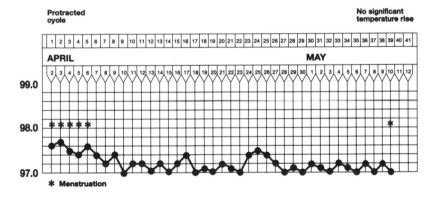

Graph 3. BBT—Anovulation

temperature drops again. If instead of menstruating you become pregnant, the temperature will remain elevated, as it was in the second half of the cycle, because progesterone continues to be produced (see Graph 2). If the temperature does not go up, you have not ovulated; this is called "anovulation" (see Graph 3). If the temperature goes up after day seventeen or eighteen in the

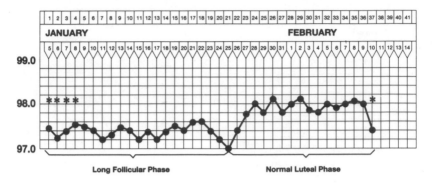

Graph 4. BBT—Long Follicular Phase and Short Luteal Phase

cycle, rather than on day fourteen or fifteen, this indicates delayed ovulation which may affect the likelihood of egg fertilization (see Graph 4). Keep in mind that this is not a way of telling directly whether or not you have ovulated. This method of measurement is just indirect, reflecting the effect of progesterone production on body temperature.

Of all the expensive and complicated methods for determining ovulation, there is none as inexpensive as the temperature chart, and the information obtained can sometimes be quite good. But frequently this chart is misinterpreted, and the patient thinks that she should wait until the temperature goes up (indicating ovulation) before having intercourse. Actually the temperature does not go up until one day after ovulation and by that time the egg is no longer capable of being fertilized, the cervix is closed, and the cervical mucus has become hostile to sperm. Thus, waiting for the temperature to rise before having intercourse is not a way of maximizing the chances of conception but is rather an excellent method of rhythm birth control. Intercourse should take place one or two days prior to the temperature rise, and with the basal body temperature you cannot predict ahead of time when you are going to ovulate. You can only show that you have probably already ovulated after it's too late to do anything about it.

Examination of the Cervical Mucus
During the Monthly Cycle

During the earliest phase of the cycle, the cervix is closed and very little cervical mucus is produced (see Figure 11 and 12). However, beginning around day nine or ten, under the influence of estrogen produced by the developing follicle, the production of cervical mucus begins to increase and the cervix begins to open slightly. When follicular production of estrogen has reached its maximum, usually around day thirteen or fourteen in a normal cycle, the cervix is gaping open and one can actually see into it because of the optically clear, watery cervical mucus flowing out (see Figure 13). Then, when the woman ovulates and progesterone is produced, the entrance to the cervix will dramatically close, and the production of cervical mucus will come almost to a standstill. What mucus is left will be sticky and tacky and will have lost its optical clarity. At this point sperm would have no chance of invading the mucus. If the physician sees a so-called "preovulatory" cervix (with a gaping opening and optically clear, abundant mucus) on day fourteen, and then the cervical opening closes the next day or two, he can be fairly certain the woman has ovulated.

Testing the cervical mucus is useful not just as a method for timing when ovulation has occurred, but rather in its own right tells us whether or not the cervix is receptive to sperm invasion. One of the commonly mentioned "causes" of female infertility is the "cervical factor." This simply means that, even at mid-cycle, the woman does not produce an adequate amount or quality of cervical mucus to permit sperm penetration.

Frankly, most of the time, this "cervical factor" is not really due to any specific abnormality in the cervix or any particular inability of the cervix to produce good quality cervical mucus, but rather is caused by inadequate hormonal stimulation in the follicular phase of the cycle. The reason I say that is that although some doctors might prefer to give cough medicine like Robitussin in an effort to "loosen up" the cervical mucus, and others will resort immediately to intrauterine insemination (i.e., putting the sperm through a small catheter right through the cervix into the uterus, thus bypassing their need to get through a hostile

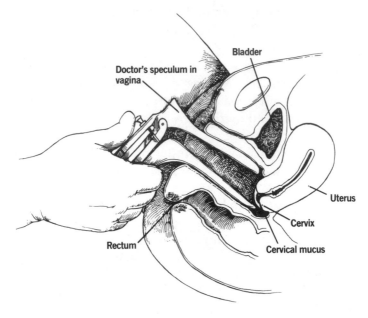

Figure 11. Pelvic examination to observe the opening of the cervix.

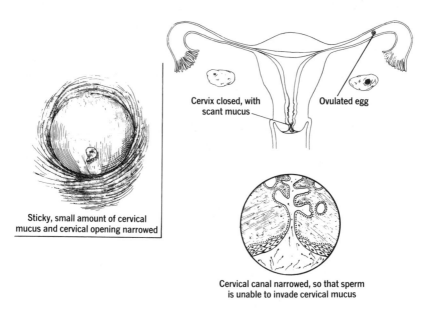

Figure 12. Cervical mucus after ovulation.

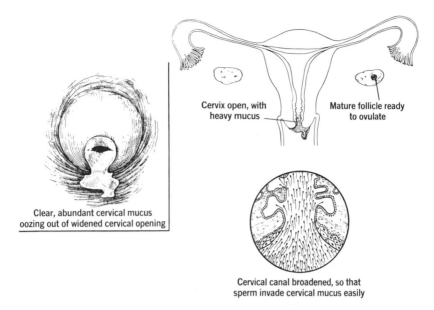

Cervix open, with heavy mucus

Mature follicle ready to ovulate

Clear, abundant cervical mucus oozing out of widened cervical opening

Cervical canal broadened, so that sperm invade cervical mucus easily

Figure 13. Cervical mucus just before ovulation.

cervical environment), I have found that stimulating the ovulatory cycle with powerful agents such as Pergonal (FSH with some LH component) not only provokes good follicle development and ovulation, but usually solves the "cervical mucus problem" as well.

Blood Hormone Tests

To do an adequate hormone evaluation of the female would require almost daily blood tests because of the changing hormone levels with each day of the cycle. Such an approach, however, is expensive and impractical. Thus, most fertility specialists rely heavily on the indirect indications of hormone balance just described. The only occasion on which hormones really need to be monitored daily is in the woman whose ovulation must be induced by a very powerful drug called Pergonal. Under these circumstances the estrogen levels in the blood must be checked every day in order to determine the proper dose. Otherwise a complicated, daily battery of hormone tests is rarely needed.

Yet, to really understand the hormonal events of your cycle reliably, let us review what the hormones would show if they were tested daily. The key hormones are FSH and LH released by the pituitary gland, and estrogen, progesterone, and testosterone (male hormone) produced by the ovary. Prolactin, the hormone usually released by the pituitary only after pregnancy (because it stimulates the production of breast milk, and inhibits ovulation during breast-feeding of the infant), is also checked because if it is being produced in excessive amounts, it can inhibit ovulation.

The Mid-Cycle Hormone Surge

The charts in Chapter 3 (Figures 6 and 7) summarize what all of these hormones are doing during the month to stimulate and inhibit each other. On day one of menstruation, FSH goes up, and stimulates the follicle to produce estrogen. As estrogen is produced by the follicle, it depresses the pituitary's production of FSH. Thus, during the first two weeks of the cycle, as the estrogen level goes up, the FSH level goes down. The rising estrogen begins to crescendo by day twelve and stimulates the pituitary gland to release a huge and sudden burst of the hormone LH, which causes ovulation. The ruptured follicle then becomes the corpus luteum, and begins to manufacture progesterone after ovulation. In the ideal twenty-eight-day cycle, this LH surge occurs at about day fourteen. At the same time the LH level goes up at mid-cycle to cause ovulation, the FSH *and* testosterone levels also go up. In fact, all of the hormones seem to surge at this mid-cycle time of ovulation.

The mid-cycle increase in testosterone (the male hormone) is usually not talked about but has a definite value for getting pregnant. As you may recall, human females, unlike any other animals, are not stimulated by the rising estrogen prior to ovulation toward wanting to have sex. In fact, estrogen has no effect on their sexual desire and that separates women from the females of every other species. That is why there is no clear indication when in the cycle sex should take place in order to create a pregnancy, because the human inclination to have intercourse is fairly constant. Unlike any other animal, the female libido is stimulated by the male hormone testosterone, just like the male libido is. The fact that this male hormone testosterone is ten to fifteen times higher in men than it is in women explains why crimes of sexual violence are almost always perpetrated by an overintense libido of the male and rarely by the female.

That slight rise in testosterone level at mid-cycle creates a subtle enhanced inclination in the female toward initiating sex at that time as opposed to any other time in the cycle. It might be viewed as unfortunate that this testosterone rise is so small because if it were greater, women would go into "heat" just like animals at the time of ovulation and we would have no difficulty timing when to have sex in order to create a pregnancy. The problem with this wishful thinking is that if the testosterone level is too high, it poisons the egg, suppresses ovulation, and literally makes fertilization impossible. The reason to be aware of this normal increase in testosterone at mid-cycle is that if a doctor gets a series of hormone tests at this time of the cycle only, he might incorrectly interpret a mid-cycle increase in testosterone level as indicating some sort of hormonal problem.

The other hormone which for some inexplicable reason surges somewhat at mid-cycle is "prolactin." This too can create confusion. An elevated prolactin level comes from a tiny, benign tumor in the pituitary gland (called a prolactin-microadenoma). It normally causes no harm except by causing an inappropriately high level of prolactin secretion, and can thus inhibit ovulation and cause infertility. In the past, women would have gruesome operations up through the roof of their nasal bone to get at the pituitary gland and remove this prolactin-secreting tumor. Fortunately, nowadays, there is a simple drug, Bromocriptine (or Parlodel), which will cause these tumors to shrink up and inhibit even the normal pituitary's secretion of prolactin.

Effect of the "Brain" on the Hormonal Cycle

If the primitive region of the brain, the hypothalamus, is not functioning properly, this complicated cycling mechanism will not work and the woman will not ovulate. This may be one reason why stress, anxiety, worry, and lack of sleep can prevent ovulation. Unless the hypothalamus is properly tuned and not burdened by anxiety, ovulation may be disturbed.

It is always troubling to hear a condescending recommendation from a physician that one should "stop worrying" because supposedly that will cure the infertility. This is a very heartless suggestion and makes about as much sense as asking an insomniac to stop staying awake and go to sleep. However, there are many examples of the impact of emotions on the menstrual cycle.

Girls who live together in college dormitories who start out in September having their menstrual periods at random times during the month, eventually, by the end of the college year, adjust their cycles so that they wind up menstruating at about the same time in perfect synchrony with each other. Women who have been placed on artificial donor insemination programs without proper counseling often suddenly develop irregularity in what previously were perfectly regular, normal cycles, thus making havoc with the doctor's efforts at timing the insemination.

"Anorexia nervosa" is an emotional condition whereby the woman is obsessed with losing weight and eats virtually nothing: whenever she looks in the mirror, she thinks she is seeing someone who is fat. This unquestionable emotional disturbance is associated with a turnoff of the hypothalamus, lack of adequate secretion therefore of FSH and LH, and often complete lack of any menstrual periods at all. So although it does no good to condescendingly tell a patient to "stop worrying," there is clearly a strong impact that emotions can have upon a normal ovulatory menstrual cycle.

Conclusions Regarding Hormones and Ovulation

It is usually impossible to determine precisely why a woman is not ovulating. The normal ovulatory function of the menstrual system relies on a very complicated and dynamic coordination of interrelating hormonal events. Whatever the cause of poor ovulation, the hormonal picture in almost all cases is too low a FSH (and often a high LH) level at the beginning of the cycle and often too much of the male hormone testosterone.

Lack of ovulation is a true disease and should not be regarded simply as a problem with becoming pregnant. Even if the woman does not want to become pregnant, the hormonal imbalance resulting from or causing poor ovulation leads to heavy buildup of a hard uterine lining that does not shed properly like the soft lining of an ovulatory woman. Not only can this lead to irregular bleeding and infertility, but over many years it can lead to the development of cancer of the lining of the womb. So the problem of not getting pregnant because of poor ovulation may go beyond the barrenness of the marriage and be a high-risk factor for later development of cancer. Insurance companies that deny payment for treatment of infertility need to be made aware of this fact (perhaps in court).

Endometrial Biopsy

After ovulation has occurred, under the influence of progesterone, the lining of the uterus becomes soft and forms what is called a "secretory" endometrium. If ovulation has not occurred, then, in the second half of the cycle, instead of a soft, spongy, secretory lining, there will be a hard, proliferative lining, indicating that no progesterone has been produced. One very indirect way of testing to see if and when a women has ovulated is, in the second half of the cycle, to examine under a microscope a tiny piece of that lining. This is called an "endometrial biopsy." The procedure is actually quite simple and can be performed in almost any gynecologist's office, but it does involve a wincing moment of pain. It is no longer very commonly done as part of the evaluation for ovulation, but it is harmless and may add to the overall understanding of the cycle.

Many years ago, I saw a patient who had been scheduled for an endometrial biopsy to be performed just before the time she was expected to menstruate. She asked whether I really thought she needed this endometrial biopsy, and I was embarrassed to realize that she was right, she didn't. That month she never did menstruate because she turned out to be pregnant.

It is always a good idea to question your physician tactfully about what he is doing and why. If he is unable to discuss his diagnostic and therapeutic decisions rationally, then you may have to look elsewhere for someone with whom you are more compatible. Certainly, I learned a lot from this patient; I was reflexively allowing her to go through a test that would give us no new useful information in helping her conceive, and in fact might have prevented her conception that month.

LH Dipstick

The most useful information you need to learn about the adequacy of your menstrual cycle and your ovulation can be learned at home without having to visit the doctor. This has been made possible by development of the "LH dipstick" technology available in your local drugstore under brand names such as Ovustick, First Response, or a variety of others from different companies. When these Ovustick tests first came out, they were laborious, cumbersome, and required about an hour at home every day. But now you can get a simple answer in the morning in just four minutes.

These LH dipstick tests do not give you the exact quantitative level of LH in your blood, but rather turn a certain color on the day that your LH surges to a high level. If you do this dipstick testing every morning, the test will be negative until the day of your LH surge when it suddenly turns positive. If you do the test a day or two later, it will once again be negative. It is obvious that this represents a simple home method for determining when you ovulate that has many advantages over the basal body temperature thermometer and cervical mucus testing.

We know from the previous chapter that ovulation should occur within about thirty-six to forty hours of the very slight beginning of the increase in LH production, and about twenty to twenty-four hours after the LH surge reaches its peak. As you will recall, LH triggers two major events. It causes the maturing egg within the growing follicle to resume "meiosis," the complicated process of reduction of the number of chromosomes from forty-six to twenty-three in order to prepare the egg for fertilization, and it also causes the wall of the follicle on the ovarian surface to thin out and eventually open up to release the egg. That is the moment of ovulation. By using the LH dipstick, you can tell the day before you are going to ovulate.

This simple test helps in evaluating your menstrual cycle by determing whether you do ovulate and whether you do so at mid-cycle in a normal fashion. So Ovustick will tell you twenty-four hours ahead of time when you will ovulate and will give you the opportunity to time your sex just like our more reproductively efficient animal friends do.

Ultrasound

All of the tests of the menstrual cycle we have discussed fail to positively visualize and clearly prove the occurrence of ovulation. Development of transvaginal ultrasound (a medical application of the navy sonar used to navigate for submarines) allows us to safely view the developing follicle or follicles without any fear of radiation damage (because no radiation as in X rays is involved) and actually to visualize the disappearance or reduction in size in the follicle, positively proving that ovulation has occurred.

Of course, this is not a test that you can do on yourself at home. The cost of an inexpensive ultrasound machine is about $60,000, and the better ones can cost up to $250,000. Nonetheless, hospitals and clinics find them so useful and so constantly in use that the cost of doing such an examination for a single cycle can be as low as $400, inclusive of all of the days of an entire cycle in which you are tested. This is a lot more expensive than a $30 LH dipstick kit, and may not be cost-effective for routine evaluation of your menstrual cycle, but it is absolutely essential for monitoring the stimulation of ovulation, and it is the most precise way of being certain of when ovulation has occurred.

An ultrasound exam can done in a matter of minutes, without discomfort. It is a very quick examination in which the ovaries, uterus, and developing follicle can be clearly seen by you and your doctor. A physician or technician who is doing the procedure simply puts a rubber glove over the "transducer," with ultrasonic lubricant placed on the tip, and then gently places it into the vagina and looks at the TV screen of the ultrasound machine. This should be no more uncomfortable than a routine pelvic exam. By placing the transducer to the right or to the left or to the center, you can see your ovaries and visualize any

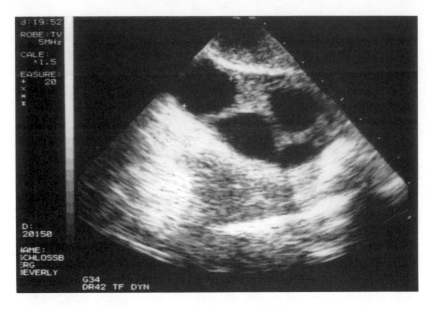

Figure 14. View of four mature follicles seen on ultrasound before ovulation.

developing follicle (see Figure 14). You can also see your uterus, either longitudinally if the transducer is held in one direction or transversely if it is held in another. Even the endometrial lining can be observed building up as the follicular phase progresses in preparation for ovulation.

On the day that you have ovulated, you'll either see a complete absence of the previously visualized follicle, a dramatic decrease in its size, or a roughening of its wall, demonstrating the formation of a corpus luteum cyst. You will also see a large amount of fluid in the "cul-de-sac" (the bottom area of the abdominal cavity behind the uterus). This is follicular fluid which has drained out of the follicle after ovulation.

Perhaps most importantly, this new technology of transvaginal ultrasound can be used to nonsurgically obtain eggs from your ovaries for in vitro fertilization (IVF), thus making IVF a completely nonoperative, outpatient procedure. No longer does a laparoscopy (see pages 107–8) or a minilap procedure (see page 311) have to be performed to obtain eggs. Furthermore, a more efficient job of obtaining every single egg can be done because visualization of the follicles is, in truth, much better with ultrasound than it would be by directly looking at the ovary through the laparoscope. Transvaginal ultrasound has thus completely transformed in vitro fertilization, as well as the GIFT procedure (in a different way), into a simpler, more readily obtainable high-technology treatment because it is so simple now to obtain the eggs without surgery of any kind.

LOOKING FOR STRUCTURAL ABNORMALITIES IN THE FEMALE

X Ray of Uterus and Tubes ("Hysterosalpingogram")

In many cases the tubes that carry the egg to the site of fertilization may be blocked or restricted in their movement. Thus, failure to conceive might be due to purely physical factors, even though ovulation may occur normally. The most obvious case in point is the woman who has had her tubes tied, i.e., she has undergone sterilization. However, many women have blockage of the tubes because of previous infections, and sometimes these are infections she never even knew she had. Even a simple case of appendicitis in youth could result in scarring around the area of the tubes which could interfere with pickup of the egg from the ovary.

One of the easiest ways to determine whether the tubes are structurally intact is through an X ray called a "hysterosalpingogram," which is slightly painful, but which is not surgical and does *not* require hospitalization. The woman is given a pelvic examination, and a liquid which is opaque to X rays (radiopoque) is injected via a cannula through her cervix. An X ray is then taken, and the doctor can see a perfect outline of the cavity of the uterus as well as the tubes (see Figure 15). If the tubes are open without obstruction, this liquid should spill freely into the

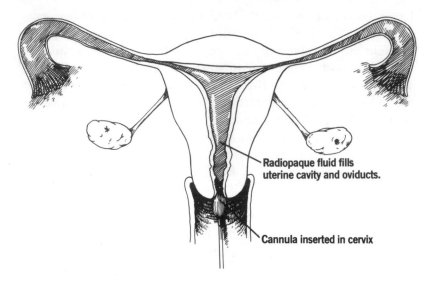

Radiopaque fluid fills
uterine cavity and oviducts.

Cannula inserted in cervix

Figure 15. Hysterosalpingogram

abdominal cavity, and this is readily seen when the X ray is taken.

It is not sufficient simply to determine that the tubes are open. The fluid must spill freely into the abdominal cavity without accumulating in pockets, which would indicate scarring outside the tube which can restrict its tentaclelike grasping of the egg by the fimbria. The tube is not simply an alley through which the egg must roll like a bowling ball to reach the womb. It is a magnificently complicated structure which must have complete freedom of movement in order to ensure that the properly prepared egg is not just wasted in the abdominal cavity.

Occasionally, however, the X ray may give an impression that the tubes are blocked when they really are not. Remember that the tiny canal that connects the uterus to the tubes has a valvelike constricting effect which slows down the sperm trying to get into the tube. Consequently the X ray contrast fluid sometimes may not go beyond the uterus just because of spasms in this area (called the "cornu" of the uterus).

Performing this test accurately thus requires gentleness on the part of the gynecologist or radiologist and a full explanation of what is happening. Otherwise, the patient's anxiety itself may interfere with the performance of an adequate X ray. Just recently I saw a patient who was referred for "blocked tubes." However, before we could operate, she became pregnant, indicating that the X rays (which seemed to indicate blockage at the "cornu") were in error and really just represented temporary tubal spasm. This is a common story.

Laparoscopy

The "hysterosalpingogram" does not always show scarring around the outside of the tubes or the presence of "endometriosis." This type of information can be obtained by actually looking inside the abdomen with a telescope inserted through the belly button (see Figure 16). This telescope, called a "laparoscope," was designed specifically to allow a very detailed examination of the inside of the abdomen. The uterus, tubes, and ovaries can be freely inspected without the necessity of making a large exploratory incision. This procedure generally has to be performed with the patient anesthetized, and therefore may require a day in the hospital. Most gynecologists perform this procedure under general anesthesia, but normally the patient can go home the same day.

Laparoscopy can reveal adhesions from previous infection that may be blocking the tubes, as well as more subtle adhesions outside the tube that could interfere with their ability to pick up the egg. Laparoscopy is also the only way of making a firm diagnosis of "endometriosis," the accumulation of normal lining tissue of the uterus in areas outside the uterus.

If there is any doubt as to the appearance of obstruction on an X ray, laparoscopy can be used as a confirmatory procedure by injecting a blue-colored liquid into the uterus through the cervix and observing through the telescope whether this fluid spills freely through the tube into the abdomen. Sometimes tubes that appear to be blocked on an X ray are shown really to be open on laparoscopy.

After this full inspection is completed, the laparoscope is removed and the tiny one-half-inch incision in the belly button is stitched in such a way that the scar is rarely visible. The patient

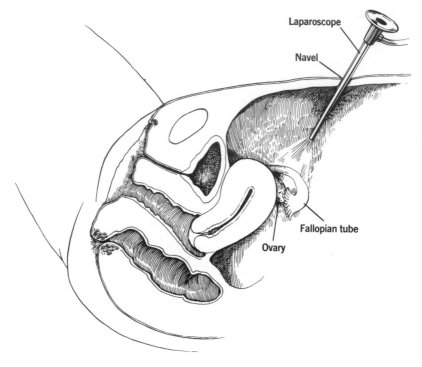

Figure 16. Laparoscopy

has only a minimum amount of pain after the operation because the incision is so tiny. She goes home the same day or the next morning.

A skilled laparoscopist can actually correct, right through the telescope, some of the milder tubal problems that may be found. He can cut through adhesions using operating instruments attached to the end of the telescope (or that he inserts through a "second puncture"). This may be all that is necessary for the tubes to be sufficiently mobilized so that their tentaclelike action can grasp the egg effectively. If denser adhesions or more formidable obstructions are found, however, the patient is often scheduled for a larger operation at a later date. But it really is quite amazing the amount of repair work that can be done through this telescope using a tiny incision and multiple puncture sites.

Idiopathic

After you have gone through all these tests, we may or may not find abnormalities, i.e., deviations from the normal findings in the average person. We may find late ovulation or we may find some "minimal lesion" endometriosis. We may find some mild tubal adhesions. This does not mean we have definitively pinpointed the cause of your infertility. Women get pregnant with absolutely no treatment who happen to have "minimal lesion" endometriosis, mild tubal adhesions, or deviations from the normal ovulatory/menstrual pattern. So unless we find absolutely no sperm in your husband, absolutely no ovulation in your cycles and no menstruation, or total blockage of your tubes, we cannot be 100 percent certain that our tests have really pinpointed the problem. But at least we have a diagnosis and having a diagnosis may be helpful to you and your doctor as you go through the stepwise approach of deciding what treatment to embark upon first.

However, in a large number of the patients we see with infertility dating back many years, none of these tests turn up an abnormality. Fertility specialists used to vastly underestimate the number of patients in whom they could find nothing wrong, because it was frustrating. Doctors would go to great length to find "subtle abnormalities." If subtle abnormalities couldn't be found in the wife, then if the husband had a sperm count under 40 million per cc (as over 40 percent of husbands do), you could simply blame it on him and call it "male factor" infertility. The fact is that we are now admitting more and more openly a high frequency of just finding nothing distinctly wrong with either partner after going through all of these tests. We call this quite openly "idiopathic" infertility. "Idiopathic" is simply the Greek word used in medical terminology to mean "we don't know what causes it."

Sometimes we can simply explain "idiopathic" infertility as being caused by age because, as we have discussed in great detail, the older the wife, the lower the pregnancy rate and the higher the incidence of infertility. But whatever rationale we want to give, after all of our testing, a large number of patients simply have no clear-cut cause for being infertile and yet they are. It is the frustration with trying to treat this large group of "idiopathic" patients (and the realization that many patients with established diagnoses may in truth also be "idiopathic" infertility) that spurred on the development and immense success of the new reproductive technologies of in vitro fertilization (IVF) and GIFT. When you simply feel like throwing up your hands because all other treatment has failed for the "specific" diagnoses that you've made, or when no specific diagnoses can be made, then bypassing the whole process via the GIFT or in vitro fertilization approach results in a high success rate and turns out in the long run often to be more cost-effective than the years of conventional therapy which preceded it.

CHAPTER 5

How the Male Works

THE MALE MYTH

Causes of Low Sperm Count

In subsequent chapters you will learn that the lower the sperm count, the lower the chance for pregnancy. However, even men with very low sperm counts can be quite fertile. Before explaining this fascinating dilemma, I will try in this chapter to give an explanation for why the husband has a low sperm count and debunk some of the myths about the causes of "oligoastheno-spermia" (low sperm count and low sperm motility).

Internal Structure of the Testicles

The testicle has two major functions: One is to make the male hormone, testosterone, which is responsible for the development of male sexual characteristics and behavior. The other is to produce spermatozoa, or sperm, capable of fertilizing the female's egg. The testicle consists of several hundred coiled

Figure 17. The testicle

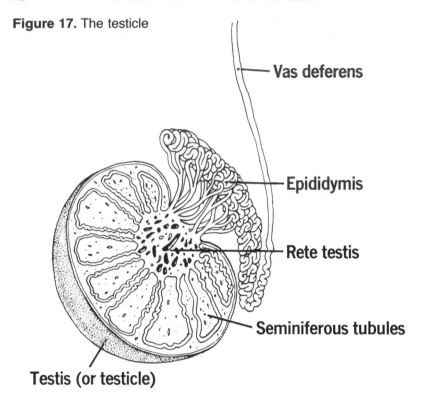

Vas deferens

Epididymis

Rete testis

Seminiferous tubules

Testis (or testicle)

microscopic tubules, called "seminiferous tubules," in which the sperm are manufactured. These tubules converge and collect into a delta (like the mouth of a river) near the upper part of the testicle. This delta (called the "rete testis") then empties through a series of five to seven very small ducts (called "vasa efferentia") out of the testicle (see Figure 17). In between the microscopic seminiferous tubules which manufacture the sperm are clumps of cells (called Leydig cells) which make the male hormone, testosterone. These Leydig cells appear to be sprinkled like pepper throughout the substance of the testicle (see Figure 18).

Whereas sperm are carried out of the testicle into the vas deferens to be ejaculated at the time of orgasm, the male hormone manufactured by the Leydig cells is picked up by tiny

Seminiferous tubules make sperm.

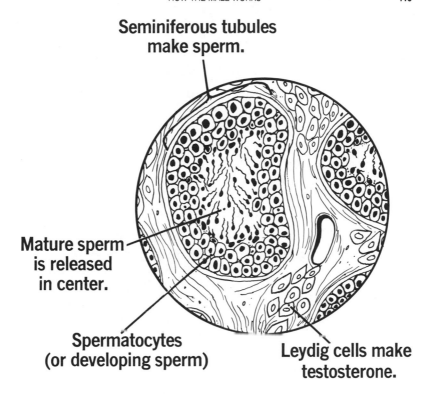

Mature sperm is released in center.

Spermatocytes (or developing sperm)

Leydig cells make testosterone.

Figure 18. The sperm factory (testicle biopsy).

veins coursing through the testicle. The testicular veins carry the male hormone into the circulation. It is because the male hormone drains into the circulation this way, rather than via the seminiferous tubules and vas deferens, that a man can undergo vasectomy (which means that his vas deferens is intentionally cut for sterilization) without altering his hormone production or sexual drive.

The Leydig cells, which produce the male hormone, are remarkably sturdy. It is very difficult for any sort of illness or disease to interfere with an adequate production of male hormone. However, the seminiferous tubules which manufacture sperm are not really very well constructed in humans and are very likely to have problems. That is why so many men suffer from infertility and yet have no lack of virility.

Both the production of testosterone (which accounts for male sex drive, beard, pubic hair, and other sex characteristics) and the production of sperm are regulated by hormones produced by the pituitary gland, which sits just underneath the brain. These pituitary hormones are in turn regulated by a "releasing factor"—GNRH—produced by the most primitive area of the brain, called the "hypothalamus." This is exactly the same GNRH that in the female permits the whole complex menstrual cycle to take place. This driving force from the brain, GNRH, acts no differently in the male than in the female, pulsing at ninety-minute intervals.

The brain thus stimulates the pituitary gland to produce and release the two hormones FSH (follicle-stimulating hormone) and LH (luteinizing hormone), just as in the female. Without FSH and LH from the pituitary gland and without GNRH from the brain, the testes in the male and the ovaries in the female would shrivel up and cease to function. The only reason for the constant production of FSH, LH, and testosterone in the male and the monthly cycle of ups and downs of FSH, LH, and estrogen plus progesterone in the female is that the ovary gives a different "feedback" message than the testicle.

In the male, FSH helps to stimulate and maintain proper sperm production. LH stimulates and maintains production of the male hormone, testosterone. When luteinizing hormone (LH) stimulates the testicles to make testosterone, this hormone, through "negative feedback," in turn causes the pituitary gland to make less LH. This "feedback" mechanism controls the level of testosterone produced by the testicle. When the testosterone level drops too low, the pituitary makes more LH so that the testicles can produce more testosterone. The brain does not regulate the amount of testosterone produced by the testes, or for that matter, the production of sperm; only FSH and LH do that. GNRH pulses occur at ninety-minute intervals from the brain and are dumb and orchestrate nothing. They just let it all happen.

Men who have severely damaged testicles (or who have no testicles at all) have extremely high circulating levels of LH and FSH. These pituitary hormones are responding to a deficiency in testicular production of hormone by reaching high levels in an effort to stir whatever testicular tissue exists into functioning at its maximum possible capacity. Many men with severely damaged testicles still have normal testosterone levels (and normal sex drive) only because their pituitary is pouring out enormous quantities of FSH and LH to drive what little testicular tissue they have to maximum production.

I had a patient who was born with *no testicles*, and who underwent a successful testicle transplant from his identical twin brother. This patient originally was a eunuch because of the absence of the male hormone testosterone. He had no pubic hair, no sexual drive, no voice change, and no growth spurt. However, the levels of FSH and LH production from his pituitary were extraordinarily high. Since there was no testosterone being produced (by virtue of the fact that he had no testicles), the pituitary was constantly being given the message that there was an inadequate amount of male hormone, and it responded in the normally programmed fashion by making excessive amounts of FSH and LH. When a testicle was successfully transplanted into him, he began to produce testosterone and sperm almost immediately and has since fathered four children. At that point his blood FSH and LH levels finally came down to normal.

Sperm Production—The Assembly Line

The testicles normally produce sperm at a phenomenal rate, so that sperm are ejaculated in seemingly extravagant numbers. Think of the unbelievable sperm wastage that seems required for male fertility. Out of perhaps 200 million sperm inseminated with one act of intercourse, only 400 ever reach the vicinity of the egg, and only a single sperm has even a 15 percent chance in any given month in a normal fertile couple of fertilizing the egg. Because male fertility in many respects is a simple numbers game, we will describe the various steps in the production of sperm and what factors, if any, influence the quantity and quality of sperm produced.

All of the cells that eventually develop into normal sperm are called "germ cells." These germ cells within the "seminiferous tubules" of the testes are lined up in an orderly array, with the most primitive early cells lying along the outer edge and the more developed sperm moving toward the center. All of these cells are held in place and nourished by a sort of formless or shapeless nuturing cell (much like an amoeba) called the "Sertoli" cell. In fact, the developing sperm sits with its head imbedded within the nurturing Sertoli cell. In the final phase of sperm production the sperm develops an oval head and a tail necessary for locomotion. When the product is complete, the mature spermatozoon is released from the Sertoli cell into the tubule and swept along toward the efferent ducts to make its escape, along with millions of others, from the testicle.

As sperm go through their development process they are passed toward the center of the tubule as though on an assembly line. In fact, the comparison of sperm production to an assembly line is quite accurate, since the sperm are passed along from one stage of production to another at an absolutely unalterable speed of sixteen days for each stage of production. The sperm go through four and a half such stages of production. Thus the total time it requires to produce every sperm is about seventy-two days. Neither sickness, testicular damage, nor hormonal manipulation can alter this inexorable rate at which the individual spermatozoa are produced. If one can imagine an automobile assembly line with a slow, steady, unstoppable movement from one stage to progressively more complex stages of production until the final car comes out for inspection, then one will have a pretty good understanding of how sperm are produced, and indeed how sloppy the results can often be. In fact, one might speculate that one reason for the extravagant number of sperm produced by the testicles is that only a small percentage will actually have all their nuts and bolts in the right place.

A deficiency in sperm production does not result from a slowing down of the speed at which the developing sperm proceed along the assembly line. This velocity cannot be changed. Rather, a deficiency in sperm production results from an absent worker, or a missing part at any one of the stages along the way. Sometimes the problem may be simply an inadequate number of the earliest precursors of sperm. Other times the continuation of sperm production to more mature stages may be blocked; this is called "spermatogenic arrest." That means that although there are plenty of sperm precursors, the normal genetic preparation to the final completed sperm cannot occur.

What Can Be Done to Stimulate
Greater Sperm Production?

Although it is very easy to stimulate the female's ovary to produce large numbers of follicles by administering FSH, or Pergonal (a combination of FSH and LH), or even Clomid, which stimulates her pituitary to release greater amounts of FSH and LH, this same effort in men has failed miserably. This seems difficult to understand, because we know that sperm production is completely dependent upon the secretion of FSH and LH from the pituitary gland. In men with sperm cells absent from the testicles, the FSH level is extremely high. Since there seems to be a normal feedback mechanism between the pituitary gland's secretion of FSH and LH and the male's production of sperm and testosterone, why shouldn't we be able to drive the testicles to produce more sperm by increasing FSH, as in the female? We are beginning to discover why our previous efforts at stimulating sperm production failed, and are learning how to conquer low sperm production in some patients.

To try to understand this question, let's first look at how we treat a rare, clinical disorder called "Kallmann's Syndrome." This is a very unusual but fascinating condition in which the man does not go through puberty because his brain never releases pulsatile bursts of GNRH at ninety-minute intervals the way it is supposed to, and consequently, his pituitary doesn't manufacture FSH or LH. As a young adult, such a patient has very little or no facial hair, no pubic hair, and an infantile-looking penis and testicles. Dr. Richard Sherins from the National Institutes of Health has studied this condition for the last twenty years, not just with an approach toward treating these patients, but with a larger goal of trying to understand just exactly how the hormones FSH, LH, and testosterone regulate sperm production, to see if this knowledge could help stimulate sperm in everyday cases of deficient sperm production.

First, Dr. Sherins started these men on injections of the hormone HCG (which has the same pharmacological effect as LH) for an entire year and found, as he expected, that they began very promptly to make normal amounts of testosterone, go through puberty, and begin to appear like normal men. However, as one also might have expected, they made no sperm. The LH simply stimulated the Leydig cells of the testicle to produce testosterone but this alone was not sufficient for sperm production. Dr. Sherins then performed testicle biopsies on these men and found something quite surprising and fascinating. These otherwise infantile seminiferous tubules which previously were going through no stages whatsoever of sperm production had developed all of the early stages of chromosome condensation and realignment that are necessary for the early sperm precursors to become sperm. The primitive "spermatogonia" had developed fully to the "pachytene spermatocyte" level very much like the development of the egg in the female just prior to the entrance of the sperm.

You'll recall from Chapter 3 that sperm cells have half of the normal number of chromosomes that the other cells in the body have; before the egg can be fertilized by the sperm, it must lose half of its chromosomes just like the sperm. LH and FSH in the female allow this to happen. However, the egg, even after the LH surge, has one final step remaining to reduce its number of chromosomes in half and prepare for union with the sperm chromosomes. That change is triggered in some mysterious way by the entrance of the sperm into the egg. It is not triggered by FSH or LH.

Administration of LH to these men with infantile testicles caused testosterone production as expected and induced sperm production right up the verge of the final meiotic division. This is very similar to what the LH surge does in women to the egg. But there were still no mature sperm, and the sperm count remained zero. After several years of being certain that sperm production could not proceed under the influence of LH only, Dr. Sherins patiently administered FSH to these men. Just the smallest amount of FSH allowed the "reduction division" to be completed and the spermatocytes matured into sperm. Sperm then began to appear in the ejaculate of these previously sterile men. Thus, it seemed that both LH and FSH were necessary for sperm production. LH could begin sperm production up to the final stage of maturation, and FSH was necessary to carry the process further to the final production of mature sperm.

After these men got their wives pregnant, Dr. Sherins stopped the FSH but continued the LH so that they could keep on making male hormone. Then something else very fascinating was discovered. Despite stopping the FSH (which seemed necessary for the final maturation of sperm), these men continued to make sperm at almost the same rate and remained fertile just by staying on LH. If they stopped LH, and then began it again, however, they only made testosterone and once again could carry sperm production only as far as the stage just before the final reduction division to mature sperm.

We can conclude from these brilliant studies that: 1) a "normal" testicle should respond to the administration of FSH and LH with a fertile output of sperm; 2) LH alone can begin sperm production but cannot complete it; 3) FSH has a very brief and limited role in allowing the completion of sperm production. At the time of Dr. Sherins's studies, we thought that if higher doses of FSH and LH were given, it did not increase the amount of sperm produced.

Men with low sperm production who do not have this extraordinarily rare Kallmann's Syndrome must have an intrinsic testicular defect, because their testicles cannot be pushed into overdrive by administering the low doses of FSH and LH that Dr. Sherins's study employed.

Indeed, the evidence is highly likely that humans, like gorillas, have an intrinsic testicular defect, some worse than others, and that oligospermia is a genetically transmitted problem found exclusively in monogamous species like ours because of the lack of sperm competition in our mating systems.

A simple understanding of these concepts of sperm production should make the reader depressingly aware of how difficult it is to improve sperm count or quality in a man with oligospermia. Many infertile men have been treated in a haphazard and unscientific manner to improve their sperm count, and none of these regimens have any proven value. That is why treatment of the female to maximize her fertility potential and use of the new reproductive technologies (IVF and GIFT) are more likely to be effective than trying to increase sperm production.

We can often push deficient testicles with much higher "megadoses" of Pergonal: Three ampules given every day for four months will raise the FSH level three-fold, and in many men abnormally high FSH levels will dramatically increase their sperm count. The problem is the high cost, and we don't yet know which men will respond.

The Reason We Need So Many Sperm

Why do we need to produce so many sperm? Why should such an enormous number of sperm be needed simply to fertilize one egg? How could nature be so wasteful as to place a requirement upon us to overproduce vast numbers of these little creatures when only one is necessary to make a baby? Why should there be so many obstacles in the female genital tract which make it mandatory for a large number of sperm to be squandered just so that one will make it? Wouldn't it be easier if nature had provided us with a simple reproductive system in which one sperm could be mixed with one egg and a baby thus formed?

There are a number of reasons for this overproduction. First, the time during which an egg in the female can be fertilized after it is ovulated is brief, about twelve hours. Therefore, it must be fertilized promptly after its release from the ovary. This requires the continuous presence of a reasonable number of sperm continually reaching the fallopian tube. It is therefore necessary for a much larger number of sperm to be available lower down in reservoir regions of the cervix to be continuously and slowly released upward. Another reason for the obstacles which the sperm must overcome is that intercourse is not a sterile process and the female genital tract must be protected against infection. The same immune and physical barriers which only allow a few lucky sperm to gain access to the egg also protect the female against invasion by bacteria. (In a test tube these barriers don't exist, and thus IVF or GIFT is currently the best solution for men with very low sperm counts.) Finally it may be that sperm production is such a complicated biological process that there will be many defective products, again as on the automobile assembly line, and only the true "gems" are allowed access all the way to the egg.

Hormone Testing for Men

If a man with low sperm count sees a urologist, he is certain to have his blood tested for FSH, LH, and testosterone, and in the majority of cases these levels will be confusingly normal despite very low sperm counts. Most of the time checking these hormone levels is not very useful in determining why the man has oligospermia or whether anything can be done about it. The reason for this confusing paradox requires a more detailed understanding of how the testicles' production of testosterone and sperm feeds back to the pituitary gland to regulate FSH and LH levels.

LH is simple. Increased production of testosterone by the testicles causes decreased production of LH from the pituitary gland, and this negative feedback results in a stable balance. Thus, if the LH level is high, it means the pituitary is working hard to overcome what would otherwise be deficient testosterone production by the testicles. FSH regulation, however, is not quite so simple.

Theoretically, FSH production by the pituitary is inhibited by sperm production from the testicle. We know that men who are born with "Sertoli Cell Only" Syndrome, meaning there are absolutely no sperm or sperm-producing precursors in the testicles, have an elevated FSH level. That is, the pituitary is getting a message that there is no sperm present in those testicles, and it is therefore secreting an excess amount of FSH. Thus it would seem very simply that if there is low sperm production because of a testicular defect, the FSH level should be high. Unfortunately, this is only occasionally the case, when the entire testicle is severely diseased. In the vast majority of cases despite severely low sperm counts, FSH is normal. Why should that be?

The fact that so many urologists do not understand this "negative feedback" system for FSH in the male causes lots of problems. Not the least of which is that they assume that a man with no sperm (azospermia) in the ejaculate, and a normal FSH, has obstruction. They assume from the normal FSH level that he has to be making sperm but the sperm simply aren't getting into the ejaculate and, therefore, he has an obstruction. Going on that erroneous basis, they often operate on these men even though in reality there is no reason whatsoever to do so. The only proof of sperm production is a testicle biopsy, not the FSH level.

Here's why. In the majority of infertile men with severe oligospermia, there is no deficiency in the total number of sperm-producing precursor cells in the testicle. The area where the problem occurs is at the point of maturation from sperm precursor (spermatocyte) into sperm. This is the point where "meiosis" or "reduction division" has to occur, so that the sperm precursors with forty-six chromosomes can be transformed into sperm with only twenty-three chromosomes. Remember, this is the same process the egg must go through when the sperm penetrates it in order to allow fertilization to occur. The number of chromosomes has to be reduced in half in order for fertilization to occur, and this process, called "meiosis," is the most difficult part of sperm production (spermatogenesis). In the majority of infertile men with low sperm counts, the problem is not an inadequate number of sperm precursor cells in the testes; the problem is some sort of genetic screwup at the point of meiosis. Thus, a man can have a very low sperm count or even zero sperm in the ejaculate and still have a completely normal FSH level.

FSH production by the pituitary is not regulated by the number of mature sperm produced by the testicles and released into the ejaculate. Rather, FSH production by the pituitary is regulated by the total number of sperm or sperm precursor cells present within the testicle, including the precursors which never get past the final stages of maturation.

Variations in Sperm Count

There can sometimes be incredible variations in sperm count observed in the same man over many months or years. Because sperm production depends upon a tremendous amount of energy as for any rapidly metabolic cells, it is subject to temporary diminution by almost any detrimental condition such as certain drugs, chemotherapy for cancer, perhaps toxins in the environment, overzealous use of hot tubs, stress, lack of sleep, or other illnesses such as pneumonia. For instance, a person with cancer is given chemotherapy, highly poisonous drugs that are designed to prevent cell division. Such toxic drugs help to kill cancer because the continued growth of a cancer depends on an extremely rapid metabolic rate of cell division. The problem, of course, is that it also affects all other cells which have a rapid rate of metabolic division. That is why on cancer chemotherapy people get extremely nauseated and vomit due to sloughing of the rapidly metabolizing cells lining their stomach and bowels. Chemotherapy obviously has the same effect on the testicle and a man will have no sperm production.

I have a patient who had undergone a successful vasectomy reversal with very high sperm counts and good sperm motility, but suddenly and inexplicably several years later, his sperm count went down to close to zero levels and those sperm that were left were no longer moving. Of course, one possibility in such a situation would be that the site of reconnection of the obstruction had blocked off, but the operation I performed on him was so delicate that I really did not think it very likely that two and one-half years later he would have suddenly gone down from a very high sperm count with good motility to near sterile levels. On the telephone, I asked him about anything that might have happened differently in his life around the time his sperm count went down.

He told me that several months earlier he had an episode of pneumonia with his temperature going up to 102°F. He had begun to take Indocin, because of a flare-up of his gout, and Zyloprim to inhibit the uric acid production which causes gout. Zyloprim is an antimetabolic-type agent. He was also taking Tenormin to try to lower his blood pressure, which had gone up because of a tremendous amount of business stress. He had no idea that any of these events could in any way be related to the sudden drop in his sperm count. After he discontinued these medications, a repeat sperm count done six months later was back up to normal. This man is a superb example of how delicate the process of sperm production is and how drugs or ill health can have a devastating effect on it.

I'll never forget a patient whom I saw several years ago suffering from eight years of infertility and very low sperm count, even though his wife had gotten pregnant shortly after they had gotten married ten years earlier. They expressed to me that the husband was an extremely tense, high-pressure executive and they honestly felt that the pregnancy early in their marriage occurred during a period when he had tremendous relief from that business-induced stress. They related to me that he got very little sleep at night, stayed up until the oddest hours preparing major reports and projects, had little time to spend with his child, and felt in a chronic state of ill health. The couple did tell me that they had just come back from a month of vacation, including a secluded week in a remote region where there were no telephones and no alarm clocks. I was about ready to tell them how inadequate our methods of treating low sperm counts are and that we would probably wind up resorting to newer technologies like in vitro fertilization to try to make his few sperm more efficient in their efforts to fertilize his wife's eggs. I then went into the lab to check his sperm count and found that it was extraordinarily high (120 million per cc) and he was indeed suddenly quite fertile.

On the other hand I have seen countless couples in whom the male, despite relatively poor health and a stressful-appearing life, has had adequate sperm production for getting his wife pregnant. Thus we can only say that sperm counts undergo an inexplicable variation. But avoidance of toxic drugs, getting plenty of rest, and staying in good health will certainly improve the sperm count in some men.

HOW SPERM REACH THE EJACULATE

Leaving the Testicles

Now we leave what used to be the very depressing issue of sperm production and go to the more classically treatable question of how sperm reach the ejaculate. There is a remarkable transport mechanism that allows these eager little sperm to exit from the male's genitals and get their crack at the egg.

After the completed spermatozoa are released into the seminiferous tubule, they flow into the area called the "rete testes," which is like a river delta near the upper edge of the testicle.

Sperm are pushed along the seminiferous tubule toward this exit point by contractions of very delicate muscle fibers. The sperm do not move on their own. After they exit from the testicles, sperm are transferred into an amazing structure called the "epididymis."

The tiny epididymis is the most common site of blockage causing male sterility. To correct such blockage requires very delicate microsurgery. The epididymis is a twenty-foot-long tube of microscopic size (one three-hundredth of an inch in diameter) which runs back and forth in loops like a strand of spaghetti, but which actually traverses a distance of only one and one-half inches. It transfers sperm from the testicle to the "vas deferens." Imagine a twenty-foot-long spaghetti strand placed on a one-foot-long serving dish. At first such a plate would appear to be filled with many different strands of spaghetti. Similarly, with its multiple curves and convolutions the epididymis appears to be a large number of tubules, but it is actually just one very long tiny tubule.

It used to be thought that the sperm require about twelve days to travel the entire twenty-foot journey through the winding length of the epididymis into the vas deferens. Now we know that this trip is very quick (about one or two days). Sperm are propelled along this highly contorted microscopic tunnel by frequent contractions of its thin muscular wall. When the sperm reach the end of the epididymis (the "tail") they move up the vas deferens and await their call to be rushed through the vas deferens and be ejaculated at the time of orgasm. Actually there is very little storage of sperm in the epididymis of the human, as compared to most other animals, where the tail of the epididymis serves as a huge storage depot. Because humans lack this storage capacity in the epididymis, once we ejaculate there is very little sperm left in the next ejaculate till several days have passed.

What Happens to Sperm in the Epididymis?

The epididymal tubule is not just a bridge between the testicle and the sperm duct. Sperm which leave the testicle are still not capable of fertilization. As they pass through the epididymis, they "mature" and thus obtain their ability to move in a straight-forward direction with sufficient velocity to fertilize the female egg. It used to be thought that sperm can only "mature" within the epididymis. Our studies now show that if sperm were to be captured from the beginning region of the epididymis, before the twenty-foot-long journey to the vas deferens, and allowed to mature with time alone, they can fertilize eggs in vitro and result in pregnancy. However, it is quite clear from years of animal studies that a remarkable process does occur in the epididymis, whereby sperm produced by the testicle which are completely unable to fertilize an egg, change so that by the time they leave the epididymis, they can.

It used to be thought that only sperm that reach the end of the epididymis, waiting to be released through the vas deferens upon orgasm, are maximally capable of fertilization. In truth, about half of the sperm located midway along the journey to the vas deferens are capable of fertilization. However, none of the sperm located in the earliest regions of the epididymis just after their exit from the testicle are capable of fertilization. Nonetheless, by surgically bypassing an obstruction in the "early" (proximal) region of the epididymis, we have found that sperm are able to mature on their own in the vas deferens and then fertilize. So "maturation" of sperm is quite necessary; but it doesn't require the epididymis. Yet, under normal circumstances, during this seemingly endless journey through the winding turns of the epididymis, the sperm mature their structure, develop their incredible swimming ability, and attain the ability to fertilize.

Sperm motility is probably the most important determinant of the male's fertility. The sperm inside the testicle can only vibrate their tails weakly and barely wiggle around. Sperm from the beginning regions of the epididymis can swim, but only in circles. Unidirectional, straightforward swimming is only achieved by sperm that have traversed a good portion of the epididymis. In looking at the semen analysis of an infertile male, it is not only the percentage of sperm that are motile that counts, but also the quality of that motility. Sperm that swim in a curve are less capable of fertilization.

Sperm remain fresh and alive in the epididymis and vas for a period of less than a month. Old age comes quickly to a little sperm, and if it has to sit around for over a month waiting to be ejaculated, it will be of no use. This does not mean that the man who has intercourse only once a month need not fear an unwanted pregnancy. There are still fresh sperm arriving every day that upon ejaculation will be capable of fertilization. However, a man who has an ejaculation only once a month will have a much higher percentage of dead, ineffectual sperm in his ejaculate, despite having a higher overall number of sperm stored up. Furthermore, sperm storage in the human is so poor that saving up for such a prolonged period is of little help in raising the sperm count.

The Fluid That Squirts the Sperm Out

Most of the fluid in the ejaculate does not come from the testicle, the epididymis, or the sperm duct. That is why vasectomy results in no noticeable change in the volume of ejaculate aside from the absence of sperm. During sexual intercourse, the epididymis and vas deferens muscles contract powerfully and propel the sperm through the vas deferens along an eight-inch journey up and out of the scrotal sac into the abdomen and finally to the ejaculatory duct, which sits just in front of the bladder (see Figure 19). The ejaculatory duct empties into the urethra, the canal inside the penis that carries the ejaculate out of the body.

Most of this fluid that pushes the sperm out comes from the seminal vesicles and the prostate gland. The seminal vesicles, located behind the bladder, expel their fluid very forcefully behind the sperm, pushing it into the urethra. The first portion of the ejaculate thus contains most of the sperm. The second portion is from the seminal vesicles, which contract violently and account for most of the ejaculatory fluid. At this time the internal sphincter of the bladder clamps down powerfully to prevent the semen from accidentally going backward into the bladder. It also prevents urine from leaking forward out of the bladder. The external sphincter, which sits just in front of the ejaculatory duct, then opens up and allows the ejaculate to enter the holding area just near the base of the penis, called the bulbous urethra. Finally the very powerful muscles around the bulbous urethra contract and squirt the ejaculate out of the penis with remarkable force. This highly coordinated symphony of complicated mus-

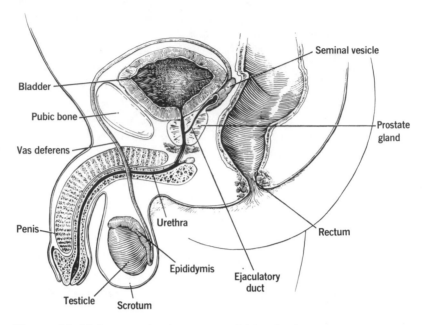

Figure 19. Male reproductive organs (side view).

cular contractions that propel the sperm from the epididymis all the way up through the abdomen and out the penis is what the male subjectively feels as orgasm.

Since the initial portion of the ejaculate contains the highest concentration of sperm, the patient who has been asked to collect semen for analysis will have an abnormally low reading if the first squirt is missed. The withdrawal method of contraception is relatively ineffective, for the same reason.

It is clear that many of the complicated fluids secreted by the prostate gland, the urethral glands, and the seminal vesicles are not really necessary except to provide a vehicle for sperm into the vagina. Though researchers have tried diligently to discover a role for the complex chemical constituents of this highly smelly fluid which carries the sperm into the vagina, they have not been terribly successful in their efforts. In fact, dilute solutions of salt water appear to be better for sperm than the semen in which they are naturally bathed at the time of ejaculation. The major function of the semen appears to be provision of a very transient alkaline environment to protect them from the harsh acid environment of the vagina during the brief moment of transition from the man's vas deferens to the woman's vagina, and until the sperm finally invade the more hospitable environment of the cervical mucus.

TESTICULAR TEMPERATURE

The testicles are located basically outside the body (in a sense) because they do not function properly at body temperature. The testes must remain at a temperature about four degrees lower than the usual 98.6°F maintained in the rest of the body. They are so sensitive to these four degrees of extra heat that if they were inside the body they would not be able to produce sperm at all.

We used to think the scrotum has a remarkably delicate temperature-regulating mechanism that keeps the temperature of the scrotal sac at 94°F at all times. Taking a cold shower causes the muscles of the scrotal sac to contract and pull the testes very close up against the body to conserve heat. On the other hand, when it is warm the scrotal muscles relax, and the testicles fall farther away from the body in order to cool off. This is an automatic reflex over which males have no control. In addition to this muscular thermal regulatory mechanism, there is a complicated network of a radiatorlike coiling of veins that brings cool scrotal blood away from the testes, which surround the arteries bringing warm blood into the testes, again helping to keep the testicles' temperature at 94°F. Alterations in this temperature-regulating mechanism may reduce sperm production and transport.

The temperature of the testicles depends completely on the temperature surrounding the scrotum. The usual scrotal temperature with pants on is 94°F. But if a man is naked for several hours in a room at 70°F temperature, the testicular temperature will go right down to 80°F or less. The scrotum allows the testicles to adjust to almost any outside temperature without the insulation from temperature change that the body of warm-blooded animals normally affords for our "internal" organs. From the point of view of temperature, our testicles are no different from cold-blooded creatures like snakes or fish. This may be important because it is quite clear that when testicles are near the body temperature of 98°F, they just can't make sperm very well.

When a man's scrotal temperature is tested it is usually in a situation when he has just taken off his pants for an examination and at that point it is usually about 94°F to 95°F. So for years it has been assumed that this range is the norm, four degrees lower than that of the body, which is 98.6°F. In truth, the testicular temperature is just determined by whatever the air temperature is inside the pants. In a nudist colony, testicular temperature would be much lower than 94°. If, on the other hand, time was spent in a sauna with a temperature set at 100°F, once again the testicles would not maintain a normal body temperature of 98.6°F. Because testicles are exteriorized, they would become the temperature of the hot tub.

Traditionally, men have been advised to avoid tight underwear, hot baths, and steam rooms. Unfortunately, not a single good scientific study has been performed on either normal men or infertile couples to see whether in a controlled, disciplined fashion these kinds of changes in habits can have any impact on sperm count. Whether a man wears boxer shorts or briefs has hardly any effect usually on scrotal temperature. Basically, and as long as underwear is worn, the average scrotal temperature is going to be around 94°F to 95°F.

However, that does not mean that the testicular temperature does not need attention. A fascinating study from Germany several years ago was designed to see whether or not increasing testicular temperature could be used as a form of male birth control. Normal, healthy male medical student volunteers literally pushed their testicles up into the fat tissue of their lower abdomens with a very tightly applied type of jock strap of their own special construction to see whether or not by truly raising the testicular temperature closer to the abdominal temperature, sperm production could be reduced. This was not adequate as a male contraceptive. The sperm count did not go down to low-enough levels to ensure protection against pregnancy. But, the fact is that the sperm count did go down.

Therefore it is still reasonable advice to avoid prolonged hot tubs, steam baths, excessively tight underwear, or anything that might conceivably raise the testicular temperature.

THE VARICOCELE SCANDAL

If your husband is sent to a urologist because of a "low sperm count," he is very likely to receive a diagnosis of "varicocele." A varicocele is a varicose vein of the testicle normally found in 15 to 20 percent of all men. That is, 15 to 20 percent of all males on this planet have a varicose vein of the testicle, and it is almost always on the left side. The reason for this is that the testicular vein draining blood back from the testicle on the right side drains directly into the major vein of the body, the vena cava, but on the left side the testicular vein drains into the kidney's vein. This type of anatomy on the left is much more likely to lead to a defect in the valves that normally prevent blood from flowing back down the veins because of the effect of gravity when one stands up. A varicose vein of the testicle is no different than a varicose vein in the leg, with which you may be more familiar. When you are lying down, you notice nothing abnormal. However, when you stand up, blood which would normally be prevented by valves from falling back down will fill up and dilate these veins so that they become readily apparent under the skin, even to the naked eye.

The standard urological line is that varicocele is "the commonest cause of male infertility," and the "most readily treatable cause of male infertility." As far back as 1952, a doctor by the name of Tulloch from England performed a varicocelectomy operation on a man with absolutely no sperm production, and then reported that within six months he was producing sperm and fathered a child. That flimsy report was picked up with incredible enthusiasm in this country in the late 1960s. It has been alleged that as many as 40 percent of "infertile men" have a varicocele. In fact, there are some urologists who find a varicocele in almost every "infertile male" they see. The literature on varicoceles and the operation to repair varicoceles for infertility is bewildering in volume and replete with success stories.

Yet nobody could explain why 15 percent of the world's fertile men have a large varicocele and yet suffer no apparent harm, or why fixing a problem on the left side should in some way correct an underproduction of sperm on both sides. I will never forget a meeting of the American Urological Association in the late 1970s, a time when everyone was gloating over the remarkable success of varicocelectomy in curing male infertility, when Dr. Rubin Gittes got up in front of several thousand urologists and stunned them with the simple statement, "I see no evidence that there is any relationship between the presence of a varicocele and male infertility."

Dr. Gittes is one of the most scientifically disciplined and clinically astute urologists I have ever known. At that time he was the Professor of Urology at the Peter Bent Brigham Hospital at Harvard and chairman of its urology department; presently he is the head of the Scripps Institute in San Diego, California. His major interest in urology did not revolve around male infertility, but his brillance in any urological area he studied was recognized by all. After the momentary shock of his comment, the pro-varicocelectomy forces marshaled their strength and vehemently argued that "years of clinical experience have demonstrated the effect of varicocele on depressing sperm production and the success of varicocelectomy in curing male infertility."

The enthusiasm for varicocelectomy continued to grow to extremes in the early 1980s. Some urologists in Europe recommended that every postpubertal boy be examined for a varicocele, and if he had one, operate on it at an early age before it had time to hurt his sperm production. This would mean an automatic operation for 15 percent of the world's teenagers. Another study supposedly demonstrated that even if a patient did not have a varicocele, the operation to tie off that testicular vein (the same operation one would perform to correct the varicocele), would increase the sperm production of any male with oligospermia, whether or not he had a varicocele. If these studies and claims were to be taken seriously, there would not be enough urological surgeons to do all of these operations. And I am sorry to say that may be the key to how such an outrageous epidemic of varicocele surgery for so-called "male infertility" ever got started in the first place.

The fact is, many urologists who treat male infertility depend heavily on varicocelectomy for their income. I used to perform varicocelectomy routinely myself. I was fooled by a "scientific" literature that was filled with enthusiasm, and by the intrinsic variation in sperm count from month to month in various patients which led to the false impression that one-third of them had an improvement as a result of the operation. However, there have now been hard, scientifically controlled studies performed by nonsurgeon endocrinologists with a special interest in male infertility and with no strong preexisting need to find varicocelectomy surgery beneficial.

In the late 1970s, Dr. Louis Rodriguez-Rigau, Dr. Keith Smith, and Dr. Emil Steinberger from the University of Texas in Houston presented the first large controlled studies which showed absolutely no difference in the pregnancy rate among couples whose husbands had a varicocele between those whose husbands underwent surgery and those whose husbands did not. This paper met with a great deal of uproar and disdain and severely hurt the reputation of these outstanding clinical scientists among urologists who just did not want to see that kind of result.

Around the same time in 1979, Nilsson from Göteborg, Sweden, reported a similar study in *The British Journal of Urology*, demonstrating no statistically significant improvement in sperm count, motility, or morphology in men with varicoceles who had surgery versus those who did not. More importantly, the pregnancy rate was even lower, but certainly not higher, in the wives of men who had the operation, versus those who did not have the operation. In 1984, Vermuelian from Ghent, Belgium, also reported no improvement in pregnancy rates in those couples whose husband had a varicocelectomy versus those who did not.

The clincher paper, however, came in 1985 in the *British Medical Journal* by Dr. Gordon Baker and his group at Prince Henry Hospital in Melbourne, Australia. They did an incredibly detailed study following 651 infertile couples in whom the man had a varicocele. In 283 of those 651 couples the man underwent a varicocelectomy, and in 368 of the couples the man did not. In both groups, 30 percent of the couples conceived by one year and 45 percent by two years. There was no improvement in pregnancy rate whatsoever in the couples in which the man had a varicocelectomy, and there was no improvement in the semen analysis either. Despite the overwhelming mounting evidence

that Dr. Gittes's statement in 1978 challenging the role of varicocele in male infertility was correct, urologists still go on performing varicocelectomies on at least 30 percent or more of men
whose wives' gynecologists refer them to a urologist.

This year I saw a patient whose wife was scheduled to undergo
a reversal of tubal ligation later in the year. Her husband, trying
to do the prudent thing and prevent his wife going through
surgery that might possibly be unnecessary, decided to see a
urologist first and make sure that he was fertile. He had a high
sperm count with excellent motility. Yet the urologist who saw
him insisted that he had to have a varicocelectomy operation,
telling him that he had a large left-sided varicocele and absolutely
had to have that surgery done before the wife could undergo
the tubal reversal operation. I thought the story sounded strange
and so I asked him to make a separate trip to St. Louis before
the planned time of the wife's operation. Not only would it have
been ridiculous to operate on his varicocele, especially with
sperm count that good, but the fact is that when I examined him
I found absolutely no varicocele.

Several years ago my office received a call from a patient who
had read my first book and just wanted to know whether the
varicocelectomy her husband was scheduled to undergo in two
weeks was necessary. It would be months before I would be
able to see them for an appointment, but I just gave her the
message that usually varicocelectomy does not benefit male infertility and there is certainly never any reason to rush into it.
She called two months later, just before she was to have her
appointment with me, to inform me that thanks to our advice
her husband did not have the varicocelectomy, and since she is
now pregnant she would have no need to see me. Interestingly,
if he had undergone the varicocelectomy, the doctor who did it
might have claimed that that was the reason she got pregnant.

One of the real problems looming is that urologists who per-
ceive the skepticism that exists about how a one-sided varicocele
operation could improve sperm production in both testicles are
now claiming to find "bilateral" varicoceles (a large one on the
left which is obvious and a much smaller, more subtle one on
the right). These men undergo a varicocelectomy on both sides
rather than just the left side and occasionally the results are
disastrous.

Several years ago I saw a thirty-five-year old couple who had a five-year-old child and were now trying for their second one. His sperm count was apparently in the low range (5 million per cc, but excellent motility). When he saw his local urologist he was told he had a "bilateral" varicocele and had a bilateral varicocelectomy performed. When I saw him he was completely azospermic (without sperm). Although normally a varicocelectomy should be a relatively simple, innocuous operation, it can also be tricky at times because in an effort to get every single vein tied off (which would be necessary to prevent any blood from flowing back into the testicles), a surgeon can accidentally tie off the spermatic artery, which is extremely small and delicate. A clumsy surgeon might even tie off the vas.

I can go on with story after story of patients without a varicocele who were told that they had one, of patients with normal sperm counts undergoing varicocelectomy, and of very large fees charged by well-known urologists for what is really an extremely simple twenty-minute operation.

Many portions of this book will not make me friends among colleagues, and many of us are tempted to accept the unscientific, clinical blundering of our colleagues in order to avoid professional damage to ourselves that ultimately results in decreased referrals. But on so many of these issues related to "male infertility" enough is enough. Drugs and hormones administered in the usual way do not increase sperm count in oligospermic men, and neither does varicocele surgery.

CHAPTER 6

ARE SPERM THE PROBLEM? HOW MANY DO YOU NEED?

THE SPERM COUNT

One of the first tests for evaluating a couple's infertility is the husband's "sperm count," or to be more precise, the "semen analysis." This is the single best method of determining to what degree the male partner is contributing to the couple's barrenness, but its meaning can be totally misconstrued. No other test for evaluating the couple's infertility is quite so simple. Yet there are immense errors and great misinterpretations of the meaning of the sperm count that can have tragic consequences. For these reasons I shall explain in detail the process of obtaining and interpreting the sperm count.

What Are Sperm?

Semen is the fluid ejaculated at the time of orgasm, and it may or may not contain sperm. It is impossible to tell by its appearance whether the semen contains sperm. For example, after vasectomy a patient has perfectly normal ejaculation and notices no reduction in his semen. Yet, looking under the microscope, you no longer see any sperm in his ejaculate.

Sperm (or spermatozoa) are microscopic creatures which look like tadpoles swimming about at a frantic pace back and forth in the semen. Each sperm consists of a head which contains all of the genetic material (DNA) of the father-to-be and a tail which lashes back and forth at an incredible speed to propel the sperm along (see Figure 20). In the ejaculate of a fertile man there are hundreds of millions of these sperm, and they usually move rapidly.

Upon first observation of sperm under the microscope, I can't help but be awestruck by the massive numbers and by the rapid, gyrating pace of their movement. Perhaps more subtle and important than the apparent frenzy of activity is the purposefulness of the movements. Despite the fact that they are all going in different directions (and so their motion appears to be haphazard and random), each one moves in a straight line with the accuracy

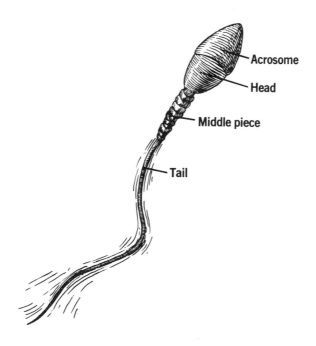

Figure 20. The basic structure of a normal sperm.

of a guided missile. In a normal specimen each sperm observed under a microscope goes straight across the field without stopping, turning around, or going in a pointless circle, and with no deviation from what appears to be a straight line. It is only the massive number of these sperm all mixed together and each going in different straight lines that superficially makes the motion appear aimless.

Does Saving It Up Help?

No matter how accurately the laboratory does the sperm count and no matter how carefully and consistently the specimen is collected by the patient, there will be frequent variations. Because of these variations, the sperm count should be repeated at least three times over the course of several months.

Since intercourse will deplete the male temporarily of some sperm, it is important to abstain from intercourse for a few days prior to collecting the specimen. Otherwise a low value will be reported by the laboratory, and the husband may mistakenly conclude that he is infertile, even though his ejaculation just prior to obtaining the collection may have had a very large number of sperm. When the couple have had intercourse the night before, this can reduce the sperm count to one-third of its normal level.

Since most couples seem to have intercourse two to three times a week, it has arbitrarily been felt that two to three days of abstinence prior to the sperm count will accurately reflect how much sperm is delivered to the wife at the time of intercourse. If abstaining for two or three days prior to collection of the specimen results in a higher sperm count, it would seem that abstaining for two weeks should bring the count up even more, and that abstinence should be a way of improving the husband's fertility. Unfortunately, abstaining for more than four or five days rarely results in any significant increase in the sperm count unless the count otherwise would have been exceptionally low.

The reason for this is that in humans (as opposed to most other animals) there is very little sperm storage in the "epididymis," the microscopic twenty-foot-long coiled tubule that carries sperm from the testicle to the vas deferens. The "tail" of the epididymis in most animals is a storage depot for huge quantities of sperm. That allows repetitive ejaculations to still contain large number of sperm. In the human, however, sperm transport through the epididymis is very rapid, and sperm storage very poor. Therefore, "saving it up" for long periods does us very little good.

The semen specimen should be produced by masturbation, with collection of the entire ejaculate in a wide-mouthed, clean jar that can be obtained from the laboratory. If the collection jar is not wide-mouthed, or if the specimen is obtained by coitus interruptus ("pulling out early"), it is easy to lose a small portion of the ejaculate. Notwithstanding the mess, this would result in great errors in the sperm count, since different portions of the ejaculate harbor different concentrations of sperm. In most men, the majority of sperm come out in the early portion of the ejaculate. Subsequent squirts after the first portion of the specimen usually contain very few sperm. Thus, if one were having a difficult time getting the bottle into the proper position and spilled an early portion of the ejaculate, the sperm count might turn out to be falsely low. Therefore, to obtain an accurate count, all of the ejaculation must be collected in one specimen container. Collection in a condom during intercourse is also not acceptable because most condoms will harm the sperm.

The semen should be examined promptly. If the analysis of the specimen is delayed more than two hours, a large proportion of sperm may have died off or lost a good deal of their motility.

How Many Sperm?

The three most important aspects of the sperm count are: 1) the actual numerical concentration of sperm per cubic centimeter, 2) the motility of the sperm (that is, the speed and the quality of the movement), and 3) the morphology (the structure) of the sperm. The number of sperm in the ejaculate is determined by looking at a tiny but measured portion of it in a counting chamber under a microscope. Then the total number of sperm in the ejaculate can be calculated. For example, if the count is 13 million sperm per cc, a relatively low count, we will have counted only thirteen sperm within ten boxes. If the count is 100 million sperm per cc (a very high count), we will have seen one hundred sperm in those ten boxes, or an average of ten sperm in each box.

Motility of the Sperm

More important than the quantity of sperm are their activity and quality. After the specimen has been counted, the percentage of all the sperm seen in any microscopic field that are actually moving and the percentage that are not moving is observed. There will always be a certain number of nonmotile (nonmoving) sperm in the ejaculate which are incapable of fertilization. Only the moving sperm are capable of entering the cervical mucus and ultimately reaching and penetrating the egg. After the percent motility is determined, the quality of that motion is observed.

There are four types of sperm movement: *Grade 1* motility means that the sperm are only wiggling sluggishly in place and making very little, if any, forward progression. These are pathetic vibratory-type motions that get the sperm nowhere. Such sperm are incapable of fertilizing the egg. *Grade 2* motility means that the sperm are moving forward, but either the speed is very slow or they do not move in a straight line, instead veering off in a curve. Normally sperm have a remarkable propensity for maintaining straightforward motion. Sperm that cannot hold their course are incapable of fertilization. Some sperm go forward a little and then, instead of continuing undaunted, stop and reverse direction. Such sperm will never make it in the ferocious arena of the female genital tract. *Grade 3* sperm are able to move at a reasonable speed with straightforward progress and accurate homing. *Grade 4* sperm advance straight ahead also, but at an extraordinarily rapid speed. Grade 3 and Grade 4 sperm are usually capable of fertilization. Grades 1 and 2 sperm generally are not. However, with very special new in vitro fertilization techniques, even these pathetic Grade 1 and 2 sperm may actually be induced to fertilize the wife's egg and result in a baby.

The average velocity of a Grade 3 sperm is about twenty-five microns (a micron = $\frac{1}{1,000}$ of a millimeter) per second. That can best be understood by realizing that the average sperm head is about six microns long and, including its tail, is a total of about twenty-five microns in length from the front of its head to the tip of its tail. That means the sperm head normally travels forward about four times its own length every second. This may seem fast and swell our male ego to think we have within us creatures that can perform such a feat. But in truth we are relatively pathetic compared to other animals. Horse sperm routinely swim at about three times that speed and bull sperm finish the race before we even leave the starting gate.

The Shape (Morphology) of the Sperm

As important as the motility is the microscopic examination for "morphology," or structure, of the sperm. In even a normal human specimen as many as 40 percent of the spermatozoa may have abnormal morphology (see Figure 21). In this respect again we are pitiful as a species in comparison to most other animals, where virtually every single sperm has a "perfect" structure. Only in the human do we find even in the most fertile males as many as 40 percent of sperm with clearly abnormal structure.

There is no relationship between abnormal sperm and abnormal pregnancy. Abnormally shaped sperm cannot fertilize the egg. The normal sperm has an oval head with a long tail. Abnormally shaped sperm may have either a very large round head, or an extremely small, pinpoint head. They may even have two heads. The sperm may be bent at the neck and misshapen, and the tails may have kinks and curls in them. None of these odd-looking sperm (which are present in large numbers even in a normal ejaculate) correlate with any genetic problem in the offspring since such abnormally shaped sperm are not capable of fertilization.

Morphology is probably even more important than motility in indicating whether spermatozoa can fertilize. The normal sperm has a head with a perfect oval shape, no crooked bend at the neck, and a straight, long, tapering tail. Very vigorously moving tails that appear to exhibit good forward progression may have a poorly shaped head or none at all. Such sperm are certainly incapable of fertilization.

Abnormal Sperm

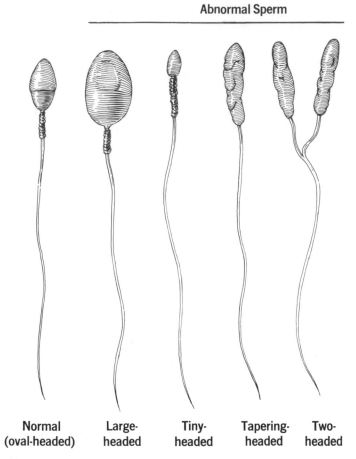

| Normal (oval-headed) | Large-headed | Tiny-headed | Tapering-headed | Two-headed |

Figure 21. Normal and abnormal morphology of sperm.

The shape of the sperm head is a very specific feature of the genetic folding of the DNA it contains and correlates very closely with its ability to fertilize. Studies from Dr. David de Kretser's group in Melbourne, Australia, and from Dr. Anibal Acosta in Norfolk, Virginia, make it very clear that the human ejaculate has only small numbers of sperm even normally that meet strict criteria for fertile morphology. If just 10 percent of sperm in an ejaculate meet these strict criteria of a perfect oval shape, the fertilization rate is good. If less than 4 percent of sperm meet these criteria, the fertilization rate is poor. Thus, you need very few perfectly normally structured sperm to accomplish fertilization in vitro.

The Amount of Semen

Most men ejaculate one-half teaspoon to one full teaspoon of semen (2.5 cc to 5 cc). The volume of ejaculate does not indicate the amount of sperm you are producing. There are some men who have very low ejaculate volumes of less than a fifth of a teaspoon, but they may have a very high concentration of sperm in that low volume. On the other hand, some men may have a very high volume of ejaculate (and think that they are making a lot of sperm) but yet have a relatively low sperm concentration.

However, there are several reasons for wanting to know the ejaculate volume. First, if the ejaculate volume is less than 1 cc (one-fifth of a teaspoon), and there are no sperm, it could mean ejaculatory duct blockage or, indeed, congenital absence of the vas, a relatively common cause of obstructive sterility in men (which today we can treat, but only a few years ago was considered hopeless). Secondly, if there is sperm present in a low volume of ejaculate, it may either be a sign of prostate problems or it may just indicate a relatively high frequency of intercourse.

In certain cases there may be no ejaculate whatsoever because all of the patient's sperm and seminal fluid are being ejaculated backward into the bladder rather than forward out of the penis. This retrograde ejaculation is a condition caused frequently by diabetes or by past surgery. In addition, certain patients on medication to control high blood pressure may have backward ejaculation of sperm into the bladder as a side effect. Such a man may mistakenly believe that he is making no sperm at all whereas in truth he may be making large amounts; they are simply not getting out.

The Appearance of the Semen—Liquid or Jelly?

Within a minute of ejaculation, the semen should normally coagulate into a tapiocalike gel. The sperm cannot be adequately counted or examined while the semen is in this coagulated blob. The main function of this "blob" is probably to prevent early leakage of sperm out of the vagina. Within ten to thirty minutes after ejaculation, the semen specimen should again liquefy.

Failure of semen to liquefy could indicate subtle infections of the prostate and seminal vesicles, but sometimes it is simply a normal variant, and subsequent semen collections on different days might present no problem. Failure of the semen to liquefy often leads to all sorts of false notions of infertility. Sometimes the patient is told that it means that the husband is allergic to himself and that his sperm are being attacked by his own antibodies.

An example of the foolishness of worrying about persistent coagulation (or nonliquefaction) of the semen is a patient who was recently referred to me with long-term infertility blamed on the persistent clumping of his semen (supposedly caused by an immune reaction). He and his wife had been trying to get pregnant for ten years. By the time their appointment with me was made, the wife had finally been seen by a superb gynecologist, who found that she not only did not ovulate every month, but that she ovulated late and that her cervical mucus was too thick. The failure of her husband's sperm to penetrate her cervical mucus thus had been blamed incorrectly on his clumping problem. The gynecologist placed the wife on proper treatment. Just before the couple's appointment to see me, I received a telephone call from the wife saying that she had finally become pregnant.

The Chemistry of the Semen

It appears that the only function of the complex, smelly chemistry of the semen is to deliver the sperm directly to the female cervix, and the function of this transporting fluid is indeed brief.

Sperm appear to be relatively safe in the vas deferens and epididymis prior to ejaculation, and thereafter have a decent prospect for survival only after they penetrate the cervical mucus. It is only in the precarious few moments when the sperm are ejaculated into the vagina that time is of the essence, and that the semen serves any purpose at all. The semen's alkalinity protects against the harsh, acid environment in the vagina that would otherwise quickly kill the sperm. The early gelatinlike blob of the semen prevents early leakage out of the vagina, and the sugar in the semen provides instant energy for locomotion. The fluid of the ejaculate is not really designed to keep the sperm alive for very long, but only to get them on their way as quickly as possible into the cervical mucus. However, before reaching the security of the cervical mucus, the semen is not a very healthy environment, since the sperm that don't make it into the cervical mucus quickly will find that the fluid of the ejaculate is actually a hostile environment after several hours.

How Many Sperm Are Really Necessary for a Man to Be Fertile?

For years it has been assumed that if a man had a sperm count below a certain arbitrary minimum, he was infertile, and a couple's failure to achieve pregnancy was caused by this "male factor." As recently as fifteen years ago it was thought that a sperm count of under 40 million per cc meant the husband was infertile and urologists gave such couples a poor prognosis for pregnancy. If the wife did become pregnant, the pregnancy was ascribed to whatever useless treatment was being administered to the so-called "infertile" husband. We now know that men with very low sperm counts can impregnate their wives, and the value of the semen analysis has been much maligned of late and great effort placed into very expensive tests such as the hamster-egg penetration test and sperm antibody tests (see pages 153–69), but these evaluations of the sperm have simply added more confusion than clarity to the picture. There remains a terribly frustrating discrepancy between the results of hamster-egg penetration tests, sperm antibody tests, and the fertilization of human eggs via in vitro fertilization (IVF) or GIFT.

A review of many studies over the last thirty-five years relating pregnancy rate to sperm counts in "fertile" and "infertile" couples indicates that the standard semen analysis (sperm count) indeed is useful in evaluating the degree of "male factor" in an infertile couple. But a low sperm count does not preclude the couple's being fertile. Male factor is quite compatible with normal fertility in a couple if the wife is very fertile. However, some cases of male factor are so severe that even with the fertile wife, pregnancy will not occur without some help. Low sperm count and poor sperm quality (oligoasthenospermia) is unfortunately, in most cases, an untreatable condition. But vigorous treatment of the wife may still result in pregnancy. Higher sperm counts in an infertile couple are associated with higher pregnancy rates. Lower sperm counts in an infertile couple are associated with lower pregnancy rates.

In the majority of infertile couples in whom the sperm count is poor, female factors also exist which prevent conception. If the wife were very fertile, she often would have become pregnant despite her husband's low sperm count, and they never would have come to see a physician for infertility. Thus pregnancy can be achieved despite very low sperm counts either by treatment of the wife, or with the new technology procedures of IVF and GIFT. The reason for this is that in vitro fertilization (IVF) or GIFT allows the fewer number of available sperm a greater opportunity for direct contact with the egg and, thus, to fertilize it.

There are cases where wives get pregnant naturally from husbands who have unbelievably low counts. In one documented case by Dr. Rebecca Sokol in 1987, a woman got pregnant from her husband despite his sperm count being less than 50,000 per cc with less than 10 percent of those few sperm being alive. After the baby was born, careful genetic tissue typing and blood typing was performed of mother, father, and baby and it was determined with 99.9 percent certainty that the husband indeed was genetically the father despite having a count so low that natural conception would seem just beyond belief. In view of cases like this, what, after all, is "male infertility" and how many sperm are necessary to be fertile?

The correlation of sperm count with fertility was originally presented by the famous article of MacLeod and Gold in 1951. These authors studied sperm counts in 1,000 "fertile" and 1,000 "infertile" couples. In the "fertile" population, the majority of men had sperm counts over 40 million per cc. Thus, over the decades it was always assumed that a normal sperm count is greater than 40 million per cc and less than that amount indicates male infertility. The weakness of the assumption that a sperm count under 40 million per cc meant "male infertility" was not recognized until the 1980s.

New understanding came from studies of sperm counts in men who were requesting vasectomy, who were clearly fertile prior to the vasectomy. In 1974, it was found that 20 percent of such "fertile" men had sperm counts of less than 20 million per cc. In 1977, Dr. Emil Steinberger's group in Texas studied the sperm counts of several thousand men about to undergo a vasectomy who had demonstrated previous fertility and found that 23 percent of these fertile men had sperm counts of less than 20 million per cc and would have been incorrectly labeled as infertile by the routine standard definitions of male infertility. It was only when the sperm count was less than 10 million per cc that they noted an increased risk of infertility in the couple.

The most shocking challenge to the notion that sperm count has anything to do with male infertility came from the work of Dr. Richard Sherins of the National Institutes of Health in 1986 who has studied men treated for Kallmann's Syndrome (see pages 117–20). After hormone treatment of these rare cases, sperm counts rarely went above the very low levels of 2 or 10 million per cc. Yet, nearly all (twenty out of twenty-two) of these men got their wives pregnant quite easily with sperm counts that were at best extremely low.

When I look at my patients who have undergone vasectomy reversal and get their wives pregnant (in comparison to those who did not get their wives pregnant), I find a distribution of sperm counts no different from that observed by Steinberger's group studying sperm counts of fertile men about to undergo vasectomy. Among the men who get their wives pregnant, about 11 percent have sperm counts under 10 million per cc, and among those who do not get their wives pregnant, 23 percent have sperm counts under 10 million per cc. Over 10 million sperm cc, there is no significant difference in the pregnancy rate at any level up to 200 million per cc.

So what is the relationship of sperm count to pregnancy rate? Even though low sperm counts can get women pregnant, the pregnancy rate is better with higher sperm counts.

In studies done in the 1970s, when the sperm count was less than 10 million per cc, only about 30 percent of the couples got pregnant using conventional treatment. But when the sperm

TABLE 1

RELATIONSHIP OF SPERM COUNT OF THE MALE TO PREGNANCY RATE AMONG INFERTILE COUPLES

Motile Sperm Count (millions per cc)	Pregnancy Rate (percent)
less than 5.0	33.3
5–10.0	27.8
10–20.0	52.9
20–40.0	57.1
40–60.0	60.0
60–100.0	62.5
Over 100.0	70.0

count was over 40 million per cc, greater than 60 percent of the couples became pregnant. There is another interesting clue to the importance of the sperm count from Dr. Robert Schoysman's study of over 1,000 oligospermic men (men with low sperm counts) in Belgium whose wives were awaiting insemination with donor sperm.

At the time of his study, Schoysman had one of the few large donor sperm insemination programs in Europe. So at that time, couples in whom the husband had either no sperm or a very low sperm count had to wait, often for many years, before being able to be inseminated with donor sperm. Some of these wives became pregnant before their turn came to undergo donor insemination, and this gave a very clear picture of what the chances would be for a woman whose husband was extremely oligospermic to get pregnant with no treatment whatsoever over a period of time.

These data were compiled from a unique group of patients who had a long history of prior infertility, who had been assumed to have "male factor" problems (whether rightly or wrongly), and were on a very long waiting list in Europe for artificial donor insemination. Couples in this group who got pregnant did so either before their name came up on the waiting list or after they had already given up on the idea of having donor insemi-

TABLE 2

1,327 OLIGOSPERMIC MEN

Motile Sperm Count	Percent Pregnancy	
	5 Years	*12 Years*
(millions per cc)	*(percent)*	*(percent)*
0.1–1	3.9	8.7
1.1–5	11.9	26.6
5.1–10	22.1	34.3
10.1–15	45.0	58.5
15.1–20	68.6	82.0

nation. The wife underwent no treatment because it was assumed to be strictly the "husband's fault." Even when the sperm count was less than 1 million per cc (as low as 100,000 per cc) with no treatment whatsoever of the husband or the wife, there was almost a 4 percent chance of pregnancy occurring within five years and close to a 10 percent chance of pregnancy occurring without any treatment in twelve years. When the sperm count was in the low range of 10 to 20 million per cc (certainly considered a low count by any infertility expert standards), over 50 percent of the patients became pregnant within five years despite receiving no treatment.

With increasing levels of sperm counts still within the low range, the pregnancy rate increased as the sperm count increased. This old but invaluable study demonstrated that while low sperm counts are associated with the possibility of pregnancy and fertility, higher sperm counts are associated with higher pregnancy rates. Male infertility was, thus, found not to be an absolute problem in the male, but rather a relative problem, which could be overcome either by marrying an extremely fertile wife, or by aggressive treatment of the wife.

The Australians, Dr. Gordon Baker, Dr. David de Kretser, and Dr. Henry Burger from Melbourne, found somewhat similar findings but in couples where the wife was treated even when the husband's sperm count was low. They compiled an elegant graph comparing the pregnancy rate per month among infertile

CUMULATIVE AND LIFETABLE PREGNANCY RATES

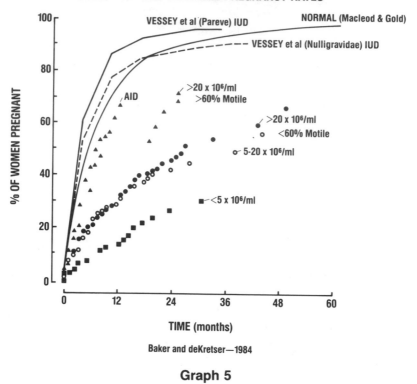

Baker and deKretser—1984

Graph 5

couples with varying sperm counts in the husband and compared it to the pregnancy rate per month of normal fertile couples (see graph 5).

By a year and a half, normal fertile couples discontinuing contraception have about a 92 percent chance of getting pregnant (Vessey and Normal curves). Azospermic couples undergoing insemination with normal donor sperm (AID) had a pregnancy rate very similar to that of normal couples discontinuing contraception but slightly lower, as can be seen in Graph 5. In infertile couples undergoing treatment who had sperm counts of higher than 20 million per cc and greater than 60 percent motility, the pregnancy rate at eighteen months was about *60 percent*, considerably less than that of either normal couples or couples undergoing donor insemination with normal donor sperm. Couples with greater than 20 million sperm per cc but less than 60 percent motility had a *40 percent* chance of pregnancy at eighteen months, and couples with between 5 and 20 million sperm per cc had a similarly depressed rate of pregnancy of *40 percent* at eighteen months. Finally, couples with sperm counts of less than 5 million per cc had only about a *22 percent* chance of pregnancy at a year and a half. This information compiled by the Australians thus clarifies an otherwise confusing picture immensely—to just what extent the husband's sperm count affects the fertility of the couple. A low sperm count does not mean the couple is infertile and can't get pregnant. It just means that it is more difficult for them to get pregnant particularly if there is a female problem as well.

COMPUTERIZED ANALYSIS OF SPERM MOTION

The standard semen analysis includes the number of sperm, its motility (the percent that are moving and the quality of the motion), and morphology (structure). Men with very poor sperm counts can still be fertile but modern studies in the 1980s have demonstrated clearly that the higher the sperm count and the greater the motility, the better the pregnancy rate. It appears that unless there is no sperm at all, husbands come in degrees of fertility and they are usually not either absolutely fertile or infertile.

One method of trying to refine the standard semen analysis to make a better prediction of the fertilizing ability of the husband's sperm is "computer-assisted analysis of sperm motion." This is simply a quantitative, automated method of grading the motility of the sperm. It has generally been felt that Grade 1 sperm, which only wiggle in place with no forward progression at all, are very unlikely to fertilize, whereas Grade 4 sperm, which move in a straight line with a rapid velocity, are indeed extremely fertile. In computer-assisted analysis of sperm motion a video camera is connected to a microscope, and the input is transferred to a TV screen and then to a computer programmed to analyze that motion. Amazing information about the velocity and the directionality of sperm is gathered that may be more reliable than just a visual impression obtained by looking down the microscope.

A printout of the actual velocity of forward sperm motion can be obtained and the percentage of sperm that are moving at different velocities. The degree to which the sperm head is moving from side to side and perhaps, most importantly, the "linearity" of motion can be measured.

The computer will automatically calculate the speed for sperm to go from Point A to Point B, and then simultaneously calculate the speed the sperm pursue in its digressions from side to side. The ratio of the distance the sperm go from Point A to Point B (a straight-line, shortest-distance path) to the actual curve that it follows is the "linearity" of motion. That means that if the sperm takes wild swings to the right and to the left as it is going forward, it has less "linearity" than if it takes small turns to the right and to the left during its forward progression.

The controlled studies of Dr. Sherins's group from the National Institutes of Health indicated that infertile men had a motility disorder characterized by having a higher percentage of cells being substantially slower in velocity and less directional in motion than sperm from normal men. The quality of sperm motion correlated much better with fertility than the quantity of sperm. However, just like with the standard semen analysis, the most sophisticated introduction of computer-based data doesn't change the basic biological fact that although good sperm parameters such as high counts, high percent motility, and high linearity yield greater pregnancy rates, poor semen parameters do not preclude fertility in the male.

Particularly, if poor sperm are assisted by being placed in a culture dish right next to the egg, poor sperm quality becomes less significant than the fertility of the female. Despite numerous studies of sperm count and semen quality, it has been impossible to establish the lowest boundaries for these parameters below which men are no longer fertile. What can be said is that the incidence of infertility increases as sperm concentrations fall and becomes most apparent below 20 million sperm per cc. Thus, the term "oligospermia" has come to describe male infertility even though we know that fertilization and indeed pregnancy can occur with very low counts well under 1 million per cc. It is simply that the lower the count and the lower the quality of sperm motion, the more difficult it is for fertilization to occur.

OTHER METHODS OF EVALUATING MALE INFERTILITY

The Hamster Test

Doctors have always been fascinated by the fact that fertilization of an egg by sperm is always species-specific. By that is meant that a dog's sperm cannot fertilize a cow egg, and a human sperm certainly can't fertilize a rat or hamster egg. In the early 1970s efforts were made to find out what it is that makes it impossible for the sperm of one species to penetrate or fertilize the egg of another species.

In nature there are certain types of crossbreeding that work. For example, the domestic bull can mate with a North American buffalo and produce a hybrid called a "cattalo," which is a fertile animal that can breed further "cattalos." A polar bear will readily mate with a brown bear, and lions will readily mate with tigers, producing an animal called a "liger," which also is indeed fertile and can produce more of its kind. The donkey and the horse have perhaps become the most famous crossbred species, resulting in a mule, an animal which carries the stronger attributes of both animals, but which is sterile and unable to produce further mules. The zebra can also mate with a horse or a donkey producing a "zebhorse," which is actually a sort of zebra-stallion that looks like a horse with stripes, or a "zebdonkey," which appears like a donkey with stripes. But once again, these animals, like the mule, are sterile and cannot reproduce. Ram sperm seems to successfully fertilize goats, but the resulting embryo invariably dies after the second month of pregnancy.

Although very closely related species can crossbreed and sometimes produce a new and even fertile species, it is impossible for the sperm and egg of not closely related species to fertilize. However, if the tough outer layer of the egg (called the "zona pellucida") were removed (i.e., the egg is denuded of its outer protective layer), then sperm from any species can penetrate and, therefore, theoretically fertilize the egg of any other species. In fact, sperm from fertile humans can indeed "fertilize" such a "denuded" hamster egg. Although this experiment might lead to speculation that some sort of monstrous hybrid could thus be formed by test-tube fertilization between species, let me assure you that none of these "fertilized" eggs have ever developed and no scientist doing this experiment ever seriously considered that such a species cross was possible.

All that has been shown is that there is a species-specific barrier to sperm penetration in the outer shell of the egg, and that removing that shell allows the sperm of a human to penetrate the egg of a hamster and initiate what appears to be the very first stages of fertilization. But in truth fertilization has not occurred. What happens when the human sperm penetrates the zona-free hamster egg is that the highly condensed DNA of the normal sperm head undergoes a process of "decondensation," forming what is called a "male pronucleus," and the nucleus of the egg undergoes "reduction division," giving off a "polar body," and forming what is called the "female pronucleus." "Syngamy," or the process of union of the male and the female pronuclei resulting in a genetically new individual, does not occur.

The ability of human sperm to penetrate a denuded hamster egg has now become a rather routine test of sperm function or "male factor" infertility. This is called the "hamster test," used by fertility experts, who have sought for the last fifty years a way of determining whether the infertility of the couple is the "man's fault" or the "woman's fault." The concept has always been prevalent that examining the sperm of the husband would reveal whose fault it was and on whom to concentrate the treatment. Disillusionment with the ability of the sperm count to rule out the male's ability to get his wife pregnant, no matter how low the count, led to the search for other ways of testing the sperm that could perhaps give us this answer better than the semen analysis.

The hamster test as well as several other tests developed out of a desire to improve upon the lack of clear-cut information from the sperm count. Hundreds of millions of dollars have been spent by various fertility clinics and andrology (male fertility) laboratories around the world to develop systems for hamster testing of infertile couples. The test is extremely expensive and an entire economy of laboratory personnel is built upon it, so that it is not going to go away easily. The test has undergone many modifications in an effort to appease critics and to try to make it more helpful.

The original report of its practical use in a human infertility clinic showed that if a large group of "zona-free" hamster eggs were placed in culture with sperm from fertile men, over 10 percent of the eggs would be "fertilized." However, if a large number of these hamster eggs were placed in culture with the sperm from men who were not fertile, less than 10 percent of the eggs were "fertilized." Some laboratories report the range of normal to be over 10 percent of eggs fertilized, some report the percent to be over 20 percent of eggs fertilized, and some report the range to be only over 5 percent of eggs fertilized. Other laboratories completely avoid this terminology and "supercharge" the sperm with a solution called "test-yolk buffer." Then, instead of counting the percent of eggs that are actually penetrated, they count the number of sperm that penetrate each egg. Then, if only a small number of sperm penetrate the egg, it is considered a negative hamster test, and if a large number of sperm penetrate the egg, it is considered a positive hamster test.

Even amongst laboratories that enthusiastically support the hamster test as an evaluation for male fertility, the percent of eggs which are fertilized varies tremendously depending upon the amount of time the eggs are allowed to incubate with the sperm and the method of preparation of the sperm prior to incubating with the eggs.

Furthermore, it should be obvious that the most difficult part of fertilization of the wife's egg for men with poor sperm is the penetration of the hard, outer shell. If you remove the most difficult obstacle to fertilization (i.e., the outer shell), then what in truth is being tested in the husband's sperm? What is being demonstrated is simply the well-known phenomenon that a human sperm and a denuded egg from another species can undergo a decondensation process which mimics, but does not represent, the earliest stages of the fertilization process.

Professor Eberhard Nieschlag, from the Max Planck Clinical Research Unit for Reproductive Medicine in Münster, West

Germany, carefully studied the hamster test in fertile and infertile men, comparing that to information obtained with semen analysis to find out whether the hamster test added any information more than what the routine semen analysis could provide. He discovered that although the hamster test did correlate with the degree of male fertility, the sperm count also correlates with the degree of male infertility, and the hamster test did not yield any additional information beyond what the semen analysis provided.

The Australian IVF clinics (which were among the early leaders and major pioneers in in vitro fertilization) have told me they were never allowed to use the hamster test since the animals cannot legally be imported into Australia because of laws protecting the livestock there. They tell me personally and openly that they thank God that hamsters were never allowed into Australia because, if so, then they also would be burdened with this headache of studying it and trying to figure out how they could justify using it in their infertility programs for evaluating the male. The average cost of a hamster test will vary from $400–$700 and the Australians just are not interested in spending that kind of money on a test of questionable value when the cost of a good semen analysis is about $35–$40.

Nonetheless, a very strong argument is made by those few remaining proponents of the hamster test that in vitro fertilization (IVF) and GIFT are such expensive procedures that in a man with questionable fertility it is useful to do whatever can be done to find out whether or not his sperm is capable of fertilization before going into an in vitro fertilization or GIFT cycle. Dr. Louis Rodriguez, along with Dr. Keith Smith and Dr. Emil Steinburger in Houston, did the first study comparing the pregnancy rate with GIFT procedures to the results of hamster tests and semen analyses performed prior to the GIFT procedure. These hamster tests were performed at an institution which does a very well controlled and meticulous job of hamster test assay. They found that the hamster test was a poorer predictor of the success or failure of the GIFT procedure than the standard semen analysis.

A patient of mine had just gotten pregnant in her first cycle of GIFT and had a prior history of eight years of infertility. She had been treated with many laparoscopies, diagnosed as having endometriosis, had hysterosalpingograms showing open tubes, and had many intrauterine inseminations, all to no avail. Finally, she had the ultimate test, the hamster test performed at a nearby university, and was told that only 4 percent of the hamster's eggs were penetrated by her husband's sperm, and that therefore he was sterile. They recommended that she undergo insemination with donor sperm. Yet on simple semen analysis, the husband's sperm count was a spectacular 100 million sperm per cc with 95 percent motility. They got pregnant easily with GIFT and I did not have to do any prior fertilization tests because we knew the quality of sperm from the semen analysis was so good.

I saw another patient, Susan, also infertile for eight years and treated for the last year and a half with intrauterine insemination Clomid and HCG at another clinic, who then went to the university and underwent a hamster test. The results were poor and so they were told their infertility was purely the man's fault and they would never be able to get pregnant without donor sperm. Yet on simple observation under the microscope, his sperm had strong forward linear motion and looked quite normal. The wife became pregnant simply on Pergonal stimulation despite clearly failing the hamster test.

Another case from several years ago demonstrates just how emotional the shaky information that this hamster test provides can become. A thirty-four-year-old couple came to see me having been trying for four years to get pregnant after a prior vasectomy reversal. I wrote in my office notes at the time that "the couple was extremely nervous and very distraught about the whole situation. One can sense the tenseness in the air as soon as you see them in the exam room." The husband had never had a child. He had undergone a vasectomy fourteen years before and a reversal of the procedure four years ago. They came in with a determination that I redo their vasectomy reversal operation because they had been told that his sperm was unable to fertilize because of a negative hamster test. In truth, his sperm counts were ranging between 11 million and 48 million with sperm motility ranging widely from 12 to 72 percent. The quality of the motility was good; the motion was forward and progressive in a straight line at a speed faster than twenty microns per second. When I examined his sperm, the count was 55 million per cc with 80 percent normal, Grade 3 motility and good velocity. My estimate simply from looking at the sperm myself was that this was a fertile specimen.

Nonetheless, the wife had been reported to have negative postcoital tests, had been on Danocrine for endometriosis, and had been on many cycles of intrauterine insemination. She was a busy, hardworking lawyer under great stress who insisted that she was ovulating completely normally and she felt the "overwhelming evidence" was that the problem was with her husband and she insisted that I operate on him to make his sperm better. She then explained that the final reason why she was so certain of this was that the hamster test done by the previous clinic she had gone to was negative and she was discouragingly told by those doctors to consider only insemination with donor sperm.

I tried to give sensitive advice and recommended that they go to a GIFT procedure with her husband's sperm, but she simply got up and stormed out of the office and her husband dutifully followed. Over a year later, I received an apology from them. They said that after a poor hamster egg test, another doctor had recommended donor insemination. The husband said that he would never forget my words as I looked through the microscope at the specimen and said, "I know fertile sperm when I see them, and these are fertile sperm."

So they underwent GIFT with his sperm and despite her extreme pessimism, she got pregnant and delivered a healthy child. Then they conceded, *"Your doubts about the validity of the results on the hamster egg test in my case appear to have been well founded."*

I have no doubt that much of what I say in this chapter and indeed in this book will stir some anger and resentment. Most books written on this subject would be designed in "handbook" format to take no particular stand on any issue, but just give lists of clinics, tests, and things to do. What I am trying to do in this book is distill all of the conflicting information, the garbage and the quality work, and give to you, the reader, not the confusion and the murky chaos of controversies, but rather the essence of what really works and what doesn't work so that you can avoid the pain and agony this last patient had to endure until their story finally ended happily.

Sperm Penetration of Cervical Mucus

One of the oldest tests, other than semen analysis, to try to determine the fertilizing capacity of sperm has been based on its ability to penetrate the wife's cervical mucus. As you already know, just prior to ovulation, the entrance to the woman's uterus, called the cervix, opens up and begins to secrete large volumes of an incredible thick fluid called cervical mucus which lies on the floor of the vagina where the sperm is deposited during intercourse. The sperm then invade this mucus, by virtue of their own motility, and indeed they must do so quickly, otherwise the harsh, acid environment of the vagina will kill them within half an hour or so. Poorly fertile sperm are not capable of invading cervical mucus.

This fact has led to the popularity of the so-called "postcoital test," in which the wife is told to have intercourse with her husband and two hours later she comes to the doctor's office. The doctor is able to aspirate a small sample of that cervical mucus and look under the microscope to see whether or not there are any sperm freely swimming in it. If there are none, it is called a "negative postcoital test." If there are many sperm present, it is called a "positive postcoital test." The significance is that if sperm are able to penetrate and swim freely in the cervical mucus, they have passed the first hurdle in the long, arduous journey toward fertilizing the egg, and the test may, therefore, give some indication of their fertilizing ability.

The problem is that if the postcoital test is highly positive and there are many motile sperm swimming in the cervical mucus after intercourse, everybody is happy. But if there are no sperm or only small numbers of them in the cervical mucus, it isn't known whether the lack of penetration is due to poor sperm, poor-quality cervical mucus, estrogen deficiency related to poor ovulation resulting in an inadequate thinning out of the cervical mucus prior to mid-cycle, or even some sort of autoimmune problem in the wife rejecting the entrance of sperm into her cervical mucus.

There are many difficulties with this test. Despite the obvious functional importance of sperm penetration of the cervical mucus, there is only a very short, precise interval during every month when a woman's cervical mucus is of the proper physical texture to permit sperm invasion. During the rest of the month, her cervical mucus represents a solid barrier to sperm penetration. Thus, if the postcoital test is not done at exactly the right time of the month, it may give a false impression that the husband's sperm is inadequate. Indeed, the usual cause for a poor postcoital test is improper timing of it on the wrong day of the month, rather than any problem with the husband's sperm.

Even if the "postcoital test" were positive, with many sperm swimming around in the mucus two hours after intercourse, a more critical question relating to the potential fertilizability of those sperm is whether they are still swimming around actively twenty-four hours later.

A more meaningful variation of the "postcoital test" is the "sperm survival test," which simply means a postcoital test done a full day rather than two hours following intercourse. In either event, it is hard to know whether the postcoital test is measuring the fertility of the sperm, or the just quality of the wife's mucus.

Despite the theoretical simplicity and attractiveness of this test for sperm function, study after study, dating from 1972 to the present, continue to cast doubt on its value either for determining sperm function or for predicting pregnancy.

In 1973, Dr. Sergio Stone, from the University of California at Irvine, took twenty-five patients with negative postcoital tests, i.e., there were no sperm at all found in the cervical mucus after intercourse, and performed laparoscopies two to three hours after they were inseminated with their husband's sperm. He then aspirated the fluid from the pelvic cavity to see if any sperm had managed to find their way up through the uterus and out of the fallopian tubes into the abdominal cavity, despite not being found in the cervical mucus. He then performed the same test on fifteen patients who had normal postcoital tests, where sperm was found in the cervical mucus. In the patients with *negative* postcoital tests, 56 percent had sperm reach the fallopian tubes and the abdominal cavity; and in those with normal postcoital tests, 53 percent had sperm reach the abdominal cavity. Thus, the postcoital test was no indication of the adequacy of sperm transport from the vagina into the fallopian tube.

In 1986, Dr. John Yovich's group in Perth, Australia, studied postcoital tests in relation to in vitro fertilization to see whether penetration of the cervical mucus could give any indication of the ability of the husband's sperm to fertilize the wife's eggs (oocytes). They found no significant difference in fertilization rate of the wife's oocytes whether the postcoital test was negative, equivocal, or positive, and this finding was the same whether the husband had a normal sperm count or a low sperm count. They concluded that the postcoital test, i.e., sperm penetration of the wife's cervical mucus, was of no value in predicting the outcome of in vitro fertilization or of the ability of the husband's sperm to fertilize the wife's eggs.

There have been various in vitro modifications of this cervical mucus penetration test. One alteration is a commercially available test kit called Penetrak. With this test kit, the physician or laboratory receives little capillary tubes properly filled with cow cervical mucus (which really does have about the same penetrating characteristics and chemical makeup as human cervical mucus) taken from a very fertile cow when she was in heat, or "estrous."

The problem with so many of these analyses on sperm function is that, as an infertile couple, you are likely to be run through at least several thousand dollars' worth of these tests on a kind of automatic "knee-jerk reflex" type basis. When it is all over you have a lot of results, but neither you nor your doctor really has a very good idea what it means about whether or not your eggs can be fertilized by your husband's sperm. Good penetration of the cervical mucus does not guarantee normal fertility potential, nor do negative results necessarily indicate infertility of the husband's sperm.

Sperm Antibodies

One of the most confusing and hotly contested areas of "male infertility" is that of sperm antibodies. This means that in some way the husband has mounted an immune response to his own sperm, or worse yet, that his wife may have a similar immunity to his sperm. This is such a controversial area and involves such a small percentage of patients that if you get tagged with this diagnosis, you're going to be in for a lot of confusion unless you take the time right now to understand what this immune system is all about. Let me explain.

We live in a hostile world surrounded by an infinite swarm of bacteria, viruses, parasites, and microscopic creatures, the most hideous varieties of which would like nothing more than to feast upon us. Our constant protection against the eternal threat of invasion by these infectious organisms is our immune system. Any living thing which our body recognizes as foreign to our own tissue stimulates the production of antibodies which specifically attack that invading organism and kill it. Our white blood cells then move into the area to dispose of the dead carcasses of bacteria and viruses that have tried unsuccessfully to get in. Frequently, bacteria and viruses do get a temporary foothold (e.g., the flu, a cold, pneumonia, or chicken pox), but it usually takes very little time for our immune systems to overwhelm them. Occasionally, we need a little help from antibiotics, but without the help of those remarkable antibodies from our immune system, no antibiotic medication would be of any use. We would be completely overwhelmed by all the bacteria and viruses surrounding us.

The AIDS disease is a perfect example of what happens if our immune system were to be removed. AIDS stands for "Acquired Immune Deficiency Syndrome." It is caused by a very unusual, very strange virus that, unlike virtually any other virus in human history, has learned that if it specifically attacks our antibody-producing cells, despite the effort of our immune system to overcome it, sooner or later we become defenseless and actually die not from the AIDS virus itself, but from any of the other swarms of viruses or bacteria that are just waiting to get in as soon as our immune system is no longer prevailing.

But sometimes the immune system can produce adverse rather than beneficial effects. If a patient has a kidney or a heart transplant, the immune system recognizes that foreign organ as an enemy and attacks it. The transplant patient, therefore, needs drugs to suppress his immune system, and this has to be very carefully monitored or the patient will die, not from the loss of the transplanted kidney or heart, but rather from infections caused by the inhibition of his immune system. Since, in a sense, a fetus, or even sperm, represents a foreign transplant, why shouldn't the female uterus think of invading sperm as enemies and set up a similar immune response? Actually, we could even go a step further and ask why the baby growing within the womb is not thought of as foreign and similarly destroyed by the mother's antibodies.

This is clearly an area of much speculation, and most of the scientific studies in this area have been contradictory. Somehow, however, the body has a remarkable and as yet totally inscrutable mechanism for recognizing that the new baby living within the mother's womb is not to be rejected or attacked by her antibodies. The same remarkable protection appears to be conferred upon the sperm so that indeed they don't stimulate an antibody response with each episode of intercourse. The question brought up by some infertility researchers is whether this immune system can sometimes be activated when it shouldn't, speculating that the infertility in these occasional cases might be due to a rejection of the husband's sperm either by himself (autoimmunity) or by his wife as a foreign invader much like a virus or bacteria. The thought that a wife might be "allergic" or immune to her husband's sperm can be staggering, and so these speculations must be analyzed very cautiously.

Although sperm antibodies are found in a few infertile women, they are also found in women of proven fertility, and the same is true of sperm antibody testing in men. Our methods for detecting these sperm antibodies in the past have been rather crude but are now improving. Still, the mere presence of antibodies to sperm in the patient's bloodstream in no way means that invasion of sperm would be stopped by them.

If sperm antibodies do affect the woman's fertility, it has been thought that this would be expressed in the cervical mucus and it could be detected simply by the failure of sperm to penetrate it. Very often when the cervical mucus sperm penetration is abnormal, the blame is placed on sperm antibodies, suggesting that at the moment of invasion of sperm into the wife's fluid, the antibodies begin to act and immobilize the sperm. In fact, such "hostile" cervical mucus is actually caused in most cases by the test not being performed at the right time of the cycle or by inadequate estrogen stimulation of the wife. Most of the time, giving either Pergonal or an estrogen supplement to the wife at mid-cycle will dramatically improve the quality of the cervical mucus and clear up whether there is truly an antibody problem causing the failure of sperm penetration.

Proceed with caution on this issue of sperm autoimmunity.

Even if sperm autoimmunity does exist and does prevent fertility, is there any treatment for it that makes any sense?

In 1982, I heard from a lady who had read *How to Get Pregnant* and related the story of how she and her husband were diagnosed as having sperm antibodies and were placed on eighteen months of "condom therapy" to "lower the antibody level." This means that she and her husband, who were trying to get pregnant, were told to use condoms for an entire year and a half in an effort to desensitize her to his sperm. She refused to be put on Prednisone because of the risk of side effects, such as pneumonia and other infections, cataracts of the eye, or even aseptic necrosis of the hip, where the hip joint collapses and is destroyed beyond repair. This woman finally stopped going to that clinic, and she became pregnant spontaneously. She wanted to tell me that she had the antibody testing done once more just out of curiosity, and it still showed she was immune to her husband's sperm, but obviously had no difficulty getting pregnant.

Sperm Antibodies After Vasectomy and Vasectomy Reversal

One of the most common causes of sperm antibodies is vasectomy, which causes an increase in microscopic pressure in the tiny tubules (the epididymis) draining sperm from the testicles into the vas, and this increased pressure in the epididymis causes leakage of the sperm with subsequent reabsorption. This leakage of sperm naturally results in the formation of sperm antibodies in from 25 to 50 percent of vasectomized men. It was speculated for many years, beginning in the early 1970s, that this might be a cause of failure of the wife to get pregnant after vasectomy reversal. Yet when we performed sperm antibody testing on the blood of men whose vasectomies were reversed in the late 1970s, we found no difference in pregnancy rate in those men who had high antibody titers (concentrations) versus those men who had no antibodies whatsoever. Therefore, I have been very skeptical about the effect of sperm antibodies on fertility. In fact, the patient who got his wife pregnant the soonest in my experience (less than one month after surgery) had the highest titer I have ever recorded of sperm antibodies.

It is true that in the late 1970s, and early 1980s, sperm antibody testing was only being done on blood, as is usually the case when one is trying to test a person's immunity to a foreign organism. For example, the popular test to determine if one is infected with AIDS is a blood test. If antibodies to the AIDS virus are found in the blood, then one knows that the patient is infected with the AIDS virus. Thus it is reasonable to expect that during the early days of research on the question of sperm autoimmunity, most of the testing to find sperm antibodies was done on the patient's blood.

Now more sophisticated testing is being done on the sperm itself (called "immunobead" testing) to determine whether sperm antibodies have been bound to the sperm prior to their getting ejaculated, thereby interfering with their ability to fertilize the wife's eggs. Ten years ago, I performed a vasectomy reversal on a man in the very early days of this more sophisticated antibody testing. This patient was told after his ejaculate was washed that his sperm were positive for antibodies attached to his sperm and interfering with motility and fertilization. Yet the very next month after he had that test performed, his wife became pregnant.

I recently received a thank you letter from a patient whose sperm count and motility had been good, but the couple was not getting pregnant and his wife was already in her late thirties and getting very worried about waiting any longer. The sperm antibody testing was extraordinarly high. This case was particularly instructive because the husband had had a previous vasectomy reversal which failed. I found epididymal blockage (blowouts caused by leakages in the more delicate duct conveying sperm from the testis into the vas) and did a microsurgical vasoepididymostomy, a much more complex operation than the ordinary vasectomy reversal (this has to be done if there has been pressure-induced anatomic damage to the epididymis). All these years, they thought that his infertility was related to sperm antibodies, when really there was simply a structurally inadequate reconnection of the ductal damage caused by the vasectomy. In fact, the wife became pregnant exactly one month after she was told that it would be impossible to do so because of the antibodies attached to her husband's sperm. What he had needed all along was a proper microsurgical reconnection of the very delicate ducts that were damaged as a result of the pressure buildup caused by the vasectomy.

A twenty-seven-year-old electronics engineer from South Africa had a history of suffering severe scrotal trauma from a land mine injury suffered while he was in the South African military. He required a very complex microsurgical reconstructive operation to correct his blockage, and five months postoperatively I was very happy to hear the report that instead of having zero sperm, he now had 21 million sperm per cc in the ejaculate with 70 percent motility. However, he and his wife were told by the laboratory in South Africa that his sperm antibody test was "positive" and that this would "make it impossible for him to get his wife pregnant." Nonetheless, seven months later, she became pregnant without any other treatment.

One year I heard from a patient whose husband had undergone vasectomy reversal, had a good sperm count, and who wanted a referral to a recognized fertility clinic in their region. I gave her the name of a highly respected gynecologist and I assumed that he would concentrate on dealing with the wife. But the doctor devastated the couple with a tirade about how "nobody" gets pregnant after vasectomy reversal because "sperm antibodies prevent fertilization." This doctor said that she would never become pregnant because of antibodies that had arisen because of his vasectomy, which would prevent a pregnancy from ever occurring. The doctor told her that the length of time between the vasectomy and the reversal operation and the resulting immunologic reaction would certainly prevent pregnancy from occurring. Happily, the couple later got pregnant with a GIFT procedure.

The question is not whether sperm antibodies exist and are measurable. That's not controversial. The question is whether these antibodies are strong enough in view of the close similarity genetically between a man and his own sperm, and in view of the normal ability of any female to allow the invasion of foreign sperm without any immunological prevention of pregnancy.

During the heyday of this fear about sperm antibodies, one of the antibody enthusiasts sent me a thirty-year-old man who had had a vasectomy and ever since then had begun to develop wandering pains in different areas of his body, "burning" eyes, pain in the penis and the joints, and overall fatigue. They thought that he might have developed an autoimmune disease caused by sperm antibodies after vasectomy. The hope was that if I performed a vasectomy reversal on him, preventing further leakage of sperm, perhaps we could lower his sperm antibody production and improve his symptoms. What was apparent was that this was an extremely neurotic man who felt forced into the vasectomy by a wife who did not want to have any more children. He could not live without her approval, but also could not survive with the thought of being sterile because of what it meant to his "manhood." There is no doubt in my mind that this man's symptoms were not part of an autoimmune disease but were rather "hysterical" and required competent psychotherapy.

MORE MODERN "IMMUNOBEAD" TESTING FOR SPERM ANTIBODIES

Nonetheless, despite all of the confusion about sperm antibodies and some of the disastrous counseling that I've referred to from the early 1980s, the late 1980s have produced newer methodology for studying a man's antibody response to his own sperm. These methodologies are simpler, more repeatable, less expensive, and more reliable. Therefore, although *sperm antibodies remain a relatively uncommon cause of infertility* and a source of great controversy, you'll need to understand these newer methods of detecting sperm antibodies because there are certain specific rare situations where the wife's immunity to her husband's sperm, or the husband's immunity to his own sperm, may indeed be a problem to be reckoned with. How do we measure these sperm antibodies and how are the newer methods improving our understanding of this otherwise muddy and confused area of infertility? In fact, why is this intense search for an autoimmune cause of infertility continuing despite a past history in the late 1970s and early 1980s which was quite negative? The field of sperm autoimmunity has been discredited by poorly performed, uncontrolled studies and very imprecise methods of sperm antibody detection current in the 1970s and very early 1980s.

How did we crudely measure sperm antibodies in the past? It's really extraordinarily simple. Blood from infertile men or women was mixed in a measured amount with sperm from known fertile donors, along with another agent such as "guinea pig complement." The number of previously motile sperm that were immobilized by this concoction were then measured, and the concoction was diluted to weaker and weaker concentrations (called titers) until finally the concentration was so weak that the effect of killing the sperm was not observed. The higher the "titer," the greater was assumed to be the amount of antisperm antibody effect. With such crude methods of antibody determination, no one ever saw the antibody, no one ever could characterize what type of antibody it was, and no one could tell what area of the sperm it was directed at, or how in any way it might have affected sperm motility. A similar type of concept was employed in the "agglutination test" except the end point was not immobilization of sperm but sticking together of sperm. Our complete lack of correlation of fertility of men with high, or low, or no antibody titers with pregnancy rate after reversal of vasectomy was based upon these tests, which were the popular state-of-the-art sperm antibody tests in the late 1970s and early 1980s.

Dr. Gordon Baker from the Royal Women's Hospital in Melbourne, Australia, concurrently with Dr. Richard Bronson from the suburbs of New York, began working in the 1980s with a more efficient, scientific method of characterizing sperm autoimmunity called the "Immunobead Test." The Immunobead Test can be performed either on the blood of the husband or the wife (the indirect Immunobead Test), or it can be performed directly on the spermatozoa of the husband. Immunobeads consist of microscopic, spherical beads attached to rabbit antibodies which are directed against any of three specific classes of human antibody. Immunobeads are thus antibodies from other animals that are specifically directed against human antibodies. It's that simple.

These immunobeads can be easily seen under the laboratory microscope if they are attached to sperm. In every type of immunobead test for infertility, the sperm act as target cells. With the direct "Immunobead Test," the husband's sperm is simply mixed with the Immunobead preparation and then viewed under the microscrope. If there is sperm antibody on his sperm, the immunobeads will attach to those antibodies and will show up very easily under the microscope. There is no longer any hocus-pocus guesswork with diluting of serum titers and seeing whether sperm die or agglutinate. With this test, there is visual proof if antibodies are attached to the sperm.

With the "indirect" immunobead test for sperm antibodies, used for detecting sperm antibodies in the blood of the husband or wife rather than directly on the sperm, normal donor sperm is mixed with the patient's blood. If there are antibodies in his blood directed against sperm, they will attach to the normal donor's sperm. Then, once again, the sperm so treated are mixed with the immunobeads, and if there are antibodies present in the blood, immunobeads will attach to the donor's sperm that has been treated with the patient's blood.

The beauty of this test is that it can characterize which of the three types of major antibodies is present and can also pinpoint where on the sperm the antibody attaches. For example, if the antibody covers almost the entire sperm, it is more likely to interfere with fertility than if it is only attached to the tip of the tail. Furthermore, if only 50 percent of the sperm have antibody attached to them, the fertility of the whole sample of sperm is not going to be severely affected. However, if over 80 percent of the sperm have antibody attached to them, then it is very possible that fertility might be affected.

Early speculations about sperm antibodies were greeted with skepticism. Serious investigators had a very difficult time finding any good correlation between elevated sperm antibody titers in the serum of infertile couples or postvasectomized men and the likelihood of the wife's getting pregnant. In fact, as it turns out, *it is only a very small percentage of couples or postvasectomized men in whom sperm antibodies may have any effect at all.* But in these few cases, using the immunobead technology, a better understanding of whether you are one of those few patients with sperm autoimmunity in whom these antibodies are actually in some way impairing your fertility can be understood.

In the cases where sperm antibodies do interfere with fertility, in vitro fertilization (IVF) and GIFT methodologies can certainly overcome the problem. For example, in studies by Dr. Pasquale Patrizio of our department, epididysmal sperm with 100 percent antibody binding had a fertilization rate even higher than cases with no sperm antibodies and an equally good pregnancy rate. *Despite being completely covered with antibodies, sperm had no trouble fertilizing in vitro and causing normal pregnancies.*

CHAPTER 7

WHOSE FAULT IS IT?

If the husband has blockage of the sperm ducts, causing no sperm at all in the ejaculate, this is the obvious cause of infertility. If the wife's tubes are blocked, that is the obvious cause of infertility. In such cases, it is easy to say whether it is the male or the female who is "at fault." But these conditions represent only a minority of the millions of couples in this country who are infertile.

It used to be said that 40 percent of infertility problems are caused by the male, 40 percent by the female, and 20 percent by a combination of problems in both. The cause of male infertility would then be broken down into such factors as varicocele, infection, obstruction, immunologic, and so on. The female would have a similarly detailed range of diagnoses. However, we now know that a clear diagnosis pinpointing the cause of infertility can only be made in a small number of cases.

LOW SPERM COUNT DOES NOT MEAN IT'S THE "HUSBAND'S FAULT"

In the majority of cases, it is really quite impossible to state for sure to what extent the husband or the wife is the cause of the problem. Consider, for example, Mr. S., from Texas, on whom microsurgery had been performed to unblock his sperm ducts. One and a half years after surgery, although he now had sperm in the ejaculate, the number of sperm was extremely low (only 700,000 per cc), and the wife had still not gotten pregnant. The assumption was that, although the microsurgery went beautifully and all the sperm he was making was reaching the ejaculate, nonetheless the amount of sperm production was just too low to realistically expect his wife to have much of a chance of getting pregnant. After several more months of agonizing over the dilemma, they decided to have artificial insemination of donor sperm. The wife was placed on Clomid to time her irregular ovulation so they could drive from their small little town to the medical center on the day before she was expected to ovulate in order to have the insemination. They were very disappointed, however, when the first month this was planned they could not make the trip because of a huge hurricane sweeping the area. They planned to try again the next month but were very frustrated when she did not get her period; they figured she was getting so tense and nervous that it was affecting her menstrual cycle. The fact was that she was pregnant, having conceived by her husband's sperm during natural intercourse during that hurricane that kept them from traveling for insemination with donor sperm that they didn't need after all. Subsequently, this couple has had several more children without any difficulty at all, despite a rather low sperm count. In fact treating the wife with Clomid was all that was necessary for them to have children.

NOT REALLY THE "WIFE'S FAULT"

It works in the other direction, too. A female patient from the same area had been through three different pelvic operations over the course of the last five years, each one of which disastrously resulted in more scar tissue than the previous one. Her fallopian tubes were completely adhesed to the pelvis and an X ray showed virtually complete blockage with only the slightest suggestive trace of a trickle of dye being able to leak through a pinpoint opening at the fimbriated end (see pages 210–11).

This patient was desperate and willing to undergo a fourth operation to try to unblock her tubes. We reviewed her laparoscopy and X rays, and discussed her case in great detail here in St. Louis and with other experts around the country. Finally, we decided that her case was simply inoperable; she could not be helped. This was a clear-cut case of female infertility caused by tubal obstruction and the only hope for her would be in vitro fertilization (IVF). Ultimately, her marriage broke up, she married another man, and then she promptly became pregnant and delivered a normal, healthy child, without any medical assistance whatsoever. This was a case of apparently clear-cut "female infertility" where it now appears in retrospect to have been the "male's fault."

RELATIONSHIP OF SPERM COUNT IN HUSBAND TO FERTILITY OF WIFE

There are so many different diagnoses that can be applied to the female, such as mild adhesions, severe adhesions, cervical mucus factor, endometriosis, luteal, phase defect, poor ovulation, luteinized unruptured follicle syndrome, and tipped uterus, among others, that the easiest way to try to attack the question of whether it is the problem of the man or the woman is simply to go by the semen analysis (and by that I mean the number and quality of sperm in the man's ejaculate). This is the most simple and objective thing to study, to see to what extent sperm is a contributing factor to the infertility. This issue of "male factor" treatment is presently the biggest problem in infertility. When we do feel the male is "at fault," unless the problem is obstruction there is nothing that can be done in 99 percent of cases to improve the man's sperm production. The only hope for low sperm count "male factor" cases is the new in vitro technology, to get those few sperm right next to the egg. Nonetheless all of the studies which I will enumerate in the rest of this chapter demonstrate that in 78 percent of male factor cases, there is also a female contribution to the infertility problem, giving hope that if the wife is treated, the couple can still get pregnant despite very poor sperm production on the part of the male.

So the question of "whose fault is it?" is more easily viewed as the question of "to what extent is the husband's poor sperm count (40 percent of infertile couples) contributing to the couple's inability to get pregnant?" In fact, does the lowered sperm count of 40 percent of these men in infertile marriages have anything to do with the infertility or is it really all the "wife's fault" except in the few cases where the husband has no sperm at all? As you will see from the fascinating studies I am about to unfold, the sperm count of the husband *does* relate to the ability of the wife's getting pregnant, whether or not she too has a problem.

Infertility has to be viewed as a problem of the couple—not as that of only the husband or the wife. This can best be ex- emplified by the difference in pregnancy rates amongst women undergoing insemination with donor sperm whose husbands have very low sperm counts versus those whose husbands have no sperm at all. Among women whose husbands were azospermic (have zero sperm), the pregnancy rate per cycle with donor sperm insemination is not much different from that of a normal, fertile couple. However, in wives whose husbands are oligo- spermic (have low sperm counts), the pregnancy rate per cycle with donor sperm was much lower. The only reasonable spec- ulation for this odd finding is that men who have some sperm in their ejaculate, no matter how low or how poor, might have gotten their wives pregnant if the wife herself didn't also have decreased fertility. However, the wives whose husbands have very low counts might never have gone to a doctor about infertility if they themselves were very fertile because they would have gotten impregnated by their husbands with low counts.

In a related study, it was found that when the husband's count was zero, only 5 percent of the wives had subtle hormonal ab- normalities. When the husband's sperm count was a little greater than zero (up to 5 million per cc), 33 percent of the wives had subtle hormonal abnormalities. When the husband's sperm count was between 5 and 20 million per cc (still in a distinctly low range), 78 percent of the wives had subtle hormonal prob- lems. In an infertile couple, the higher the husband's sperm count, the less likely it is to find a completely "normal" wife. The lower the husband's sperm count, the more likely that low sperm count is the sole cause of the infertility.

THE TRAGEDY OF NOT TREATING THE WIFE BECAUSE THE HUSBAND IS INFERTILE

The overriding message in all of the extensive studies done on male factor infertility is that the biggest tragedy amongst these couples where "male infertility" is involved is that treatment of the couple is delayed, sometimes for years, while the urologist is going through countless unnecessary tests and futile treatment programs to try to raise the husband's sperm count, thinking that in some way it is going to make the wife get pregnant.

To concentrate strictly on trying to improve the man's sperm count is exactly the wrong way to deal with male factor infertility in a couple trying to have a baby.

One couple came to me years ago because of the husband's very low sperm count, and at that time the relationship between low sperm count in the husband and infertility in the wife was not yet established. He had a small varicocele and so I performed a varicocelectomy on him. This resulted in no improvement in sperm count. I treated him with Clomid for many years, then with Pergonal and HCG for many years. Nothing improved his sperm count. He had less than 5 million sperm per cc and only 10 percent motility with most of those sperm showing very poor forward progression and only a few of them looking normal. I feel very badly that I wasted so much time treating the husband fruitlessly, but all of his treatment was part of many studies performed which wound up demonstrating that routine, non-megadoses of hormonal manipulation will not increase the man's sperm count. When the wife was treated with Pergonal to stimulate her ovulation, she got pregnant in the first cycle, and since that time has had two more babies. Their family is complete, and several years ago, he asked me to perform a vasectomy on him.

Years ago I remember seeing a man in his twenties who was the son of a close friend. He and his wife had been trying to get pregnant for a year and they were told by the wife's doctor that the husband's sperm count was "sterile." When I examined him his sperm count was consistently, on three different occasions, only about 5 million per cc and only 20 percent of the sperm showed adequate motility with forward progression, indicating the ability to fertilize. He also had a large varicocele and I recommended a varicocelectomy. Because he had a very busy work season ahead, he decided to put this surgery off for a half year and, fortunately, during that time his wife became pregnant without either of them undergoing any treatment at all. (Because I have a long waiting list, I have had many such patients awaiting varicocelectomy who got their wives pregnant before I had a chance to do the surgery.)

Several years ago, I saw a couple who I thought for sure would require a GIFT procedure. He had terrible-quality sperm but yet had managed to impregnate his first wife and had two children without any problem. In his new marriage, however, his present wife was unable to get pregnant and they were told it was because of his terribly low sperm count. Yet he argued quite convincingly that he had no difficulty getting his first wife pregnant and indeed paternity testing proved beyond a shadow of a doubt that those two children from his first marriage were his.

He had even gone through a bilateral varicocelectomy operation nine months earlier by another doctor, all to no avail. His sperm count was ridiculously low and his wife was not getting pregnant. His first wife was clearly an extremely fertile woman and his second wife was not. Despite all other infertility treatments not working for her, when we put them through our GIFT program, she got pregnant in the first cycle.

One of my patients sent a good friend of hers to me who had been told in no uncertain terms that the husband's "hamster test" was negative and, therefore, his sperm could never fertilize. They went through several cycles of donor insemination and still didn't get pregnant, verifying my suspicion that there was a problem in the wife all along. But before I could institute treatment in the wife, their adoption proceedings came through and they managed to get a beautiful little baby and stopped worrying about trying to conceive. A half a year later, they came into my office to let me know the wife's pregnancy test was positive, without any medical intervention whatsoever, despite a sperm count that was moderately low and a "hamster test" that the "experts" had told her precluded the possibility of her ever getting pregnant.

Finally, I can't tell you how many of my vasectomy reversal patients (who fly in from all over the world for this procedure and to whom I don't have ready access because they come from far and wide) have what appears to me to be an adequate semen analysis after surgery, but whose local doctors tell them they will never get pregnant because of sperm antibodies in the husband caused by the original vasectomy. It takes great effort to convince these local doctors that sperm antibodies are not a problem and that indeed there must be a fertility factor in the wife that needs to be treated in order for her to get pregnant. There is naturally going to be an incidence of infertility in the female population in the age group of thirty to forty that approaches 25 percent. It is easy to hide behind a simple-minded, not scientifically based diagnosis of "male infertility" and completely neglect treatment of the wife.

The cases in my records over the last ten years of patients who have gone through unnecessary and ineffective treatment of the husband while completely disregarding the problem of the wife are too numerous to adequately cover. One patient who came to see me had a sperm count of 14 million per cc with 70 percent excellent quality motility with good forward progression and morphology. However, his wife had never had regular periods and had literally never ovulated. Yet her gynecologist told her it was strictly her husband's problem because his sperm count was "low." So her gynecologist sent her husband to a urologist who was only too happy to perform a varicocelectomy for a "small" varicocele which, in truth, I am certain was not a varicocele at all. At the time they were seeing me for a second opinion they had even been advised to have artificial insemination with donor sperm. Yet she became pregnant quite easily on Clomid without ever having to go through donor sperm insemination, which, as you now know, would probably not have led to a pregnancy for them because the problem was hers (see pages 129–35, 146, and 196–97).

One of the most amazing cases I saw was a man with 90 million sperm per cc and 85 percent excellent quality, progressively forward motility whose wife all her life had periods lasting forty to sixty days on an irregular basis and clearly had never ovulated in her life. Yet the local urologist started the husband on testosterone, telling him that the hormone would improve his fertility. Of course, the testosterone might make his muscles get bigger (the reason many athletes illegally use it), but it certainly lowered his sperm count drastically, rather than raise it. Going off this ridiculous steroid treatment brought his sperm count back up to normal.

Twenty years ago the male contribution to the infertility of the couple was never seriously considered. In my previous book, I gave the humorous account of a rather enormous, macho football player who came in to see me with his meek, accepting wife. He looked like he was going to tear me apart when I told him that his low sperm count could be contributing to their infertility. He leaned forward with a stare of anger and disbelief saying, "What do you mean, my sperm ain't okay?" After I assured him that I felt that he was not the only one to blame and that it was a problem of the couple, he calmed down a little bit, but proceeded to blame his wife for feeding him too much fish and vegetables and not enough meat and that he was sure that was the explanation for his sperm count problem, which must assuredly be her fault rather than his.

That episode occurred at a time when no one really wanted to take a serious look at the male causes of infertility and always assumed, in the sexist society we lived in then, that it was the female's fault. As you may recall, Anne Boleyn, the mother of Queen Elizabeth of the Sixteenth Century, had her head chopped off by the king, her husband, because she kept giving birth to only girls. He never even began to consider that the problem was simply that his Y sperm (which would have led to conception of a boy) never fertilized her eggs, but only his X sperm did. It was truly his sperm that were misbehaving rather than her eggs.

But now the problem has been reversed from one of paying no attention to the male to one of concentrating so much on the male factor that the woman's contribution to the infertility problem of the couple is often erroneously disregarded. For example, one couple's story was that he had a relatively low sperm count of 9 million per cc but with 60 percent excellent quality motility and excellent structure (morphology), indicating that I felt he had good enough sperm to fertilize her eggs. However, she had had prolonged periods coming at sixty-to-seventy-day intervals and had never had any indication that she ovulated. She also had acne problems all her life, with excess facial and body hair, as well as extremely oily skin consistent with high male hormone levels related to her poor ovulation. I had explained to her that although the husband's count was not as high as one might like, I felt that treating her problems would most likely lead to a pregnancy. Apparently, she held inside her a deep fury about this because she could not accept the possibility that their infertility as a couple might in some way be related to her rather than to her husband. I told her if there were anything we could do to raise her husband's sperm count, I would most assuredly do it and I was not trying to "get her husband off the hook." But she could not accept that and indeed eventually went on to try insemination with donor sperm at a different center and continued not to get pregnant.

Thus, when the husband has a poor sperm count, it does not automatically mean that that is the sole cause of the couple's infertility.

CHAPTER 8

LOW-TECH SOLUTIONS

HOW LONG DOES IT TAKE TO GET PREGNANT, OR WHEN DO WE KNOW TO LOOK FOR HELP?

Couples who have had infertility for many years know they have a problem and need medical help. But what about the couple that has been trying to get pregnant unsuccessfully for six months? When should they begin to worry? Even for those who are not infertile, pregnancy does not usually occur in the first month of trying. When my wife and I decided to start our family, it took a full six months before she finally conceived. We know people who were not able to achieve pregnancy for several years, never bothered to consult a doctor, and eventually had their children. So when should you begin to worry that you might not be able to have children? Is there a particular time beyond which you should fear that you may be infertile and seek medical attention? All potential parents-to-be will need a little lesson in statistics from this section to understand the similarity between becoming pregnant and rolling dice. That's the only way you will know when to start worrying.

Getting pregnant is basically a game of odds. Some couples are simply likely to get pregnant sooner than others. If infertile couples had three hundred years in which to breed, it seems almost certain that eventually without any treatment most wives would become pregnant. But the usual breeding period for families is no more than fifteen years, and so the odds need to be considerably improved. When a couple has waited as long as six months to a year without achieving pregnancy they will probably begin to fear they are infertile, and are likely to become frantic. Yet many of these couples may not be infertile at all, but merely victims of statistical chance, having no less likelihood of pregnancy occurring with each given month than the couple that was fortunate enough to get pregnant at their first attempt.

Probability of Conception Per Month in Fertile Couples

What is the probability in any given month of a normal, fertile couple's achieving a pregnancy? Years ago I posed this question to several authorities on population. At that time most of them considered it a very difficult question to answer with accuracy. Yet it is critically important to understand the natural incidence of pregnancy month by month in a fertile population, so that the couple having difficulty with conception can understand whether or not they really have a problem.

A century ago we knew from studies in England that young women get pregnant sooner and more easily than older women. The incidence of infertility in women twenty-five years of age was 7 percent, and the incidence of infertility in women thirty years of age was approximately 13 percent. At thirty-five years of age, 20 percent of women were unable to have children. By age forty, 32 percent of women were unable to get pregnant. Modern statistical data is remarkably similar.

About 40 to 50 percent of women achieve pregnancy within the first four months of trying. Are the women who are not yet pregnant after four months of trying any less fertile, or any less likely to achieve pregnancy in subsequent months, than those who have already been lucky enough to conceive? After two years, about 9 percent of women still have not yet conceived. Are the 9 percent of women who have not conceived after two years a hard-core group with severe infertility problems, or do they just represent a statistical inevitability which may be erased with the next monthly cycle? How many couples who have not yet gotten pregnant are really worrying for nothing? In how many "infertile" couples would just waiting and doing nothing result in a pregnancy without the expense and trouble of medical treatment? On the other hand, when is complacency likely to be tragic in overlooking a problem that won't resolve itself without treatment?

Think of fertility in these terms: If a man were to flip a coin three times in a row, and it lands on tails each time, he might think that his particular coin is more likely to land on tails again the next time. Of course this is not true. Each time the coin is flipped there is a fifty-fifty chance of its landing either heads or tails, regardless of the past history. To really understand the likelihood of conception with each passing month (and when a couple perhaps should start worrying), do not be concerned too early by unsuccessful flips.

Modern studies have shown that with the most fertile population of patients (those who eventually went on to raise large families) there was only about a 20 percent chance in any given month of the wife's becoming pregnant. If she was not pregnant after six months, the chance that she would become pregnant in the seventh month was still 20 percent. Studies of artificial insemination from Dr. Robert Schoysman in Belgium in the 1970s have shown that with each succeeding month the chance for pregnancy is no less in *normal* women who have not yet conceived than in those who were lucky enough to become pregnant in the very first month. This should be of some comfort to those couples whose fertility tests have been normal, but simply have not yet achieved pregnancy. But there must be some point beyond which the couples who remain not pregnant are a "selected" group who are less fertile than those who got pregnant earlier and who therefore don't have a 20 percent chance each month, but a much lower chance, perhaps 5 percent or 1 percent, and who therefore need help.

After What Period of Time Does Not Getting Pregnant Mean We're Infertile?

The studies in Belgium involved absolutely *"normal" young* (under age thirty) women whose husbands were clearly the problem because of *zero* sperm in the ejaculate. The series began with 632 such fertile young women. Very fertile donor sperm was used to inseminate each female just prior to ovulation each month until she became pregnant. In the first month, 130 of the 632 women became pregnant (20.57 percent). In the second cycle, 103 more women became pregnant (16.29 percent). In the third monthly cycle, 81 more women became pregnant (12.81 percent). Thus a total of 49.67 percent of the 632 women starting in this series achieved pregnancy within the first three months. In the fourth month, 54 more women became pregnant (8.54 percent). In the fifth month, 40 women became pregnant (6.32 percent). By six months, a total of 73 percent of the patients had become pregnant. It is at this point that the other 27 percent of the women might have been tempted to give up.

However, if we figure the percentage of pregnancies for each month only among the women who were still trying to conceive that month, there is a strikingly constant probability (20 percent) of pregnancy each month. Of the 632 patients undergoing insemination in the first month, 130 became pregnant, 20.57 percent of those inseminated. Of the 502 remaining women inseminated in the second month, 103 became pregnant, or 20.47 percent. This left 399 women who underwent insemination in the third month. Eighty-one of them became pregnant, or 20.3 percent. However, this represented only 12.8 percent of the original 632 women. In the tenth month, only 3 percent of the total women starting this program became pregnant, but the pregnancy rate among the women who were actually inseminated was still 20.21 percent. By that time there were only 94 women out of the original 632 who had not yet achieved pregnancy. Yet in that month 19 women, or 20.21 percent, conceived. In the eighteenth month after the beginning of this study, 5 women (less than 1 percent of those originally entering the study) became pregnant. However, by that time only 23 women were remaining who had not yet achieved pregnancy, and the 5 who became pregnant that month represented 21.75 percent of those remaining.

Thus it would appear that even though the majority of fertile women became pregnant within the first six months of trying, and only a tiny minority required as long as eighteen months or two years to become pregnant, nonetheless we can see that with each succeeding month, each normal young woman still had a 20 percent chance of becoming pregnant. When women who required many months to conceive by donor insemination came back to have their second child, many became pregnant within just a few months. In addition, some women who had achieved pregnancy very early with their first child required a much longer time to become pregnant with the second child, despite no obvious change in their fertility. If the conception rate in a large group of normal young women trying to achieve pregnancy in a given month is 20 percent, it is a mathematical certainty that a small number of them will not obtain their goal until several years have passed.

The problem with drawing broad conclusions from this study is that these were *young* women who should have an extremely low risk of infertility (1 to 4 percent), and the donor sperm was extremely fertile. What about women in their late twenties or thirties with their husband's sperm (of unproven fertility)? If they have not achieved pregnancy after a year, what is their chance of ever getting pregnant in subsequent months without any help?

Dr. Gordon Baker from Melbourne, Australia, studied "life-table" analyses of pregnancy with couples undergoing artificial insemination with donor sperm (AID) and found a curve quite different from that of couples who had been infertile for several years and trying to get pregnant. Patients undergoing donor insemination just kept getting pregnant with the same frequency each month and showed a higher pregnancy rate per month than "infertile" couples with normal sperm counts. Thus, although young couples with normal sperm may have reason to keep on expecting a 20 percent chance of pregnancy for up to several years, eventually what is left are those patients who have a very low expectation of pregnancy with future attempts. In older patients in their thirties, this hard-core group of truly infertile couples with a lower chance of pregnancy per month (1 to 5 percent) might be revealed after only a year of trying unsuccessful attempts at getting pregnant.

Dr. Charles Westoff of Princeton University, using a similar mathematical approach, has worked out the probability of conception with each month for "fertile" couples of various ages.

TABLE 3

LIKELIHOOD OF PREGNANCY IN FERTILE WOMEN— HOW LONG SHOULD IT TAKE?

Age	Probability of Conception per Month (percent)	Average Time to Conception (months)	Probability of Conception Within a Year (percent)
Late thirties	8.3	12	65
Early thirties	10	10	72
Late twenties	15	6.7	86
	20	5	93
Early twenties	25	4	97

For women in their early twenties—and presumed to be highly fertile—the monthly probability of conception is thought to be between 20 and 25 percent, in the absence of contraception.

For somewhat less fertile women, in their late twenties and early thirties, the monthly probability of conception is lower: between 10 and 15 percent. Around 72 to 86 percent conceive within a year.

Once the monthly probability of conception is figured out, the doctor can compute the chances of a fertile couple's achieving pregnancy within six months, one year, or two years. For young women in their early twenties, the monthly probability of conception is generally between 20 percent to 25 percent. By four months about 50 percent of women in this age group will have achieved pregnancy (assuming a 20 percent chance with each month); about 94 percent will be pregnant within the first year. For women in their late twenties and early thirties, however, the probability of conception is somewhat lower, in the range of 10 to 15 percent each month. In such a group only about 70 to 85 percent will achieve pregnancy within the first year. However, those who have not become pregnant within the first year might still have the same 10 to 15 percent chance of becoming pregnant in each succeeding month. They should not give up simply because they did not become pregnant in the first year.

However, as women get older (in their thirties), the monthly chance of conception is much lower, and for them numbers like 8 percent per cycle are *very theoretical*. In this older age group, a failure to get pregnant after a year is likely to mean their monthly chance of natural conception is so low (not 8 percent but perhaps 1 percent or less) that waiting any longer without treatment would be foolish.

This discussion of pregnancy rates in "normal" fertile women demonstrates that fertility is not an absolute, easily definable quality. Even in a group of young women with uniformly normal fertility, many will have a long wait before they achieve their pregnancy. It is a simple mathematical inevitability.

So when should the couple begin to worry and when should they seek medical attention? It is difficult to know whether a particular couple's conception probability per month is 20 percent, 15 percent, 10 percent, or 1 percent. The older the couple, the greater is the likelihood that a year of infertility means a much lower chance of future conception.

There is one ironic statistic which has to be a bit sobering to any fertility specialist. In a large population of young fertile couples, about 60 percent will have achieved pregnancy by six months and 80 percent by twelve months. Only 90 percent of such fertile couples will have achieved pregnancy by one and a half years. This means that in the six-month period following the first year of no pregnancy, only 10 percent more women will conceive. But remember that this group represents a full 50 percent of the 20 percent of couples who did not achieve pregnancy in the first year. Thus half of those young couples who had not achieved pregnancy by one year will have succeeded by a year and a half, without any medical intervention whatsoever. The physician who does nothing more than evaluate such couples and provides no treatment will theoretically achieve a 50 percent pregnancy rate in the following six months. Thus, for young couples in their twenties with no obvious problem like tubal obstruction or azospermia (no sperm), several years of not getting pregnant might be needed before concluding that treatment is necessary. Their problem may simply be a mathematical one requiring nothing more than optimism and patience. For couples in their thirties, however, it is not so clear, and not getting pregnant in a year might very well indicate a low chance of future pregnancy if help is not sought.

Pregnancy Rates with Untreated Infertility: Common When Patient Is Young and Duration of Infertility Is Less Than Two Years

In 1983, Dr. John Collins of Dalhousie University in Nova Scotia analyzed the pregnancy rates over four years of 597 couples who were "treated" for their infertility and 548 couples who were *not* "treated." He was trying to determine what percent of "infertile" couples got pregnant with no treatment at all (where "treatment" meant strictly conventional, old-fashioned approaches like surgery for adhesions or endometriosis, and drugs like Danocrine and Clomid). The pregnancy rate in the treated group (41 percent) was not much greater than that of the group that received no treatment (35 percent). (It would be wrong to conclude that treatment did not work because clearly the patients who received treatment had the severest problems. Also, infertility was defined as only *one* year or more of trying previously to get pregnant. So don't *over*interpret the meaning of his study.) What his study *did* underscore was the large number of younger couples (35 percent) who thought they were infertile on the basis of only one year of not getting pregnant, but who obviously were not infertile and got pregnant with no treatment at all.

I saw a couple with a very poor sperm count who had been trying for a full year to get pregnant with no success. The wife then was placed on Clomid by another physician and underwent intrauterine inseminations (to be discussed in the next chapter) on a monthly basis for six months. She never got pregnant with this treatment and no sperm were seen in the "postcoital" exam. Because of his extremely low sperm count the husband had even undergone a bilateral varicocelectomy by another physician nine months earlier. Yet he had had two children in a previous marriage despite poor sperm. Because of the relatively short duration of infertility, and because the wife had already been through almost a year of conventional treatment with no success, and because his sperm count was so extremely low, they had been put on a waiting list to undergo in vitro fertilization. But when the time came for her procedure, she was already twelve weeks pregnant despite receiving no treatment.

A year later I examined a woman with severe adhesions and complete blockage at the end of her fallopian tubes from previous inflammatory disease. She had undergone surgery for this a year and a half earlier, and postoperatively X rays showed the recurrence of scarring but with a very slight pinhole opening at the end of one of the tubes. Because the tubes were so severely damaged-appearing, it was suggested that she undergo in vitro fertilization; while she was on the waiting list at the beginning of March she too became pregnant. She delivered a healthy baby and quite clearly was not really infertile despite the poor appearance of her fallopian tubes on X ray.

Another couple who had been trying to get pregnant for only two years were very busy at both their careers, tied up intricately in the financial world with a very hectic schedule, and were anxious to hurry up and get this infertility problem taken care of. Although she was not yet thirty, the fact that she had been on fourteen months of fairly intensive conventional therapy, including Clomid, with good evidence prior to going on it of having a complete lack of ovulation, estrogen, and progesterone, it was decided to try to schedule a Pergonal regimen sometime in the future, whenever they could work it into their timetable. The very next month she called to explain that they would not have to find time for a Pergonal regimen; she had missed her period and was pregnant.

Getting Pregnant Without Treatment
Despite Many Years of Prior Infertility

I recently saw a thirty-five-year-old woman who had been trying for five years to get pregnant, whose husband's sperm count was completely normal, and who had gotten pregnant quite easily when she was twenty years old. But she had that pregnancy terminated. Now, fifteen years later, she desperately wanted a child. At this point in her life she had gone through two years of testing, ovulation timing, and intrauterine inseminations at a fertility clinic with no success. Although she was somewhat overweight, her tests were normal. Nonetheless, it was decided to put her on the list for having a GIFT procedure. However, by the time I saw her, she was already several days late on her period, and sure enough, she turned out to be pregnant.

Another example of a patient with infertility of very long duration who got pregnant without treatment was a very intense woman in her thirties who was erroneously told that she had not gotten pregnant because her husband's hamster test was negative, indicating that his sperm were not able to fertilize. Nonetheless, after twelve cycles of artificial donor sperm insemination she still did not get pregnant, and I had to assume a very strong likelihood that there was a subtle problem with her. Nonetheless, all of her tests came out normal. She decided to discontinue donor insemination. They adopted a child, and several months later, without treatment, she became pregnant. For whatever reason, many couples speak of a tremendous relief of tension associated with the decision to just "quit," and they may ascribe their subsequent pregnancy after years of infertility to some undefined psychological benefit derived from "taking the pressure off."

The issue of whether stress and emotions can cause infertility is in itself a highly emotionally charged, controversial problem which will inflame many infertile couples. Doctors have certainly been fooled into thinking that varicoceles and minimal lesion endometriosis can cause infertility, although now we certainly know they do not. It would be just as easy therefore for cases like those just described to convince us perhaps erroneously that emotions and stress cause infertility and that the relief of that stress will result in the likelihood of a spontaneous pregnancy.

However, up until now, there have been no controlled scientific studies to determine whether in some way stress and emotions could be causal factors of infertility.

A large percentage of patients, particularly younger ones who have not been infertile for more than a year or two, will get pregnant spontaneously without any treatment and may not have really been infertile in the first place. In fact, often the second baby comes without a long waiting period, indicating that it was just a statistical odds game as to when this couple's chance for the sperm meeting the egg and implanting would occur. It is even more humbling as a physician to recall the less common cases when infertility has been of relatively long duration and yet pregnancy still occurs before we have a chance to work any of our medical wonders. It may be related to emotions or it may simply just be related to the fact that infertility is rarely an absolute condition and every couple has a certain percentage chance per month with active intercourse of getting pregnant. For some couples that chance per month is just a lot lower than for others.

PROPER TIMING OF INTERCOURSE

Some people who complain of infertility have a simple problem of infrequency of sex at the appropriate time in the cycle. Simply improving the timing and techniques of intercourse may be sufficient to allow pregnancy, without medical intervention and therapy. Animals, of course, always know just when to time their intercourse, because their periodic rise in estrogen, just prior to ovulation, is what induces their desire to have intercourse. They have sex only during this obvious period when ovulation is imminent and pregnancy is most likely to occur. Humans are interested in sex at almost any time of the month, and we cannot be assured of the proper timing that benefits all the other animals in the world except humans.

Position and Method of Intercourse

A thirty-six-year-old man was referred to me a long time ago for a low sperm count. He and his wife, who was the same age, had been trying without success for five years to have a baby. She had had very careful gynecological evaluations, which showed regular ovulation, no blockage in her tubes, and no endometriosis. The blame for their infertility was placed on her husband's low sperm count. Their sex life was active, vigorous, and frequent enough to have easily allowed impregnation during the fertile time of her cycles. The only unusual aspect of their intercourse was that she was in the habit of getting up within a minute of ejaculation and going to the bathroom. There was thus considerable leakage of his semen out of her vagina. They had not stopped to think that this might be a problem. If his sperm count were higher, this habit of theirs would probably not have made any difference. I asked her to lie down for a full half hour after ejaculation and only then get up to go to the bathroom. Two months later she called, full of excitement, to tell me that after years of trying to conceive, and going through several thousand dollars' worth of testing, she was finally pregnant.

There are all kinds of positions in which couples may prefer to copulate, and these preferences may vary from month to month. In fact, modern sex books and magazine articles boast of all the different types of positions and contortions that the sexually active couple can utilize to increase their gratification. For the average couple all of these different positions will not have any effect on fertility, but a couple with a marginal sperm count just cannot afford to lose any sperm by leakage out of the vagina. The position of intercourse that allows the greatest contact of the semen with the cervical mucus is the simple traditional approach with the woman on the bottom and the man on the top. A woman will need to stay in this position for thirty minutes after ejaculation, because any sperm that have not gained access to the cervical mucus within a half hour will not be able to do so later.

When to Have Intercourse

More important than the position of intercourse is the frequency
and timing of intercourse. Many couples are so anxious about
having intercourse at exactly the right time that they may abstain
for a whole week or more prior to the evening when the wife
thinks she should be ovulating. The doctor is usually the culprit
in this over-rigorous scheduling of sex, and the wife may feel
that they must abstain until the gynecologist gives her the go-
ahead. This kind of overattention to regulating the precise night
during which intercourse will be allowed can create so much
anxiety that often ovulation itself may be delayed by the emotional distress and its effect on the primitive region of the brain
which regulates ovulation.

A long time ago, a man, somewhat frantic, came to my office
and begged that I see him as a patient. He simply couldn't take
the strain anymore, and was hoping there was something I could
do to help. He and his wife had been trying to have children
for a year. Six months earlier she had consulted with her gynecologist, who had her do basal body temperatures, which was
fine. Then he told her to abstain from intercourse for five days
before her temperature went up, and only then, *after her temperature went up*, to have sex. Of course, as explained in Chapter
4, this is the method you use to *avoid* getting pregnant. Worse
yet, when she was given this directive her cycles became totally
unpredictable, lasting twenty days one month and forty-five days
another. Her basal body temperature charts were difficult to
interpret, but the couple tried to read into each little temperature elevation the possibility that she was about to ovulate.
They did not realize that what the chart was showing was that
she had stopped ovulating altogether. Sometimes, because her
periods were becoming so irregular, instead of abstaining for
five days, they would abstain for as long as a week and a half.
She had no idea what was happening, but was still trying in
some way to pinpoint ovulation. Her original overanxiety about
not conceiving during the first six months coupled with the
rigidity of their sex life during the next six months (not to mention
its infrequency) was about to lead to a divorce.

I saw both of them together, and explained that they should
in no way gear their sex schedule to a chart. I advised them

simply to have sex whenever they wanted. With her history of irregular periods, I assumed there was likely to be some ovulatory disturbance. Much to my surprise, her first month's temperature chart after I saw her showed a prompt ovulatory rise on day thirteen. That month, her cycle was twenty-seven days, the first normal cycle she appeared to have had since discontinuing birth control pills one year earlier. The very next month, she was afraid her periods were getting irregular again, because she did not start to menstruate at twenty-eight days. In truth she was pregnant.

With other couples, the problem is that they really do not have an active enough sex life. In fertile couples who have intercourse less than once a week, only 16 percent conceive within the first six months of trying. In fertile couples who have intercourse once a week, 32 percent conceive within the first six months. In fertile couples who have intercourse twice a week, 46 percent conceive within the first six months, and in those who have intercourse three times per week, 51 percent conceive within six months. And while the recommendation of having intercourse whenever one likes is sometimes modified for certain patients with low sperm counts, in general the more sex the better.

I have seen quite a few patients who were able to have sex only on the weekend because of heavy work schedules during the week, often involving traveling. The penalty of success in a career is sometimes a schedule so busy that intercourse, in an otherwise workable marriage, is either sporadic, or at best once a week. It takes no particular medical education to calculate that in these patients the chance of having sex at the fertile preovulatory day is one-third that of couples who have sex every other day. Furthermore, if the woman's cycle has a duration of twenty-eight days, then she is likely to be ovulating on the same particular day of the week in any given month. Thus, she may be unfortunate enough to be regularly ovulating on a Wednesday, once every four weeks, when her husband is always out of town. Of course, many couples who have sex only on the weekends have no problem impregnating, because the wife's ovulation may be occurring at that time.

Sometimes the problem with infrequent intercourse is not just a business schedule which keeps the partners apart at the appropriate time of the month, but rather a lack of interest in having intercourse more frequently. An example is a couple who had been trying unsuccessfully for several years to have children. When they told me they were having intercourse only once every two weeks, I explained to them that this was considerably less than average, and they were a bit surprised. The husband was a very hardworking fellow who usually got home too tired to think about anything but a little quiet conversation and going to sleep. Their frequency of intercourse then did increase, and she became pregnant. Thus, although a rigid schedule for intercourse is unrealistic and anxiety-provoking, at least the frequency and approximate timing of intercourse may need to be guided somewhat by an understanding of when the sexual act is more or less likely to lead to pregnancy.

Basal Body Temperature Charts

The time-honored method of determining when the woman ovulates used to be the basal body temperature charts discussed in an earlier chapter. This is such a cumbersome bother that it is no longer recommended for couples who have enough on their minds already. Nonetheless it is fascinating to realize that if a woman were to take her temperature the first thing in the morning before the slightest activity and chart it, by virtue of a 0.5 to 1.0 degree Fahrenheit rise in temperature that occurs somewhere in the cycle, she can tell that that is when she is beginning to make progesterone, indicating that ovulation occurred about a day earlier. For years this was one of the cheapest and most reliable methods for evaluating a woman's ovulatory cycle.

But the problem was that physicians often mistakenly told the wives that they should wait until their temperature goes up and then have sex. By waiting until your temperature goes up, you are actually performing rhythm birth control, because by the time the progesterone level is elevated, the cervical mucus has become sticky, the cervix is closed, you have already ovulated about twenty-four hours ago, and the egg is no longer able to be fertilized. Thus the basal body temperature chart is a cheap although cumbersome way of documenting when you ovulate in the cycle, but it cannot predict for you ahead of time when you are going to ovulate and therefore it cannot ever be used as a basis for "timing" intercourse.

LH Dipstick Test

There are two methods for timing intercourse that work extremely effectively, one inexpensive that can be done at home and one very expensive that is carried out in the doctor's office or in the hospital. The cheap, at-home method is the "LH Dipstick" test on urine, and the expensive method is to go to the doctor's office or the hospital and have a vaginal ultrasound performed daily until ovulation. With the "LH Dipstick" test, simply go to the local drugstore and purchase any one of several brands such as Ovustick or First Response. Every year the test becomes more and more simple, and it will require less than four or five minutes in the morning. Instructions are clearly and easily printed with every kit, and there is also an 800 number to call for any questions. The drug companies marketing these products provide excellent information and help for any questions that you might have.

To use the LH Dipstick test for determining ovulation, begin around day eight or nine of the cycle and collect a small portion of your first-morning urine. Using the directions that the particular test kit gives you, test the urine for the presence of the hormone LH. About twenty-four hours prior to ovulation there will be a high concentration of LH.

Although the test itself is extremely simple and relatively cheap, it utilizes a complex new biotechnology called "monoclonal antibodies" to detect the presence of LH in your urine. But all you have to do is watch for a simple color change on the dipstick or in the liquid being tested. This color change does not tell you how much LH is in your urine; it will only react when there is a *large amount of LH*, indicating an LH surge. If this test is done every day, beginning day eight or nine of your cycle, assuming you do ovulate, eventually the test will turn positive and ovulation can be expected to occur twenty-four hours later.

The time to have intercourse is not *after* ovulation, but preferably within the twenty-four-hour period *prior* to ovulation so that the sperm will be ready and waiting in the cervical mucus and in the fallopian tube when the egg is released. The advantage of the LH test over the basal body temperature test is that a woman can know ahead of time when she is going to ovulate and can therefore time intercourse properly to make conception most likely to occur. If you wait until after you ovulate, then all that you are really doing ironically is minimizing your chances of getting pregnant.

Daily Transvaginal Ultrasound

The other, more expensive way of determining when you ovulate for timing of intercourse (or for that matter for artificial insemination) is daily ultrasound exams. In years past doctors had no direct visual way of knowing for sure that a woman ovulated. Our methods were all indirect and only inferred ovulation. Now, with ultrasound we can actually watch the follicle grow until it reaches mature size of 2 cm or more (four-fifths of an inch or greater), and then we can watch it disappear, indicating that ovulation has taken place. If you are undergoing intrauterine insemination with washed sperm, you would want to have the sperm placed in the uterus right after ovulation after the follicle disappears (because the sperm would go up into the fallopian tube immediately). On the other hand, if you are simply trying to time intercourse accurately, you would just need ultrasound to tell you that your follicle is getting big enough that it might ovulate in the next day or so. In that event, you begin to have sex when the follicle is big and mature looking, and then you can stop having sex (if you so desire) once you have proof on ultrasound that ovulation has finally occurred.

I merely mention these methods of "timing" intercourse for those special couples who have travel obligations, in whom frequent intercourse is impossible, or for whom the husband's sperm count is so low that it would conceivably lead to sperm depletion. For the vast majority of patients, it is much smarter to pay no particular attention to the time of ovulation other than to try to diagnose its quality. Happy, relaxed couples whose lives are not terribly overcluttered tend to have sex naturally somewhere from two to three or more times per week spontaneously and joyously. If you have sex at that frequency, and if your ovulation is normal and your cervical mucus is normal, then there is likely always to be some sperm available in the fallopian tube for fertilization. After intercourse sperm are probably able to fertilize the egg for two or three days. If you are having sex three times a week, that means that the odds are very good that whenever you happen to ovulate, there is likely to be some sperm present.

CLOMID (CLOMIPHENE CITRATE)

For ovulation to occur, it is not sufficient merely for the pituitary gland to produce its stimulatory hormones FSH and LH. It must produce these hormones in a specifically synchronized, properly timed fashion. The first requirement for proper ovulation is an adequate amount of FSH stimulation in the very beginning of the menstrual cycle. If there is an inadequate production of FSH by the pituitary gland on the first day of menstruation, the early follicle may not get an adequate growth start, and this sets the stage early in the cycle for poor ovulation. The object of administering the drug Clomid is to increase the pituitary's production of FSH so that the follicle gets a good boost in the early stage of the cycle.

History of Clomid

If the follicle gets this necessary boost by an early increase in FSH, it will develop properly and release enough estrogen around mid-cycle to trigger the pituitary gland on day fourteen to release LH, which causes the follicle to rupture and ovulate. A high level of FSH production by the pituitary gland, stimulating the follicle to grow in the early portion of the menstrual cycle, is the key to successful ovulation. The purpose of taking Clomid is to ensure that a high FSH level does occur in the early portion of the cycle.

Clomid has traditionally been given on days five through nine in the cycle only. Nowadays some doctors prefer days three through seven, and still others give it for longer (i.e., days three through ten). It is just needed for these critical five to eight days after the menstrual bleeding has stopped, when maximum FSH stimulation is necessary. After that, Clomid is no longer needed. It has already done its job and has set the stage for the proper subsequent hormonal clockwork to take place.

Ironically, Clomid (a synthetic estrogen with very little estrogen effect) was originally introduced as a potential oral contraceptive (that's right, a birth control pill). Many decades ago researchers had hoped that this estrogenlike drug with no estrogen effect would suppress the pituitary's production of FSH and LH, just as modern birth control pills do. In fact, in some animals that is exactly what Clomid does. Clomid, one of the most widely used fertility drugs in the world, was originally designed to produce *infertility*. Many great biological discoveries are sheer accidents, and the discovery of the fertility-enhancing property of this remarkable drug, which has brought so much happiness to couples who would otherwise not have had children, was an accident. Rather than prevent ovulation as was originally intended, the pill has the opposite effect in humans —it stimulates ovulation.

The way this happens is quite fascinating and still not completely understood. The estrogenlike activity of Clomid does not suppress the pituitary the way estrogen itself normally would in the early half of the cycle. Rather, it blocks the pituitary's recognition of your body's own naturally circulating estrogen. It thus gives the pituitary the false message that your ovary is not making estrogen, and this causes the pituitary to increase its FSH production dramatically.

How and When to Take Clomid

The physician will usually start with a relatively low dose of one pill per day (50 mg) from day five to day nine of your cycle. If this does not cause you to ovulate properly, he may increase the dosage to two pills per day (100 mg), or possibly even to as high as four pills per day (200 mg). Women respond differently to Clomid and this is why your doctor will usually start with a low dose, since starting with very high doses might overstimulate the ovaries. If a low dose is effective, he will stick with it. If that dose is not effective, then he will increase it. However, Clomid is generally a very safe drug and the risk of overstimulation of the ovaries is not great at all. Usually, Clomid causes the follicle to develop so well that it makes enough estrogen around the mid-cycle to stimulate the body's own LH release with subsequent ovulation. However, sometimes if the LH surge is not adequate a shot of HCG (similar to LH) is given on day fourteen to help.

A major problem with Clomid is that it not only prevents the pituitary from recognizing the body's own estrogen, but it also prevents the cervix and endometrial lining from recognizing estrogen. Clomid is an "anti-estrogen," and therefore it blocks the effect of estrogen on the cervix and frequently makes the cervical mucus too sticky to allow sperm penetration. The attempted solution to this problem has been to give a small daily dose of estrogen on days ten through fourteen of the cycle (simply in the form of 10 to 20 micrograms per day of ethynyl estradiol) as an extra boost to the cervix. Although this sometimes improves the very poor cervical mucus seen in Clomid cycles, it often just delays ovulation more and counteracts the stimulatory effect of Clomid. The basic problem with Clomid is that it does not have a "clean" effect. On one hand, it stimulates ovulation by increasing FSH early in the cycle. On the other hand, it counteracts the effects of estrogen on the cervix and the endometrium, and possibly on the egg itself.

The benefit of Clomid is that it is such a mild drug it can be prescribed without the need for close monitoring. The incidence of twins in clomiphene-treated women is only about 6 percent. Triplets, quadruplets, and quintuplets are extremely rare with this relatively gentle and mild fertility agent.

The "hyperstimulation syndrome" with Clomid is usually very mild and is rarely dangerous. It is a safe, easy-to-prescribe drug.

At least 70 percent of women who are not ovulating at all can eventually be induced to ovulate with Clomid but less than 30 percent of them become pregnant, despite years and years of treatment. Thus, most of these patients need to go to more involved treatment such as Pergonal or GIFT.

Clomid is used not only to induce ovulation in women who are not ovulating, but also to improve the quality and the regularity of ovulation. Women who ovulate on day eighteen, nineteen, or twenty without therapy will normally ovulate on day fourteen when taking Clomid. Women who have a short or inadequate luteal phase (which means that after they ovulate, their corpus luteum does not make enough progesterone and they menstruate too soon) will also become regulated on Clomid. The mechanism is always the same: Increased pituitary release of FSH in the early portion of the cycle ensures proper development of the follicle and sets the stage for the precise synchrony of hormonal events to occur during the rest of the cycle.

Clomid is probably the most popular drug used for enhancing fertility because it is so simple to administer, and patients can take it with very little supervision. But it is certainly overused, and many patients have been on Clomid literally for years and years with no pregnancy. The doctor may add an HCG injection at mid-cycle, or perform artificial insemination with the husband's semen, but generally if Clomid does not produce a pregnancy in the first several months, it's not likely to do so over the next several years.

OVARIAN DRILLING

One rather crude form of therapy used in the past for women who did not ovulate was the actual surgical removal of a portion of their ovaries. This barbaric-sounding approach actually had a significant success rate. Although not recommended today because of the excellent drugs available to induce ovulation, such surgery was moderately successful in the past, and tells us a little bit about why these ovaries do not ovulate. The only important and documented hormonal change in nonovulating women who have undergone this old-fashioned "ovarian wedge resection" is that their blood testosterone levels drop dramatically. This suggests that high production of testosterone by the ovary is one of the reasons why follicles are not forming properly and not ovulating. A wedge resection is a bit like hitting an ovary over the head and temporarily preventing it from making hormones. When the male hormone production of the ovary is thus stopped, ovulatory cycles frequently resume. The problems with this surgery were that it caused potentially harmful scar tissue around the ovary, and that it did not solve the problem permanently. Most patients failed again to ovulate after a certain period of time had passed. Thus, "ovarian wedge resection" has certainly become a treatment of the past.

On the other hand, a form of surgery which accomplishes the same effect, but without the scarring and mess caused by "ovarian wedge resection" is ovarian "drilling" (with a laser) through the laparoscope. It is known that the nonovulating ovary is usually smooth and round with a tense, filled-out capsule, quite unlike a normal "fertile" ovary which has a completely wrinkled, prunelike appearance. The reason that the poorly functioning ovary is so tense and smooth in its outer capsule is that hundreds of partial follicle cysts never got past the early follicular phase of development. This is either caused by an inadequate level of FSH in the first half of the cycle leading to nonovulation, or by an increased level of the male hormone, testosterone, inhibiting early follicle development, or both. In either case it is a vicious cycle. Once the ovary stops ovulating properly it makes too much testosterone, and this in turn continues to prevent proper ovulation. By drilling holes in all of these little partially developed follicle cysts, draining the ovary just like "wedge resection" unwittingly did in the 1960s and 1970s, the testosterone level drops precipitously, and often ovulation resumes. This can be accomplished simply at the time of diagnostic laparoscopy with a laser.

BROMOCRIPTINE, OR "PARLODEL"

Occasionally a lack of ovulation is caused by increased levels of a hormone called "prolactin," which is released by the pituitary, normally after the delivery of a baby, to allow breast-feeding. "Prolactin" directly stimulates the breasts to make milk. It also prevents ovulation. (You'll remember that the !Kung tribesmen of the Kalahari Desert in Africa have children only once every four to five years because the women breast-feed their young constantly around the clock for about four years.) Breast-feeding stimulates the pituitary gland to secrete more and more prolactin, and this hormone has two effects. First, it stimulates the breasts to make milk. Second, it inhibits the release of FSH and LH, and thus prevents ovulation. So, normally, prolactin is only secreted in large amounts during breast-feeding, and it inhibits ovulation.

In some patients a small and often undetectable pituitary tumor may cause the prolactin level in the blood to be increased in a non-breast-feeding woman and thereby make her infertile. A drug called Bromocriptine, or "Parlodel," dramatically suppresses the pituitary's production of prolactin in these cases, and ovulation ensues promptly after its administration. Bromocriptine is not useful in other cases of infertility and is not a cure-all fertility drug. However, it is an exciting treatment for those few women who are found on routine screening for infertility to have increased production of prolactin.

In the past, the small pituitary tumor causing the increased prolactin was removed by neurosurgeons through an incision in the roof of the nose. This was rather difficult, painstaking, and risky surgery, but it was necessary because Parlodel, though available in Europe, Canada, and Australia, was not available for political and bureaucratic reasons in the United States. Eventually Bromocriptine was accepted by the FDA for usage in the United States, and since that time pituitary surgery for increased prolactin levels has been very unusual. Even large prolactin-secreting tumors usually shrink up readily when the patient goes on Parlodel. Most of the time the tumor is too small to even be detected, but nonetheless an increased level of prolactin virtually always comes down to normal when the patient takes this drug.

Bromocriptine can have some aggravating side effects like nausea, dizziness, and headaches if given in normal doses too rapidly without a gradual buildup. However, this problem can be prevented by starting with a low dose of one half of a 2.5 mg tablet once a day; then going to a full 2.5 mg tablet once a day; and finally to two full tablets per day, once at night and once in the morning.

Prolactin, like testosterone, and virtually all the hormones secreted during the menstrual cycle, has a normal rise at the time of the LH surge. Often the prolactin level may seem to be on the upper limit of normal only because it is supposed to go up at mid-cycle, when estrogen, the LH, FSH, and even testosterone also peak. Giving Parlodel to "normal" women to prevent this normal mid-cycle surge of prolactin enjoyed some faddish popularity for a while as a possible overall fertility enhancer, but this is no longer in style, and the drug is reserved for true, constant elevations of prolactin level.

DANOCRINE, OR SURGERY, FOR ENDOMETRIOSIS

Among some doctors "endometriosis" is considered the major cause of infertility. Endometriosis has enjoyed unprecedented popularity as a diagnosis, and surgery for it has built many fine homes for doctors who are enthusiasts for operating on this condition. In truth, endometriosis is a more controversial condition than some would give it credit for, and although it is an extremely frequent diagnosis associated with hospital and surgery bills for infertility-related procedures, its relationship to infertility is highly mysterious and the treatment of it is questionable. First, let's review what endometriosis is.

What Is "Endometriosis"?

Normally when a woman menstruates, the lining of her uterus is shed and most of the blood is extruded through the cervix, which opens up at the time of menstruation. At the same time that the menstrual blood is shed out into the vagina, a small portion of it is shed backwards through the fallopian tube into the abdominal cavity. This is so-called "retrograde menstruation." If the endometrial tissue, or menstrual flow, that goes back into the abdomen catches hold and endometrial cells start growing in the abdominal cavity, that is the beginning of "endometriosis."

There have been dozens of theories offered for how the presence of endometriosis might cause infertility. Most of these reasons are quite mysterious and lack definite proof. One general term that has been used by its proponents is that the presence of endometriosis in a woman's pelvis creates a "hostile" pelvic environment which prevents pregnancy. Under this assumption, a doctor seeing the smallest lesion of endometriosis in an infertile woman may want to surgically remove it or else put her on some sort of drug that will cause the endometriosis to dissolve.

There is no question that the presence of endometriosis is associated with a greater likelihood of poor ovulation, lack of ovulation, or "luteal phase defect." However, controlled studies have demonstrated that women who have "moderate" or "minimal" lesion endometriosis that is treated have no greater pregnancy rate than women who go with no treatment at all. So the question comes up whether endometriosis actually causes infertility or is in some way caused by some other factors that are associated with infertility. If that were the case, then removing the endometriosis would do nothing to improve the woman's fertility.

The question you have to ask before embarking on some of the rather severe treatments for endometriosis (which can be costly and indeed delay rather than hasten your possibility of getting pregnant) is why does this retrograde menstrual flow of endometrial tissue actually take hold in the lining of the abdomen? It is more likely to take hold in a woman who has poor ovulation, or who doesn't ovulate at all, for the following reason: During the second half of a normal ovulatory cycle, progesterone is secreted and this softens the lining, makes it more spongy, and in medical terms makes it "secretory." This allows for a clean menstrual slough of the endometrial lining once the period begins. Remember that an "unopposed estrogen effect" seen in a woman who doesn't ovulate (who only has estrogen buildup because the follicle never turns into a corpus luteum and never produces progesterone) is likely to cause a continual buildup of endometrium lining in her uterus to the point where many years later she is more likely to get cancer of the endometrium than a woman who had ovulated normally.

Women on birth control pills always notice that their periods, although heavy prior to going on the pills, become much lighter and usually more comfortable after going on the birth control pills. The reason for this is that most birth control pill formulations have an excess of progesterone over estrogen. You get a softening of the uterine lining without a great deal of estrogen buildup and so the periods are very light. It is for this reason that women who have been on the birth control pill have a much lower incidence of cancer of the endometrium later in life than women who never took it. In the same respect, women who ovulate normally have a lower incidence of cancer of the endometrium later in life than women who didn't ovulate. The simple point is that the progesterone secreted normally in the second half of the ovulatory cycle causes the endometrial tissue to soften up for a clean bleed, and indeed prevents endometrial tissue from developing an estrogen-mediated overbuildup. For this same reason, progesterone deficiency is associated with a greater incidence of endometriosis.

In fact, one of the old treatments for endometriosis was to place the woman on high doses of progesterone, and this treatment was actually quite effective. Over a prolonged period of time progesterone eventually caused her endometrial lesions to disappear. It is for this same reason that women with endometriosis were told, ironically, that their condition could be best cured by getting pregnant, since pregnancy produced superhigh levels of progesterone of nine months and this cured the endometriosis.

Thus it seems more likely that endometriosis is caused by a relative estrogen excess or a relative lack of progesterone related to an inadequate luteal phase or poor ovulation. That is why the hundreds of thousands of operations that have been performed to remove little endometrial lesions, and the hundreds of thousands of women placed on Danocrine to shrink up their little endometriosis lesions have not caused any higher pregnancy rate than no treatment alone.

Endometriosis of the Ovary

There is one exception to this, and that is endometriosis located in the ovary. For whatever reason, when surgery is performed either through the laparoscope or through older operative techniques to ablate (vaporize) endometriosis lesions of the ovary, pregnancy rates were quite dramatically improved over what one would expect from no treatment at all. The question is whether ablation of an ovarian "endometrioma" in some way improved ovarian function and allowed for better quality ovulation. A common theory is that ablation of ovarian endometriosis reduces whatever toxic effect the endometrioma might have on the ovary. However, a theory that may be more plausible is that ablation of the ovarian endometrioma works very much like the "ovary drilling" operation mentioned earlier. In any event, ovarian endometriosis does seem to respond to ablation, but treatment of endometriosis anywhere else in the pelvis seems to not result in a significantly increased pregnancy rate.

Danocrine for Endometriosis

There are two therapies for attempting to shrink up the endometriosis, medical and surgical. Medical therapy for many years used to be the administration of continuous birth control pills, which resulted in a strong "progesterone effect" which eventually caused the endometriosis tissue to become more "secretory," shrink up, and disappear. This treatment became less popular in the late 1970s and 1980s, however, with the development of the drug Danocrine.

Danocrine is probably not much more effective than progesterone in shrinking up endometriosis lesions, but the problem with progesterone is that it often caused the lesions to grow somewhat larger before they finally shrank away. Progesterone was said to have caused an "artificial pregnancy" effect which caused lesions to shrink up over a long period of time, while Danocrine was said to have caused an "artificial menopause effect" which caused the lesions to shrink up more quickly.

Danocrine is simply a male hormone, a testosteronelike derivative, which has very little male hormone effect. By giving Danocrine to a woman you inhibit her pituitary gland from making FSH and LII, and this puts her into an artificial menopause. Her ovary stops functioning completely, and she stops making estrogen and progesterone. By causing the ovary to cease functioning, and removing the estrogen hormone that is stimulating the continued development of endometrial tissue, the woman no longer menstruates and her endometriosis gradually shrinks away.

Danocrine has some unpleasant side effects in that it does still have some male hormonelike effect, and women complain of oily skin, acne, and an increased appetite developing while in this "pseudo-menopause." Theoretically, when the Danocrine is discontinued after three or six months, the endometriosis is then gone, and in some mysterious way the woman now can get pregnant. In fact, studies have shown that the pregnancy rate in women taking Danocrine is actually a little less than in those who did not take it, probably because they could not possibly get pregnant while on the Danocrine. In any event, Danocrine may cause the endometriosis to shrink up, but it has not been shown to be responsible for any dramatic increase in pregnancy rate, probably because it is not attacking the heart of the problem.

Surgery for Endometriosis

Surgery for endometriosis is extremely popular. In fact, in the late 1970s and 1980s it would be very difficult for a woman to show up at a fertility clinic asking for infertility help without getting a diagnosis of endometriosis, and subsequently some sort of surgery for it. It was overdiagnosed because insurance companies would readily pay for the procedure without any questions. The second reason is that an endometriosis lesion as tiny as one millimeter was actually given the respectability of a title called "minimal lesion" endometriosis. Lesions so minuscule that they were almost (and sometimes actually) imaginary were quite respectably signed out on the hospital chart as "endometriosis." The only tragedy would be if a woman underwent an unnecessary, major, open abdominal operation to remove these little endometriosis lesions. More commonly, and quite harmlessly, these endometriosis lesions are ablated either with electrocautery or a laser through the laparoscope. The woman is going to undergo laparoscopy anyway for diagnosis, so if a tiny lesion of endometriosis is spotted there was no harm done in cauterizing it. The benefit is that the insurance company would pay for the procedure, and doctors often fooled themselves into thinking there would be a higher pregnancy rate.

With these comments I will not earn any friends among doctors treating endometriosis; but most scientifically minded doctors in the field of infertility will verify that endometriosis has finally run its course. Although an endometrioma of the ovary probably does require surgery, the other treatments for endometriosis in an effort to supposedly cure infertility are as far-fetched in benefit as they are commonly and popularly oversubscribed.

SURGERY FOR BLOCKED TUBES AND PELVIC SCARRING

In about 10 percent of infertile couples there is either scarring of the outside of the fallopian tubes or scarring on the inside causing complete blockage. Scarring on the outside, referred to as adhesions, can "tie the tube down" and make it difficult for it to pick up the egg from the surface of the ovary at the time of ovulation. Such scarring is usually caused by previous pelvic infections either from venereal disease, a ruptured appendix, or bowel disease. If the infection causing these adhesions was very severe, it could result in total blockage usually at the fimbriated end. This total blockage of the tube at the fimbriated end means that the tubal secretions can no longer flow out into the abdominal cavity, and the tube tends to dilate up much like a balloon with fluid. This kind of blocked condition at the end of the fallopian tube is the commonest cause of tubal blockage, and is referred to as "hydrosalpinx." Surgery either through the laparoscope or by opening up the abdomen is necessary to treat this type of infertility problem.

It is important to make a clear distinction between the cases where adhesions merely inhibit the motion of the tube but the fallopian tube is "open," and those cases where the fallopian tube is completely closed, i.e., "hydrosalpinx." In the cases where the fallopian tube is open, usually the mucosa, i.e., the internal lining of the fallopian tube, is adequate to pick up the egg from the ovarian surface, and can nourish the egg for fertilization. Thus, all that is required is to cut, or "loosen," the adhesions that are holding the tube down and preventing its proper movement. The chances for pregnancy after surgery to free up the scarring in these women is 60 percent.

However, when the end of the fallopian tube is actually blocked, this is usually associated with fairly severe damage to the inside lining of the tube, and the ability of the tube to pick up the egg from the ovary and nourish it is severely damaged. Therefore, despite very nice surgical operations for opening up the end of the tube and creating a new, beautifully flowered fimbriated end, the pregnancy rate for solving this kind of obstructive problem is only about 20 to 25 percent. It was actually this low pregnancy rate with surgery for "hydrosalpinx" that led initially to the clinical development of in vitro fertilization, completely bypassing the necessity of even having the fallopian tube at all.

Surgery for "Hydrosalpinx": Why Some Get Pregnant and Others Don't

Patients with hydrosalpinx could be divided into two groups: those with severe mucosal damage noted at the time of surgery, and those with relatively preserved mucosal tissue with good cilia remaining. In those patients with healthy-looking mucosa, correcting the blocked hydrosalpinx with surgery (opening up the end of the tube) results in a pregnancy rate of over 70 percent. However in those with very poor mucosa that was obviously destroyed by the infection, the pregnancy rate is under 5 percent. What this all boils down to is that surgery for tubal blockage and/or adhesions carries a very good pregnancy rate if the mucosal lining of the tube is relatively undamaged, but carries a miserable pregnancy rate making surgery not even worthwhile if the tubal lining is severely damaged.

Surgery can be performed either through an open incision or, as is becoming somewhat more popular, attempts can be made through the laparoscope. The advantage of doing surgery through the laparoscope is that the patient has much less pain and usually goes home the next day. However, the operation through the laparoscope can be more tedious, more demanding, and can require as long as four to six hours for an operation that would otherwise perhaps require only an hour.

Some surgeons prefer to use a laser for freeing up the adhesions and opening up the end of the tube because it has a tremendous twenty-first-century appeal, but actually standard electrocautery with a small electrode works just as well with no increased risk of scarring and with no difference in pregnancy rates. In fact, probably the world's leading expert in this type of female surgery, Dr. Victor Gomel from the University of British Columbia in Vancouver, prefers not to bother with a laser, and gets absolutely beautiful results using simply micro-scissors and electrocautery with a small electrode. Many patients are very impressed when their doctor tells them that he used a "laser" to perform their surgery, but for this type of surgery *the laser has absolutely no advantages over standard laparoscopic or microsurgical instruments.* It just has a high-tech-type sound to it that is misleading to the patient.

One of the biggest questions today is whether patients with hydrosalpinx should undergo surgery to open up the ends of the tubes, or whether they should simply go straight into an in vitro fertilization program. You will get different viewpoints from different fertility doctors depending upon their area of expertise. Since I have expertise in both areas I may have some sound advice for you to follow. If the hysterosalpingogram X ray demonstrates what looks like good "rugal folds," suggestive of an unscarred, undamaged, relatively healthy lining to the fallopian tube, then surgery to open the blockage would not only give a very good pregnancy rate compared to in vitro fertilization, but require only one procedure for all the babies you might ever want, rather than require multiple repetitions of a procedure such as with in vitro fertilization. On the other hand, if the hysterosalpingogram shows a very smooth-looking surface to the lining of the fallopian tube with no prominent "rugal folds," then I would recommend not going through surgery to open the tubes, as it will most likely be a complete waste of your time and money. If that kind of severe damage is apparent on the X ray, then your best alternative is to go straight to in vitro fertilization.

If there is even the slightest trickle of radiopaque dye getting through the tube and going into the abdomen, such patients should have a high pregnancy rate with corrective surgery, and that would be the priority before thinking about in vitro fertilization. The advantage of corrective surgery if it works is that only one operation is needed. With in vitro fertilization a woman may have to go through many cycles before getting pregnant even once. Despite my enthusiasm for going quickly to the new technology and not wasting time with older approaches that over many years can create a tremendous drain with a low yield, I believe the result is certainly high enough in selected cases of obstruction and adhesions to go ahead with conventional surgery in preference to in vitro fertilization and save in vitro fertilization for those cases where conventional surgery is not at all likely to yield a pregnancy.

When I was invited to the Soviet Union in 1988, to perform microsurgery and survey the possibility of setting up in vitro fertilization and GIFT programs there, I was shown many X rays of women with tubal blockage and was able to select the ones who would be likely to benefit from surgery, and save all of the others for the day when the Soviet Union would be in a better position to offer in vitro fertilization to these women. It is very important to recognize that you shouldn't just take a dismal outlook toward surgery for hydrosalpinx. It is simply important to distinguish between those cases of "hydrosalpinx" that have a high pregnancy rate with surgery and those that have a low pregnancy rate. This can be accomplished by carefully reviewing the hysterosalpingogram X rays for the quality of the mucosal lining of the tube.

Surgery for Adhesions

One final word of caution is in order for women whose tubes are not completely blocked but simply have external adhesions. I am absolutely amazed at the women with severe adhesions of the fallopian tubes which have either not been corrected with surgery, or for whom surgery was considered virtually impossible, who are nonetheless able to get pregnant. The most stunning example I can think of is a woman on whom in vitro fertilization was attempted in 1989. She had undergone several mutilating operations which had removed almost all of her ovarian tissue and created a tremendous amount of scar tissue that almost completely encased and blocked off her fallopian tubes. A hysterosalpingogram demonstrated the barest trickle of dye through a terribly scarred tube, and laparoscopy just revealed that the tubes were completely embedded in scar and one could barely see contrast material coming out of a hidden peephole in the end of the tube. It appeared that there was very little hope for this woman without in vitro fertilization.

With incredibly high doses of Pergonal she was able to form just two follicles, one mature and big-looking, and one smaller. Using transvaginal ultrasound, we were able to needle these follicles, and got a relatively immature egg out of the small one, but were not able to retrieve an egg from the one big follicle stuck in this massive scar tissue. The immature egg obtained did not fertilize in vitro with her husband's sperm, but the couple was instructed to have intercourse that night just in case by some kind of miracle the egg from the other follicle might have gotten picked up by her extremely damaged fallopian tube. There was no embryo to replace in the uterus because the retrieved immature egg did not fertilize. Nonetheless, she became pregnant in that cycle, indicating that the single follicle that had been stuck with the needle must have released an egg into that scar tissue. It was somehow or other picked up by her severely scarred fallopian tube, and she got pregnant.

The reason for giving this example is that very often filmy adhesions of the tube are given the entire blame for the woman's infertility, but yet the woman may have ovulatory problems that are neglected and are in fact the major cause of the infertility. This particular woman obviously got pregnant because she was made to ovulate from the tiny amount of ovarian tissue she had remaining. Despite massive scarring that should have prevented the tubes from normally picking the egg up, somehow or other the egg was picked up by the fallopian tube and she became pregnant. Thus if there is any leakage of dye whatsoever out of the fallopian tube during a hysterosalpingogram X ray, one has to be skeptical about whether the cause of infertility is truly these adhesions, or perhaps an ovulatory defect. The adhesions may only be secondary bystanders.

CONCLUSIONS

The purpose of this chapter is to review what I consider to be conventional infertility treatments (including just watchful waiting for those people who are younger and whose infertility has not been of terribly long duration). Many of these conventional approaches such as clomiphene citrate, Parlodel, or surgery are

going to help certain patients get pregnant and need to be understood. On the other hand, it is important not to spend so
many years on treatments of dubious outlook, such as varicocelectomy for the husband, different drug treatments to try to
improve his sperm count, ablation of endometriosis of the wife,
years and years of Clomid, or Parlodel in women who don't have
elevated prolactin, or just going for years with simpleminded
saving up of intercourse to the time of ovulation, that can lead
to tremendous emotional pain and cost, and still not get a couple
closer to getting pregnant.

There are people who have gone through years of conventional
treatment, always under the assumption that in vitro fertilization
or GIFT would be a last resort. But in truth many waited too
long for the procedures that would have given them the highest
pregnancy rate, and they reached a point of emotional and economic exhaustion.

CHAPTER 9

Artificial Insemination by Donor Sperm and Sperm-Banking

If the husband has no sperm and this problem cannot be successfully treated, one solution is for the wife to have "artificial insemination" with "donor sperm," termed "AID" (*artificial insemination by donor*). To many couples this may seem undesirable, but in fact it is no different than adoption. It is simply a matter of "adopting sperm." You're adopting the baby at a much earlier stage, that is, prior to conception. Artificial insemination, using the sperm of a well-selected anonymous donor, is the most realistic and sensible solution for couples in which the husband's infertility cannot be cured. In fact, it has tremendous advantages over classic adoption, for parental bonding and child development.

IS IT MY BABY?

There has always been a heated debate about where a child's personality and abilities come from, his environment or his genes. After counseling hundreds of couples who have undergone artificial donor insemination (AID) and having seen the results over the last fifteen years, as well as having studied rather extensively the early childhood development research coming from the Harvard and the Ypsilanti early childhood projects, I have some definite views that could be of benefit to couples who are facing this issue of whether to have donor insemination. It is obviously preferable for almost any couple to do whatever is possible to allow them their own genetic baby using the husband's sperm. However, if such a solution is not at hand, consider seriously the following observations.

The divorce rate among couples who choose to elect artificial insemination with donor sperm is less than 1 percent, even though the general divorce rate in our population is over 50 percent. This is not because in some way the decision to have a baby by donor insemination holds the marriage together. Rather, couples who wind up choosing this route have a solid relationship and a good basis of communicating with one another. Couples who have any flaws or weaknesses in their ability to communicate on tough issues usually will not elect donor insemination. Couples who do elect donor insemination are a select group that have an extraordinarily solid marriage. They can deal with a potentially divisive issue and come to a common understanding nonetheless that makes them both happy. So if a couple decides to have donor insemination because the husband's problem is unsolvable, it is a very good sign that the marriage is going to remain solid.

Couples will frequently ask how the baby will do when its genes come only half from the mother and half from some stranger. Very often they will express the viewpoint, "Well at least if we go this route, as opposed to adoption, the baby will be 'one-half ours.' " This outlook is a strong reason *not* to have donor insemination.

My observation has been that when the husband and the wife both accept the baby as being 100 percent theirs, and take the view that the genetic contribution is of no significance, then the father-infant bonding is completely normal.

Although there is a controversial view held in some circles that a child's personality, intelligence, and athletic ability are basically genetically transmitted and there is only a partial contribution from parental rearing, evidence from most AID couples and from the early childhood projects argue strongly against this commonly held genetic bias. In truth, the child's personality, intelligence, and even athletic skill (though not size, hair color, eye color, or body build) are overwhelmingly related to how he was raised in the very first year or two of life.

Children in the first year and a half of life are in many respects like parrots. They learn by copying what they see around them. A personality tends to emerge more clearly as a sense of individual identity around the age of a year and a half when language skills first become readily apparent. The way in which a non-genetic offspring mimics his or her rearing father, regardless of genetic origin, is so striking that these parents are sometimes shocked and do double takes when a friendly neighbor (who knows nothing about the child's genetic origin) comments admiringly on how the child is the spitting image of his father. In couples who elect donor insemination, most of the time the father's bonding with the infant is no different than if it were his own "genetic" child.

The interesting thing is that the courts take a similar view in ruling on cases where a husband might allege that his wife got pregnant by having an affair with another man and that the child his wife bears is not really "his." The courts define the father as the person who is living with the woman and are not terribly concerned about whose sperm fertilized the mother. (Of course the courts have a different agenda in that their major concern is establishing a responsible father to handle financial arrangements for the child's future care.) Still it is of interest that the official legal view does not contradict what the latest studies on early child development demonstrate.

It is true that we have all witnessed how a two-year-old's personality, intelligence, and skill level are quite predictive in many cases of how that child will eventually turn out as an adult, and this observation leads many to conclude unquestioningly "it's just all genetic." That viewpoint is enhanced even further among parents who are in one way or another unhappy with how their child had turned out. Even though it may be "their own genetic child" (they blame the result on "genes," assuming that the child just had the bad luck of getting the parents' worst genes), because it takes away any possibility that they would have to blame themselves and their rearing efforts. So there is tremendous attractiveness for being able to allow genetics to shoulder the responsibility for how a child turns out, but these "genetic" arguments can raise fear among couples who are considering artificial insemination with donor sperm.

Nonetheless, couples electing to have donor insemination should make sure that the sperm come from the healthiest, most intelligent possible source, and that there is some matching up of hair color, skin color, eye color, and body build. A good artificial insemination program therefore will pay close attention to these selective characteristics so that the couple may get as close a physical match to the husband as possible, to remove from them any doubt that sperm from a truly undesirable character was being used.

MAKING THE ARRANGEMENTS AND SELECTING THE DONOR

Artificial insemination was first successfully used in women by the famous physician John Hunter in England in the eighteenth century. In 1890, Dr. Robert Dickinson of New York was the first to use donor sperm for women whose husbands had untreatable infertility. This early use of artificial insemination with donor sperm was carried out in great secrecy. However, it has now become so popular that more than 30,000 babies are born every year in the United States as a result of it. Patients are accepting it when there is no other solution, and most of the psychological, social, and legal fears about it have disappeared.

In 1964, Georgia was the first state to issue legislation that guaranteed that a child conceived in this manner will be considered legitimate. Oklahoma passed a similar law in 1967, as did Kansas in 1968, and all other states followed suit. Even prior to these legislative decrees, common law provided some protection for the legitimacy of such children. Unless it is proved that the husband had no access to the wife, any child born of her is considered to be his by the law. Whether or not the husband is the true father, he is the legal father of any child born to his wife while they are living together.

From a medical point of view, artificial insemination is extraordinarily simple. A sperm specimen obtained from the donor is drawn up into a syringe, and then simply squirted into the vagina near the cervix. Since the sperm are only capable of fertilization for up to forty-eight hours in the female reproductive tract, and since the egg is only capable of being fertilized within twelve hours of ovulation, the insemination must be timed appropriately just before ovulation.

Prior to the wife's undergoing artificial insemination, the doctor will always have both wife and husband sign a special consent form which states: 1) that any children produced by artificial insemination will be their own legitimate children and their heirs; 2) that they waive forever any right to disclaim such a child as their own; and 3) that the nature of the agreement will make it confidential among the husband, the wife, and the doctor. The agreement will state that the husband and wife rely upon the judgment and discretion of the doctor to choose a donor whose physical and mental characteristics are compatible with those of the husband, or they may choose the donor themselves from an information sheet supplied by the sperm bank. They then must agree that they understand the doctor cannot be held responsible for any physical or mental characteristics of any child so produced. At the moment of conception the husband must automatically accept the child as his own.

Selection of an appropriate sperm donor is certainly the physician's heaviest responsibility in artificial insemination with donor sperm. Obviously the donor has to be healthy and very fertile. Skin, hair, body build, and eye color should match the patient's husband as closely as possible and their blood types should be completely compatible. All donors have to be checked for the presence of hepatitis, AIDS, or venereal disease.

Because of the possible six-month incubation time of the AIDS virus, frozen sperm is virtually always used today as opposed to ten years ago, because it allows the donor to be observed for six months after the collection of the sperm, and have a repeat blood test for AIDS. Only if his blood test for AIDS is still negative six months after donating the sperm is his sperm used for donor insemination. Furthermore, the donor is screened for any history of genetic disease in his family. Even the history of diseases that are only partially genetically transmitted, such as diabetes, would generally rule him out as being accepted as a sperm donor.

Once the donor is accepted he is generally asked to abstain from intercourse for two or three days and then to provide a specimen in a clean, sterile container. The specimen is carefully cultured for bacteria such as gonorrhea or chlamydia and the remainder of the sample is prepared for freezing and storage.

In the past it has always been thought best for the sperm donor to be anonymous. When a couple requests a particular donor who they know as a close friend it has been thought that problems could arise if the genetic father is known to the couple. With a greater openness in our society, and a better understanding of the relative lack of significance of genetic contribution as opposed to rearing, some physicians (though not the majority) are becoming more open in carefully selected couples for allowing insemination of sperm from donors who are well known to the couple.

In fact, at present most sperm donors are medical students or interns, usually of high intelligence, who are readily available to the medical community for sperm donation and are paid for their services. Just as the identity of the donor would never be revealed to the couple under these circumstances, the couple's identity is never revealed to the donor.

Because of the requirement that anonymous donors' sperm be frozen in order to make certain that they don't become AIDS positive over the ensuing six months before their sperm is used, and because of the meticulous detail that couples using donor insemination have a right to expect regarding the characteristics of the donor, many physicians are turning more and more to formally operated and carefully regulated frozen sperm banks. One of the very best sperm banks in the United States is the Southern California Cryobank located at Century City Hospital in Los Angeles, California. They make shipments of sperm all over the world, and are presently the largest sperm bank in North America. They provide a detailed pedigree of every single donor, including race, hair color, eye color, skin color, body build, religious preference, nationality, degree of education, and even hobbies. In truth, all that really makes a difference is that there be no history of genetic disease, that the donor not have hepatitis, AIDS, or venereal disease, and have a reasonable match of inherited appearance. The other issues such as level of education achieved, hobbies, and interests are simply a way of assuring future recipients who might have any lingering doubts about the possibility of any broad genetic transference of intellectual ability or personality.

There are so many cases of short parents having tall children that are genetically their own, of dark-haired parents having a red-head for a child, that all of us are aware of the importance of "recessive" genes expressing themselves unpredictably in children that are genetically their own. In fact, even if there is a perfect matching of donor to the recipient, the child may have a very different appearance because of these recessive genes.

Another important selection that a sperm bank must perform is to make sure that the donor is fertile and that his sperm is properly frozen so that when the thawed specimen is sent to the physician doing the insemination, its fertility has not been hurt by a poorly performed freezing process.

The sperm bank should also make sure that no particular donor is overused. Population scientists have made it very clear that if a particular donor were to be used in more than ten different couples around the United States, there would be an ever so slight risk of a future unknown first-cousin marriage if the off-spring of any of these families were to ever meet and get married. The temptation for a poorly organized sperm bank would be to use a particular donor over and over again and thereby avoid all of the expense related to the selection of new donors. Despite the increased cost, it is important that the sperm bank resist any such overuse of its donors, and that is why only the most reputable sources for sperm (either a commercial sperm bank or a local university sperm bank) should be used.

There was a great deal of publicity in the early 1980s associated with the institution of a "Nobel-Prize Sperm Bank." This bank was started in the San Diego area by a very old, former Nobel prize winner (who has subsequently died) who received his prize for inventing the transistor. It was his firm belief that intelligence was genetically transmitted and that the future of our society depended upon sperm from these most intelligent men being used for donor insemination. His sperm bank was never really taken very seriously, and never caught on. As one of my patients put it: "If genes do have anything to do with superintelligence and winning Nobel Prizes [which I don't believe they do], then we should be using the sperm from Nobel-Prize winners' *fathers, not from the Nobel winners themselves.* By and large the children of Nobel Prize winners are not any more distinguished than children born from parents with less illustrious minds."

The brain of modern man is really no different from the brain of Cro-Magnon man, who lived 40,000 years ago in caves and drew crude paintings on the wall. The human brain has been able to take us as far as we have come not because of inborn abilities (such as most animals are born with), but rather because of its remarkable flexibility and capacity to learn. If I were born 40,000 years ago in a Cro-Magnon cave, I would not be a so-phisticated microsurgeon or in vitro fertilization (IVF) specialist. Nor would I have developed the complex language abilities that have allowed me to write this book. My brain would have developed in other directions appropriate to allowing me to figure out how to survive in an entirely different, more primitive world. If a brutish Cro-Magnon man living in caves and huddled over a fire were to be born today, and reared by parents who encouraged the spark of curiosity, enthusiasm, and intellectual challenge, he would be just as likely to win a Nobel Prize as the child of anyone else born today.

AZOSPERMIC VERSUS OLIGOSPERMIC HUSBAND

Frequently the husband has a very low sperm count, one which would have a very small chance of ever resulting in conception, but at least there are a few sperm present. Male infertility is such a frustrating condition to deal with that more and more physicians are recommending artificial insemination with donor sperm to wives of husbands who are merely oligospermic and not completely azospermic (no sperm at all). The major warnings I have to make about this practice are that 1) the wife might very well be able to get pregnant with the husband's poor sperm if she is treated to the fullest, and also that 2) the pregnancy rate using fertile donor sperm in such women is much lower than in women whose husbands have no sperm at all.

This may be a little confusing, so let me explain it again in terms of what was discussed in Chapter 7. In 1982, the artificial insemination program from Bordeaux, France, reported that when donor sperm was used to inseminate women with husbands who were completely without sperm (azospermic), the pregnancy rate per each insemination cycle was 11.6 percent. However, in women undergoing donor artificial insemination whose husbands were merely oligospermic (i.e., had a low sperm count) the pregnancy rate per cycle was only 4.9 percent. Overall, 61 percent of women whose husband's were azospermic became pregnant with donor sperm, but only 29 percent whose husbands were oligospermic became pregnant with donor sperm. Why should the husband's sperm count in any way affect the likelihood of the wife's getting pregnant using perfectly fertile donor sperm?

The reason is that if the wife were not herself infertile, the husband even with a low sperm count would have possibly gotten her pregnant. The fact that she had not gotten pregnant yet with a husband who had some sperm even if a low number indicated that she too was likely to have a problem. Otherwise, they might never have reached the fertility clinic, and rather would be one of the 10 percent of fertile couples requesting vasectomy whose sperm count is below 10 million. This finding was verified by physicians in the Netherlands who noted a long-term pregnancy rate with donor sperm of over 95 percent when the husband was azospermic, 73 percent when the husband's sperm count was between 2 and 10 million, and only 62 percent when the husband's sperm count was greater than 10 million.

You will recall from previous chapters that although the chance of getting pregnant is higher when the husband has a high sperm count, very fertile women seem capable of getting pregnant when the husband has extremely low counts, as long as there is just some sperm present. Thus if you are undergoing insemination with donor sperm because of a "low sperm count" rather than a "zero" sperm count in your husband, it is important that every effort was made first to get you pregnant with his sperm using the newest technology; and secondly, even using donor sperm, you are likely to require other treatment as well in order to increase your chances of getting pregnant.

HOW IS IT DONE?

The woman's ovulatory pattern is determined either by basal body temperature charts, cervical mucus production, dilation and closure of the cervix, or more efficiently by ultrasound or LH dipstick testing to pinpoint the time of ovulation so that the sperm can be introduced on the best day or days. Sometimes the precise timing of ovulation becomes difficult because the emotional stress placed upon the wife affects her hypothalamus to the extent that she may ovulate late, or she may even fail to ovulate at all. For this reason the approach of the physician is very important. If the wife is terrified by an inadequate understanding of what is being done, she may very easily stop ovulating altogether. Usually daily ultrasound or LH dipstick monitoring by the patient herself is the best way to determine the proper day for insemination.

Because of the difficulty of pinpointing the exact time of ovulation under the psychological stress of artificial insemination, or because the wife herself may also have a fertility problem, the physician may place the wife on Clomid, or Pergonal and HCG, to induce good ovulation at a predictable time. Women treated with Clomid are more likely to ovulate right at midcycle, around day fourteen or fifteen, despite the emotional stress that might otherwise interfere with their cycles. On Pergonal and HCG, ovulation is almost sure to occur two to three days after HCG. Using this approach, a number of doctors have reported a higher pregnancy rate within a fewer number of cycles than when the time of ovulation is not artificially controlled. For whatever reason, pregnancy rates with AID are generally higher when ovulation is stimulated.

Regardless of whether ovulation is induced with drugs or allowed to proceed spontaneously, the woman must still be monitored, usually by ultrasound and LH testing. With a "natural cycle," the doctor will inseminate her on the day before expected ovulation and again one or two days later if her follicle has not yet disappeared on ultrasound.

When Pergonal and HCG are used to stimulate the wife in an artificial insemination cycle, she is followed with ultrasound and estrogen monitoring (see pages 258–63), and is inseminated the day after HCG is administered, which should be the day before she ovulates. Nonetheless, she is checked with ultrasound monitoring and if the follicle doesn't disappear when expected, she is inseminated again two days later.

The procedure is somewhat different when the sperm is washed and placed directly into the uterus. Under these circumstances, the cervical mucus reservoir is being bypassed, and the best time for placing the sperm into the uterus is therefore when there is already an egg clearly waiting in the fallopian tube. Therefore, if the sperm are being washed and placed into the uterus (see pages 230–43), the physician will continue to check the ovaries with ultrasound and will perform the insemination on the day that the follicle disappears indicating that an egg has been ovulated and is waiting in the fallopian tube.

Pregnancy rates in the past with artificial insemination of donor sperm have varied from 6 to 20 percent per cycle. The higher pregnancy rates per cycle were obtained in programs that pinpointed the insemination very accurately, were willing to work on the weekends, and able to do several inseminations until it was absolutely certain that at least one of the inseminations was done around the time of ovulation. With the simpler and more accurate methods of more precisely timing ovulation that are now available, pregnancy rates with artificial insemination of donor sperm (AID) in wives of azospermic men should be between 15 and 20 percent per cycle, equivalent to the pregnancy rate per cycle in a typical fertile couple having regular and repeated intercourse.

The actual technique of artificial insemination is simple and entirely painless. The patient is placed in routine pelvic exam position and the vaginal speculum is inserted (just as though she were having a Pap smear). The donor's semen is then either squirted against the cervix into the recesses of the vagina (like natural intercourse) or placed in a plastic-type cap which is then put over the cervix and allowed to stay in position for a half hour to three hours. Alternatively, sperm may be injected directly into the cervical opening, or "washed sperm" (see pages 246–49) may be placed directly into the uterus.

I prefer to have the husband inject the sperm rather than the doctor since it is not a complex medical procedure. If the husband physically injects the sperm, it is a symbolic indication of his total acceptance of the idea, and his complete bonding with the child born from this procedure. Whichever method is used, the patient is usually requested to remain in position for at least one half hour, allowing plenty of time for the sperm to be secure in the cervical mucus. After that first half hour most of the sperm that would have any chance of reaching the egg will have already entered, and the patient is then allowed to leave.

PREGNANCY RATES WITH DONOR SPERM

In most artificial insemination clinics, 90 percent of the women who eventually get pregnant do so within the first six months. This has led to the erroneous notion that if the woman is not pregnant within six months it might be wise for her to give up, since she is not likely to become pregnant with future inseminations. Pregnancy rates with artificial insemination should be as good as normally occurring pregnancy rates in an otherwise fertile population. The failure to conceive after six cycles does *not* mean that the chances for pregnancy in subsequent cycles are poor. Among fertile couples with a 15 percent chance of pregnancy per cycle only 85 percent will have conceived in the first year.

Nonetheless, it is clear that with each successive cycle in which pregnancy does not occur, the couple is likely to become more and more despondent because of the energy placed in each attempt. Furthermore, after a period of time with no pregnancy, in an older couple or in a couple where there may be some female factor as well, those who have not gotten pregnant yet may represent a remaining group who have a lower chance of conception per month than a theoretically normal fertile population. For such a couple to go through two years of artificial insemination without a pregnancy may be asking too much.

GIFT WITH DONOR SPERM

Fortunately, there is a dramatic solution now available for couples who have gone through many cycles of donor insemination without a pregnancy. Their chances of pregnancy can be dramatically increased to 60 percent per cycle by employing the GIFT technique with donor sperm. IVF and GIFT will be discussed in detail in the next few chapters, but having read thus far you already have a good idea of what this involves. GIFT simply means the placement of sperm (in this case from the donor) and eggs from the wife, after ovulatory stimulation and needle aspiration, directly into the fallopian tube of the wife. This bypasses virtually all obstacles in the normal fertilization process, including proper egg maturation and sperm and egg transport to the site of fertilization. In women who have gone through more than a year of artificial insemination cycles every month with donor sperm (AID) and yet no pregnancy, GIFT with donor sperm will provide a 60 percent chance per cycle of pregnancy, which is four times the conception rate that could be expected with standard artificial insemination (AID) in a couple who are not suspected of having any infertility problems.

Why should the pregnancy rate using GIFT and donor sperm be so high in couples that clearly have not gotten pregnant after many normal cycles of donor insemination? Most likely the reason is that with guaranteed fertile sperm (where there is no male factor implicated at all), the pregnancy rate with GIFT, bypassing all the hurdles in the female's reproductive tract, is somewhere between 50 and 60 percent per cycle. When sperm is not of such good quality, the pregnancy rate with GIFT would be much lower. Furthermore, remember that when the husband is azospermic, the chances of the wife having a detectable infertility problem are less than 5 percent. Thus we are dealing with "idiopathic" infertility in which we suppose there must be a female factor, but it is completely undetectable. By performing GIFT these problems are bypassed, and in retrospect pregnancy rates this high in such a group using donor sperm should have been anticipated.

FROZEN SPERM AND SPERM BANKS

All men dream from time to time about the possibility of immortality. Science-fiction novelists frequently toy with the idea of human beings being placed in a deep freeze just prior to the moment of death, to be revived perhaps two hundred years later, at which time science may have better treatments for illnesses and a way of prolonging life indefinitely. Life is in a sense a series of chemical events proceeding irreversibly toward death, and these chemical events cannot take place at $-400°F$. Thus if an organism can be "safely" placed in a deep freeze, it could be preserved until a future century, and revived with subsequent warming.

Of course, freezing large animals would kill them immediately because of damage created by crystallization of water within their cells during the freezing process. However, it has been known since 1776 that human sperm are remarkably resistant to the damaging effects of freezing. In that year an Italian scientist exposed spermatozoa to freezing temperatures and noted that, after warming, some of them regained their motility. It was speculated then that frozen semen might be used not only in breeding the finest farm animals but also for saving the sperm of a man going off to war so that his wife might have a child from him even though he had already died on the battlefield.

Although these crude, early studies established that sperm could survive freezing and thawing, the sperm were so terribly damaged that there was no possibility of practical application. But in 1949 British scientists discovered completely by accident that if a relatively common chemical, glycerol, is added to the semen before it is frozen, the majority of the sperm survive freezing and thawing uneventfully. The researchers who made this discovery were so surprised to find live, healthy sperm in large concentrations after thawing that they had to go back to their laboratory shelf to find out which of the chemicals acci- dentally added to their sperm suspension was the one that pro- tected the sperm against freezing. They finally discovered that it was glycerol. It took very little time after their remarkable discovery for frozen-sperm banks to rapidly find acceptance in the field of cattle breeding, and today the vast majority of calves born in the world are the result of artificial insemination from frozen bull semen.

In 1953, four years later, it was demonstrated that frozen and thawed human sperm could result in pregnancy and the delivery of normal babies. The first human sperm bank was established the next year. Doctors originally thought that, using this method of freezing sperm, a husband with a very low sperm count could have as many as fifty ejaculates frozen, stored, and combined for use in artificial insemination of the wife; they hoped that with such a large number of sperm, the wife would be more likely to get pregnant. These hopes were dashed by the discovery that sperm from infertile men tolerate the freezing process very poorly. There is so much sperm death caused by freezing, even with glycerol, that a decent specimen could never be obtained for inseminating the wife. Doctors have since come to understand that some men's sperm tolerate freezing better than others'. Even men whose sperm usually would freeze well have variations from ejaculate to ejaculate. Sometimes their ejaculates freeze and thaw without any significant loss, and at other times they freeze and thaw very poorly.

Sperm freeze better than most other cells because there is so little cellular water content. The sperm head is basically an extremely compact, dense arrangement of DNA with much less water content than any other cell. Therefore, there is very little intracellular ice crystal formation to damage it. Nonetheless, even sperm require some sort of "cryoprotectant," in this case glycerol, whose function is to pull water out of the cell and to get inside it to act as a sort of "antifreeze," to prevent ice formation of any water still remaining inside.

The technique for freezing and storing the sperm is extremely simple. A fresh semen specimen is collected in a sterile container and several drops of glycerol, equal to one-tenth of the volume of the specimen, are added to the jar. The semen and glycerol must be very thoroughly mixed together. This mixture is then drawn up into a straw, and held over the vapors of liquid nitrogen to freeze it. Then it is inserted into the liquid nitrogen bath for permanent storage. When the time comes to thaw the frozen sperm, the plastic straw is simply removed from the liquid nitrogen bath, and either placed in warm water for one minute or left on a table at room temperature to thaw. There has been an improvement in "cryoprotection" by adding test yolk buffer to the glycerol and freezing the sperm in a more carefully controlled, programmed, slow freeze approach.

If the donor's sperm tolerate a freeze-thaw test well, then most of his samples (though not all of them) are likely to survive indefinitely in liquid nitrogen. There have been births of normal children from sperm that have been stored well over ten years.

There is no increased risk of birth abnormalities over a normal population. Whatever harm may come to sperm from freezing, either in the sperm's structure or ability to fertilize, there does not appear to be any increased risk of defective children. Extensive experience both in cattle and in humans has now documented that artificial insemination with frozen sperm from sperm banks is safe. Literally hundreds of thousands of normal pregnancies and births in humans from this technique have been reported in the scientific literature.

Fertility, however, is lower with frozen than with fresh semen specimens. A specimen might start out with 80 percent motility and after thawing have only 40 percent motility. In fact one study in the 1980s by Dr. Sander Shapiro and his group from the University of Wisconsin found an 18.9 percent incidence of pregnancy per cycle with artificial donor insemination using fresh semen, but only a 5 percent incidence of pregnancy per cycle using frozen thawed semen. Fresh semen was three times as likely to induce a pregnancy in any given cycle than frozen semen. For this reason despite the convenience of frozen semen, until the AIDS epidemic, most artificial donor insemination (AID) programs preferred fresh rather than frozen sperm.

Dr. Emil Steinberger's group in Houston, Texas, later found that if the wife had perfectly normal hormonal testing and regular ovulation on day fourteen in twenty-eight-day cycles, the incidence of pregnancy per cycle with frozen semen did not differ much from that with fresh semen. However, if there was any irregularity whatsoever in the wife, then in these cases the pregnancy rate was dramatically reduced using frozen semen as opposed to fresh semen. He concluded that it was the combination of a problem with the sperm caused by the freezing, and a problem with the wife that resulted in a lower pregnancy rate rather than just a problem with the frozen sperm alone.

Further analysis from several centers in 1989 solved this problem in a simple quantitative fashion. They demonstrated as expected that the total number of motile sperm was reduced dramatically in frozen thawed sperm as opposed to fresh sperm. However, if the total number of sperm that were used for insemination was increased, particularly if only the most fertile donors were accepted, pregnancy rates would not be significantly less with frozen than fresh sperm in donor insemination. Thus, greater total numbers of sperm were needed with frozen sperm in order to achieve a pregnancy rate per cycle equivalent to fresh sperm.

The biggest problem is with women over thirty-five years of age, in whom everyone who has ever studied donor insemination has noted a dramatic decrease in pregnancy rate despite using completely normal donor sperm. This effect, as predicted by Steinberger's work, is more apparent with frozen sperm than with fresh sperm unless much larger numbers of frozen sperm are used to make up for the decrease of fertility in frozen semen samples. In this era where frozen sperm will be the only sperm available the best recommendation for the woman who has not gotten pregnant after a reasonable number of trials of donor insemination, and particularly if she is over thirty-five, is just to go to GIFT using donor sperm.

The major benefit of sperm-banking at the present stage of our knowledge is to create easier and more convenient programs of artificial donor insemination in cases where the husband's infertility is not treatable. Freezing of sperm for donor insemination is mandated today by the need to AIDS test all potential donors for six months *after* sperm collection and *before* insemination to ensure that no AIDS-infected sperm is used.

CHAPTER 10

Sperm Washing, Intrauterine Insemination (IUI), and Pergonal

I am now ready to explain the simpler types of treatment with the new technology, which are based on scientific information covered in the earlier chapters of this book. The simpler, new-tech treatments include washing the sperm to increase their fertilizing capability, placing the sperm nonsurgically past the cervix so as to bypass the cervical mucus barrier, and ovarian hyperstimulation with powerful drugs like Pergonal to improve the recruitment and maturing of eggs for ovulation and fertilization.

These techniques of sperm washing and ovarian hyperstimulation with Pergonal must also be employed with any GIFT or in vitro fertilization (IVF) procedure. Learning about these new techniques is a stepping stone toward complete understanding of in vitro fertilization and GIFT.

SPERM WASHING

Ironically, semen, the fluid in which the sperm is normally transferred to the female at intercourse, is the worst possible environment for sperm. Not only does sperm in an ejaculated semen specimen die rather quickly (anywhere from two to eight hours later), but in it sperm cannot undergo the rapid movement necessary to fertilize the egg. Furthermore, semen is, in a sense, a toxic substance in that if it is injected in volumes greater than 0.5 cc directly into the female's uterus, it causes violent cramps. So, while in the semen sperm are completely incapable of fertilizing the egg, semen placed directly into the female anywhere other than the vagina not only interferes with the fertilization process but can make the woman quite sick.

CAPACITATION

In the early days of infertility treatment, it used to be thought that if a man had a low sperm count or if the woman's cervical mucus were of poor quality, the semen specimen could be placed directly into her uterus, past the cervix, and thus bypass the cervical mucus barrier. What was quickly discovered instead is that she gets violent cramps of the uterus, and there is virtually no possibility of pregnancy occurring. Not only is semen toxic to the uterus, but it is also inhibitory to sperm. The inhibitory effect of semen on sperm is called "decapacitation," and the removal of sperm from the semen into the fluids of the female tract results in their "capacitation." Semen is actually toxic to sperm and can't be allowed to get past the vagina. The purpose of the cervical mucus is not only to slow down the sperm so that there is a constant reservoir of smaller numbers of sperm periodically going up into the fallopian tube. Another equally important purpose of the cervical mucus is to remove the sperm from the semen, and to keep the semen out of the uterus.

As early as the early 1960s (before the tremendous proliferation of knowledge about in vitro fertilization) it was thought that before sperm can fertilize, it has to reside for a certain period of time outside of the semen and within the "fluids of the female tract." This requirement for residence of the sperm in the female tract before fertilization could occur was called "capacitation." Sperm taken directly from the male animal and placed in the female animal would never cause her to get pregnant unless time were allowed for this "capacitation" process. It used to be thought that in some mysterious way the capacitation process required that sperm reside specifically within the female before they could fertilize, and it was felt that this would be a major limiting factor for the successful application of in vitro fertilization (IVF).

Now it is known that the capacitation process can occur in any of a dozen types of tissue culture fluids ("media"), and that the key factor in capacitation is not the specific nature of the fluid, but rather simply getting the sperm removed from the "decapacitating" effect of the semen into any other fluid that will still nourish them. The specific type of laboratory culture "media" the sperm are placed in after removal from the semen doesn't seem to matter much.

In natural fertilization, the exit of sperm from the semen into the cervical mucus and then into the uterus is what allows the sperm to capacitate. Once sperm enter the fallopian tube, their "capacitation" allows an explosion of increased motility that will be necessary for sperm to penetrate the egg. Only then can the "acrosome" (the enzyme-laden "warhead" that covers the front two-thirds of the spermhead) become capable of releasing its enzymes that allow the sperm to drill a hole through the outer "corona cells" and "zona pellucida" of the egg.

Thus, when sperm are removed from semen and placed in virtually any tissue culture fluid, two noticeable things happen. First, there is a tremendous increase in the velocity and character of sperm movement which increases the force of sperm propulsion twenty-fold (see Figure 22). Second, the acrosomal membrane, which holds the enzyme contents of the acrosome tightly sealed on the outside of the sperm head, becomes capable of dissolving and thereby releasing the acrosome's chemicals, which are necessary for drilling a hole through the zona pellucida of the egg. The tremendous increase in motility which occurs when the sperm are capacitated is called "hyperactivation," and the release of acrosomal contents is called the "acrosome reaction."

Simple sperm "washing" with common laboratory culture media has a dramatic effect on increasing the motility of the sperm. This increased motility results in a twenty-fold increase in "hydrodynamic power output." This augment in thrust is a necessary

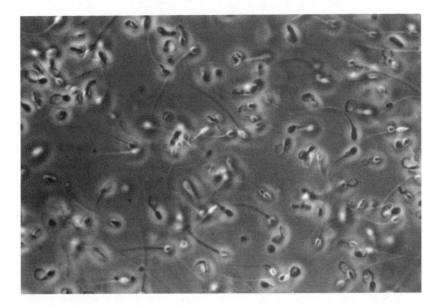

Figure 22. Microscopic view of tremendous increase in the velocity and the force of sperm propulsion after sperm are capacitated in culture fluid.

ingredient for penetration of the outer egg investments and allows penetration of the extremely resilient zona pellucida. This shifting of sperm into "high gear" is reserved for a time when there is imminent need for maximum thrust. These improvements in sperm function necessary for fertilization can all be accomplished in a test tube by simple sperm-washing methods without the need for any period of residence in the female tract.

Sperm washing is extremely important in the new technology. Whether for in vitro fertilization (IVF) in a test tube, placement of sperm and eggs together into the fallopian tube (GIFT), or simply insemination of the husband's own sperm into the wife via the cervix, prior washing of the sperm with the methods which are about to be described tremendously increases their motility, prepares them for the acrosome reaction, and dramatically enhances the efficiency of their ability to fertilize.

METHODS OF SPERM WASHING

Sperm washing is performed with nutrient fluid, or culture media, that is essentially no different from the media used to nourish the sperm and the egg during in vitro fertilization or GIFT procedures. The detailed requirements of these fluids for nourishing sperm, eggs, or for that matter any other cells one wants to culture will be of more interest in the context of the chapters on GIFT and in vitro fertilization (see Chapters 11 and 12).

Simple Sperm Wash with Centrifugation

The simplest method of sperm wash is merely to mix the semen with culture media (in a ratio three parts media to one part semen) in a test tube and then centrifuge it. By spinning the centrifuge tubes containing this semen–culture media mixture for about five minutes, the sperm all go to the very bottom in what is called a "button," a small, dense mass of millions of pure sperm completely separated from the relatively large volume of fluid that it came from (see Figure 23). The "supernatant" is the large volume of sperm-free fluid remaining over the "button."

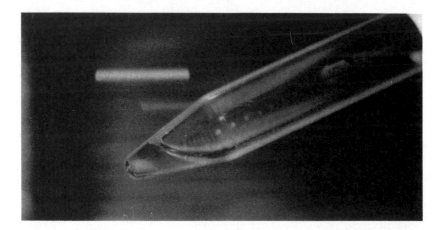

Figure 23. "Button" at the bottom of tube containing hundreds of millions of sperm after the semen is centrifuged.

This "supernatant" fluid is then taken off of the top with a pipette, or narrow tube, leaving the button at the bottom of the test tube intact. Then more culture media is added to the pure sperm and mixed thoroughly. This mixture of sperm and culture media is then spun in the centrifuge once again for five minutes. Once more there is a visible button of pure sperm on the bottom of the centrifuge tube and on top is pure culture media containing the extremely tiny residual amount of semen that had been left in the first button. This supernatant is then pipetted off the top again, and a small amount of fresh culture media is placed once more over the button and thoroughly mixed.

The end result of this simple "washing" technique is that the sperm are completely separated from the semen and now reside in pure culture media. Each time the sperm are centrifuged there is the risk of traumatizing them from the tremendous pressure applied by the spinning process. For this reason most laboratories have decided that two spins do minimal if any harm to the sperm and yet do get the sperm "clean" enough.

There are a number of problems with this very simple washing technique which make it not very suitable for in vitro fertilization (IVF) or GIFT procedures. With this simple technique, the live and dead sperm are not separated, and any white blood cells, bacteria, or debris that were present in the semen will still be present in this washed specimen. And while putting this type of washed sperm specimen in the uterus (intrauterine insemination) can be effective, most likely putting a lot of dead sperm and white blood cells in the culture dish next to the egg, or in the fallopian tube, could interfere with fertilization. For that reason better methods have been developed for removing the most motile and fertile portion of sperm from the washed specimen.

Swim-Up Technique

Probably the commonest method used to separate the most motile sperm for in vitro fertilization and GIFT is the "swim up." With this approach, after the sperm has undergone a simple wash, instead of just resuspending the button in fresh media, a small amount of culture media is gently placed on top of the button (usually about ⁴⁄₁₀₀ of a teaspoon). Then the test tube is put in an incubator or waterbath and kept at normal body temperature of 37°C, or 98.6°F. The most actively motile sperm actually swim up out of this solid mass of millions of sperm from the button into the media that has been overlayed on top of it. The more sluggish or nonmoving sperm, and the white blood cells and debris, are more likely to remain trapped in the button.

After about an hour the media that was overlayed on the button is pipetted off and used (see Figure 24). The rest of the button is simply discarded. After the swim-up technique, under the microscope the overlayed fluid shows very few dead sperm, and hardly any debris or white blood cells, and almost a pure preparation of highly motile sperm.

However, it is not always that simple. If the sperm quality in the first place was very poor in a couple with a severe "male factor" problem, even the man's best sperm may be very sluggish and slow about swimming up out of the button. In cases like these, more time (an hour and a half to two or three hours) is necessary in order to give these weaker sperm the best possible chance of swimming up. Even then, if the sperm are extremely weak, there may be a very poor swim-up preparation simply because so many of the dead sperm are getting in the way of the few live sperm.

The other problem with the swim-up technique is that sometimes the dead sperm or debris can just float up spontaneously, albeit more slowly than the active sperm, and a completely pure preparation of strictly the most fertile motile sperm is not achieved. Also, in the process of doing the swim up, many of the motile sperm that were simply not able to work their way to the top of the button and get into the supernatant can be lost.

With any method of sperm washing that tries to separate the good from the bad sperm, there will be a dramatic loss of large numbers of sperm. Nonetheless, despite these disadvantages, in most cases the swim-up technique gives a good preparation of capacitated sperm with improvement in percent motility and removal of much of the inactive sperm, debris, and white blood cells.

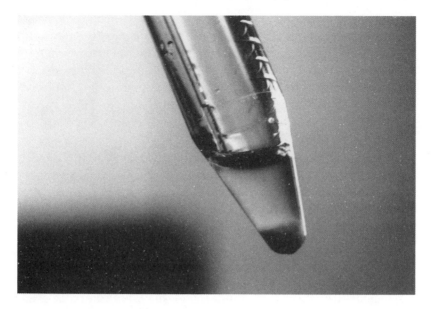

Figure 24. Pipetting supernatant after sperm have been allowed to swim up out of the pellet.

Migration Technique

The technique originally used by Steptoe and Edwards in England for separating sperm from the semen and trying to use only the most vigorously motile sperm is called the "migration" method. With this approach no centrifugation is necessary and there is no risk of harming the sperm from the tremendous g forces necessary to "spin them down" to the bottom of the tube. With this approach, about one cubic centimeter of raw, unprocessed semen is placed at that bottom of the centrifuge tube, and a small volume of pure culture media is gently overlayed on top of it. They do not mix because there is a great difference in their densities.

The preparation is placed in the incubator and motile sperm swim from the semen directly up into the culture media no differently than sperm deposited at the time of intercourse would swim out of the semen into the cervical mucus. After about an hour or longer, the culture media is then pipetted off the semen. As with the swim-up technique, you will find mostly vigorously motile, capacitated sperm in the media. The only problem with this method is that although the sperm are saved the trauma of centrifugation, there is a loss of much larger numbers that never make it out of the semen.

Migration/Sedimentation Technique of Jondet

When I visited Paris in the mid-1980s and saw my friend Professor Michael Jondet (one of the most innovative sperm scientists in the world, whose father was one of the scientists who developed the original methods for sperm freezing in the late 1940s), he was very excited to show me a simple, ridiculous-looking test-tubelike device that he had just invented (see Figure 25). This little tube that Jondet and his co-workers in Paris designed has a small central well at the bottom and a balcony-like rim around the top of the small central well. The tube is filled with pure culture media, and raw semen is placed in the circumferential balcony surrounding the central well. The tube is then placed in an incubator. Naturally, the most active sperm swim out of this balcony into the culture media above (no differently from what I described in the last section). The difference is that after the migration of sperm out of the semen into the culture media, most of them swim right over the edge of the balcony and fall down into the central well, which acts more or less like a trap. After two hours, when one takes the culture media out of the central well, almost like magic he discovers a magnificently pure motile preparation of sperm that have never been centrifuged.

When I came back from Europe and explained what I saw to some of the in vitro fertilization (IVF) clinic directors in the United States, they couldn't seem to understand how this simple little tube could work the way it does. Jondet's explanation was very simple. During the migration technique of Steptoe and Edwards the sperm that swim out of the semen into the culture media above are not specifically striving to continue coming out of the semen. They just go up and they also go down. This is true of the swim-up technique as well. Large numbers of motile

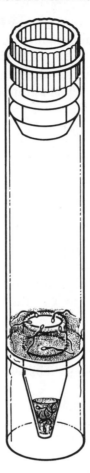

Figure 25. Migration sedimentation tubule of Jondet, which allows the most motile sperm to "jump over the edge of the balcony" into a collecting well at the bottom.

sperm are lost because they are not simply constantly trying to swim up out of the button or the semen that they came from. Rather, they are simply actively moving and that active movement in any random direction takes the most active ones out into the culture media. But just the same as they are moving up ("migrating") they are also moving down ("sedimenting").

So at the same time the "swim up" effect is taking place and the most motile sperm swim out of the button or out of the semen, sedimentation is also pulling them down by gravity. With Jondet's remarkable little tube, after the sperm swim out of the semen, as they "sediment," a large number fall off of the edge of this balcony and will remain trapped in the bottom of the central well of the tube. Only the most motile sperm that were able to swim out of the semen will be able to sediment down into the well. The less motile sperm will remain in the balcony.

This brilliant and simple method of Jondet's allows the removal of the most motile sperm by swim up and prevents excessive loss of sperm by trapping those that do swim up as they fall back down again, and it completely avoids the potentially damaging effect of centrifugation. This approach is more popular in Europe and South America than in the United States, simply because the Jondet tube is distributed by a European company. Nonetheless, they are available in the United States now through a distributor in Minneapolis, and this migration/sedimentation technique of Jondet may one day become popular everywhere.

Percoll Density Gradient

For over twenty years laboratories and blood banks have known how to separate white cells and red cells from blood with simple "density gradients." Most of these early density gradients were "radiopaque" fluids used in X-ray-type work to prevent the penetration of X rays and thus highlight whatever organ they are placed in. Their application in the cell biology laboratory therefore might first seem shocking, but these density gradients have now become one of the most effective methods of separating the most highly motile, fertile sperm from the ejaculate, and starting the capacitation process going probably more efficiently than any other method of sperm separation. This is called the "percoll" density gradient method for sperm separation.

Percoll is an extremely dense fluid which has a heavy weight but what is called a low "osmolality." That means that the individual molecules are very heavy, but there is a very low concentration of those molecules in a pure preparation. This would make percoll very toxic to any cells that were suspended in it because the "osmotic forces" of this low osmolality fluid would cause water to enter the cells and make them swell and die. One of the basic principles of biology is that any fluid that mixes with body fluids or cells must be the same osmolality (i.e., the same number of molecules per cubic centimeter) as that of body fluids (which is about 280 to 300 molecule equivalents, or milliosmols per cc). Therefore, before the percoll can be used for separating sperm, it must be mixed with a culture media that has an osmolality twenty times that of the body fluids. This results in a percoll solution that has the same number of molecules per cubic centimeter as body fluids, i.e., is "isosmotic." Once this is done, the percoll is no longer toxic and can be readily used for sperm separation.

With this technique three different layers of varying concentrations of "isosmotic" percoll are placed in a centrifuge tube: 95 percent percoll is placed on the bottom of the centrifuge tube; 75 percent percoll is placed carefully on top of this bottom layer (without allowing any mixing of the different layers); and 50 percent percoll is layered carefully on top of that. It is critical not to allow any mixing because sperm separation does not occur simply by virtue of going through the percoll. Sperm separation occurs by virtue of going through the "interface" between the various percoll density layers.

One cubic centimeter of raw uncentrifuged semen is then placed on top of this series of percoll density gradients, and the centrifuge tube is then spun for a full forty-five minutes. During this process something quite remarkable happens.

As the sperm are pushed down through the percoll gradients by centrifugation, poor quality sperm, as well as white blood cells, debris, and bacteria, are trapped in the upper interfaces (see Figure 26). The poorest quality sperm and white blood cells are trapped in the uppermost interfaces between the semen and the 50 percent percoll, and between the 50 percent percoll and the 75 percent percoll. Only the most motile, perfect sperm are able to get all the way down through all three interfaces to the bottom of the centrifuge tube. If such high-quality sperm are not present in the semen then the best sperm that are available at least should be able to get into the 95 percent percoll. If the sperm sample is a good one, a button will form at the bottom of the 95 percent percoll and will contain almost 100 percent perfect sperm without any debris, white blood cells, or poorly

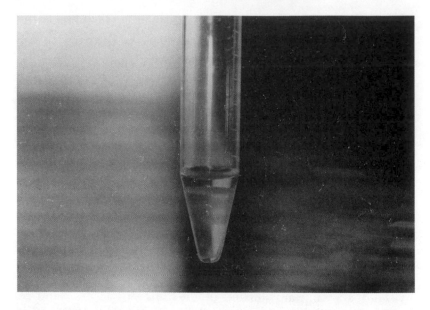

Figure 26. Dead sperm and white blood cells are trapped at higher levels of a "mini percoll" density gradient, and only the most fertile sperm reach the bottom of the tube.

motile sperm. The various interfaces between the other densities of percoll will form cloudy layers where the poor-quality sperm or white blood cells were stopped.

With the pipette, only the button is taken (if there is no button, the 95 percent percoll will be taken) and placed in another centrifuge tube with fresh media. We then wash the percoll out of this sperm twice. At the end of this procedure, despite several centrifugations, extremely hyperactivated, capacitated sperm, and very few (if any) poorly motile sperm or debris, are left. This method seems to get the purest preparation possible.

How does this miracle occur? There are two speculations: Different cells have different densities and different weights, and the least dense cells layer off on top of the gradients. Cells that weigh more per volume are denser and will "sink through" a density gradient under the pressure of centrifugation, while lighter or less dense cells will not sink through. The sperm head is nothing more than a highly compact, extremely condensed concentration of DNA (chromosomes) with a highly dense acrosome mounted on the front of it. Naturally, therefore, sperm are likely to go farther through the density gradient than white blood cells or debris. That's obvious. But, in addition, the most fertile sperm may be denser than the less fertile sperm, and therefore go right to the bottom while less dense sperm remain trapped in the upper interface.

Another speculation is that the most motile sperm have the greatest ability to penetrate an interface of two different density gradients because the constant movement makes them more likely to break through the surface tension and less likely to get caught. Under the influence of centrifugation, the most highly motile sperm would be more likely to penetrate to the bottom of the test tube than inactive or nonmotile components of the semen. It's obvious that if you throw a feather into the water it is likely to float on the surface, whereas if you throw a billiard ball into the water it will sink immediately to the bottom. Clearly, a less dense object is more likely to be caught higher up on the density gradients and not sink to the bottom than a dense object. However, if the feather had a vibratory mechanism in it that allowed it to stir up the surface tension of the water, that too would make it more likely to sink when tossed into the lake than a feather that simply fell flat on its back and had no motion of its own. It is likely that one of these two theories, if not both, are the explanation for the remarkable ability of the percoll gradient to separate out the most highly motile, highly fertile, morphologically normal sperm.

Now that you have learned all about how we wash the sperm, getting it out of the toxic atmosphere of the semen, producing a *natural* enhancement of their fertilizing ability by speeding up the process of "capacitation," you will want to know about other little magic tricks that can be done to the sperm that may enhance their fertilizability even further before they are put back inside of you or placed in culture with your eggs.

DRUGS AND AGENTS USED TO INCREASE SPERM MOTILITY IN VITRO

Caffeine, 2 Desoxyadenosine, and Pentoxyphyline

Caffeine is the most common pick-me-up'er prevalently used in our society. Many people have a hard time just getting up in the morning without their cup of coffee. It belongs to a class of chemicals called methyl xanthines that are metabolic stimulants. If these metabolic stimulants can wake us up in the morning, perhaps they could wake up our sperm as well. The three most commonly experimented with agents for trying to "wake up" sperm by enhancing their metabolism are readily available caffeine, 2 Desoxyadenosine, and Pentoxyphyline. Careful studies have demonstrated that these agents do sometimes enhance sperm motility dramatically, but more often only modestly. Nonetheless, there is no controversey that sperm motility is enhanced. Thus far nobody has been able to demonstrate, however, any increased fertilization resulting from this enhanced motility. It is probable that the increase in motility caused by these metabolic stimulants is just not dramatic enough to have any effect on the fertilization rate.

The motility of the frozen-thawed sperm was improved with caffeine, but there was no increase in fertilization caused by that enhanced motility. Similarly, disappointing results have been noted with the use of 2 Desoxyadenosine and Pentoxyphyline. However, Dr. John Yovich in Perth, Australia, still holds out some hope for Pentoxyphyline if the timing is right. He found in very preliminary studies that if Pentoxyphyline is added to the washed sperm too soon, the enhancement in motility lasts for only a brief period of up to one hour, and that is the time the sperm must be immediately added to the egg if increased fertilization is going to be noted. Nonetheless, despite his enthusiasm there is a feeling among many investigators that efforts to chemically stimulate weak sperm in order to enhance the possibility of fertilization may simply be whipping a dead horse. Only the future will tell.

Calcium, Calcium Ionophores, and Creatine Phosphate

When sperm are capacitated, their membranes suddenly become susceptible to the influx of calcium, and this is what helps trigger hyperactivated motility and begins the acrosome reaction. Dr. Gabor Huszar from Yale University's sperm physiology laboratory found that by adding calcium to the culture media, sperm motility increased dramatically. When he added a "calcium blocker," motility was decreased dramatically. Thus it was very clear to him that calcium in the sperm-washing media (calcium is present in almost all medias that are used in in vitro fertilization or sperm washing) can enhance sperm motility. He did not find that magnesium or other ions had the same effect. The effect of calcium was quite specific. As with the other sperm motility stimulants it is not yet known whether there is any practical value in terms of increased fertilization rates.

Test-Yolk Buffer

One of the most common agents used to increase sperm's fertilizing ability is a disgusting-looking yellow fluid called "test-yolk buffer." Originally this test-yolk buffer (a large proportion of which is slightly heat-treated raw egg yolk) was used for low-temperature preservation of sperm without freezing. Unwashed sperm in semen can be preserved in a refrigerator without freezing for at least two to three days if mixed with this "test-yolk buffer." If this is used in combination with glycerol for sperm freezing, it also gives better results than glycerol alone.

Sperm that have been stored at this low temperature with test-yolk buffer for just twenty-four hours tend to have a higher fertilization rate after washing and in vitro fertilization than sperm prepared without this method. In other words, not only does the test-yolk buffer allow prolonged cold preservation of sperm, but it also enhances the ability of sperm so preserved for twenty-four hours to fertilize. Of course, after the semen has been stored with test-yolk buffer it must be carefully washed in the fashion described earlier. Indeed when sperm is first extracted from the test-yolk buffer solution it has slower motility than sperm that was not preserved this way. Eventually the motility picks up and the fertilization rate is high.

The question is, how does twenty-four-hour storage of semen at cold temperatures in this hideous solution improve the sperm's ability to fertilize? It appears that incubation for eighteen hours in test-yolk buffer causes removal of certain fatty components of the sperm membrane, particularly cholesterol. When the test-yolk buffer is washed out of the sperm with the standard two-step sperm wash technique, the fatty components of the sperm membrane are removed, which increases the percentage of acrosome-reacting sperm.

But this is still not a magic solution for poor sperm. All of the methods described for chemically stimulating the fertilizability of sperm seem to offer some hope for the future but there is no definite proof that any of them enhance the pregnancy rate over the effect simply obtained by capacitating the sperm through the washing techniques described in the earlier part of this chapter.

INTRAUTERINE INSEMINATION (IUI) OF WASHED SPERM

Now that you have learned about the remarkable things that can be done in the laboratory to "improve" the motility and the fertilizability of the sperm, not to mention the benefit of just getting it out of the semen, what can be done with this washed and improved sperm to increase the chances of getting pregnant? Obviously these methods of sperm washing are necessary for in vitro fertilization (IVF) where eggs are fertilized in a test tube. An egg can't simply be fertilized by using unwashed sperm in semen. And a GIFT procedure can't be performed without these sperm-washing techniques because a pure suspension of semen can't be placed in the fallopian tube without expectation of anything but terrible results. The sperm simply have to be removed from the semen and placed in culture media in order to perform GIFT or in vitro fertilization.

The Concept of IUI

Is there some way the improvement in sperm quality resulting from the washing can be used to achieve pregnancy simply by inseminating this sperm back into the vagina or uterus? This notion became extremely popular in 1982 when it was first introduced by Dr. Val Davajan at the University of Southern California Medical Center, along with Dr. Richard Marrs who had started one of the earliest in vitro fertilization programs in this country. They were trying to see if, by placing washed sperm directly into the uterus (IUI) and bypassing the cervix and cervical mucus barrier, they could accomplish results equivalent to in vitro fertilization but with obviously much greater simplicity. Since their initial report there has been an explosion of interest in this approach, and virtually every infertility patient goes through a series of IUI's (whether rightly or wrongly) before she takes the step up toward in vitro fertilization or GIFT.

The idea behind this approach is a very good one. This procedure can be performed easily in the office without any surgery, anesthesia, or sedation whatsoever. The patient feels no different than she would from a pelvic exam, and a complicated laboratory setup is not necessary. It is logical to expect a higher pregnancy rate because such greater numbers of viable sperm will reach the uterus with this technique than with normal intercourse. That is why it is so popular and so widely used. But in truth pregnancy rates with this procedure are not great. Many pregnancies have resulted from this procedure, but there have been virtually no adequate controlled studies to see whether the intrauterine insemination of washed sperm increases the pregnancy rate over what would have resulted simply from normal timed intercourse.

Results with IUI (and Pergonal)

The enthusiasm for the technique increased in early 1984 when Dr. Geoffrey Scher from the Northern Nevada Fertility Clinic presented fourteen couples with long-standing infertility associated either with poor cervical mucus, male infertility, or unexplained infertility. The women were all stimulated with Pergonal to create greater ovulation, and washed "capacitated" sperm were placed through the cervix into the uterus at the time of ovulation. Five of these fourteen women got pregnant (35 percent); and on the basis of that extremely small uncontrolled study a lot of people got very excited that there would be a simple dramatic solution to infertility problems using the sperm-washing technology. The question, however, is whether just stimulating ovulation alone with Pergonal and allowing timed intercourse would have resulted in the same pregnancy rate for that small group of patients. Did the intrauterine insemination of washed sperm help? And could such a high pregnancy rate per cycle be sustained in a larger sampling of patients? Since then, studies have shown much lower pregnancy rates with this approach (less than 8 percent per cycle) in most centers.

Dr. Yovich in late 1986 reported that out of 426 cycles of patients only 40 got pregnant (9 percent). During the same time period with equivalent patients undergoing GIFT, 30 percent became pregnant. The GIFT procedure is generally four times more likely to result in a pregnancy in any cycle than IUI and Pergonal. For infertility not related to tubal blockage, intrauterine insemination with Pergonal is cheaper and simpler but much less likely to yield a pregnancy than GIFT.

The results with intrauterine insemination and Pergonal have been disastrous when the husband's sperm had poor-quality motility. The pregnancy rate for most "causes" of infertility are 8 percent per cycle with intrauterine insemination, but intrauterine insemination on its own without Pergonal yields much lower pregnancy rates. It is only its combination with ovulatory stimulation that seems to result in a respectable 8 to 10 percent pregnancy rate per cycle. Intrauterine insemination alone timed to the wife's cycle is not likely to improve the chance for pregnancy unless combined with ovarian stimulation, preferably with Pergonal.

Timing the IUI

How is intrauterine insemination timed? Unlike natural intercourse, with intrauterine insemination the object is to put the sperm in the uterus after ovulation, when the egg is already waiting in the fallopian tube. Bypassing the normal cervical mucus barrier, the sperm are likely to go on up into the fallopian tube and out the peritoneal cavity in just a matter of hours. Therefore, the intrauterine insemination is best not to be done on the day of LH rise as with timed intercourse. It is better to wait until the day the follicle disappears and then have the insemination performed.

WHEN TO GIVE UP ON IUI (AND PERGONAL) AND GO TO GIFT OR IVF

Many couples go through months and even years of intrauterine insemination never knowing when might be the appropriate time to go on to GIFT or in vitro fertilization (IVF).

Intrauterine insemination (IUI) without Pergonal or some form of ovarian stimulation has such a low pregnancy rate that it probably isn't worthwhile considering. When intrauterine insemination is combined with ovarian stimulation, unless the sperm is really poor, the pregnancy rate per cycle is about 8 percent. Whether a woman should go through two cycles of ovarian stimulation and IUI, or twelve cycles, before considering GIFT or IVF is difficult to answer. Pergonal stimulation and its monitoring represents almost one-third of the cost of a GIFT procedure. Furthermore, it represents a tremendous expenditure of time and energy, including showing up every day for an ultrasound and blood test.

Thus, for the low pregnancy rate of 8 percent, and the tremendous amount of time and cost going into it, my personal recommendation is to go to a procedure that gives a higher yield (such as GIFT) if three cycles of Pergonal and IUI have not yet resulted in a pregnancy. Other physicians may suggest that you go through six cycles, eight cycles, or twelve cycles; it is a matter of personal judgment.

There have been many happy patients who have gotten pregnant with Pergonal and IUI. I do not mean to cast a negative pall on this technique because it avoids surgery, anesthesia, and a lot of laboratory expenses. In fact, before the GIFT procedure was developed (1985–1986), an 8 percent pregnancy rate per month was quite sensational, and certainly as good as in vitro fertilization (IVF) was at that time. In 1984 there was no option of going to a GIFT procedure, and it was certainly preferable to use Pergonal and IUI to IVF if the fallopian tubes were normal.

The husband of one couple treated with this technique was a man I met up with in the wilderness of Alaska. We were camped out at a small lodge which he had helped to develop hundreds of miles from the nearest road, surrounded by beautiful mountains and a lake scene so serene that you only see it in posters. He told me he had tried unsuccessfully for thirteen years to have a child and wanted to know my opinion. When you are sitting by a fire roasting marshmallows after having had a couple of glasses of wine, such subjects come up readily.

Back home, after looking over their records showing that he had an extremely high-quality sperm count with good motility, and that his wife was menstruating regularly and had perfectly normal fallopian tubes, I looked them straight in the eye and told them that I thought we would be able to get them pregnant. But they would have to be patient and willing to come back over and over and over again for multiple cycles of treatment because she might not get pregnant on the first cycle, she might not get pregnant on the fifth cycle, and she might not even get pregnant on the tenth cycle. What I had in mind was Pergonal and IUI. We didn't even know about GIFT then. With his sperm quality being so good I figured on an 8 percent chance of pregnancy per month.

They flew all the way down from Alaska (having to rearrange important business plans and totally disrupt their life) for six cycles of treatment over a year's time. Still she was not pregnant. Finally, on the seventh try, after over a year of many visits, she finally got pregnant and delivered a beautiful baby girl. A few years later they came back to St. Louis again. But this time she got pregnant with the very first cycle of Pergonal and IUI.

Since sperm washing and intrauterine insemination techniques don't seem to be very effective, unless combined with ovarian stimulation (preferably with Pergonal), we will devote the last portion of this "transitional" chapter to how we stimulate your ovaries with Pergonal.

OVARIAN STIMULATION WITH PERGONAL

A common cause of failure to achieve pregnancy is poor quality ovulation. Even when ovulation does occur, there may be a subtle, barely detectable defect in follicle maturation which makes the egg less fertilizable. Some fertility doctors are of the opinion that they can detect "sub-optimum" ovulation by noting a slow, late-rising basal body temperature, a short (less than fourteen days) luteal phase, or poor cervical mucus at mid-cycle. But often physicians just can't be sure there is anything clearly wrong with a cycle, and yet there may be a problem that could hamper the proper preparation of the egg for fertilization. Remember from Chapter 3 that the FSH stimulation in the follicular phase and the LH surge that induces "ovulation" accomplish a lot more than just "ovulation." The early FSH stimulation makes the egg grow, forms its protective outer "zona pellucida" covering, and then makes the follicle surrounding the egg fill with estrogen-rich fluid, while the estrogen in turn prepares the uterine lining and the cervical mucus for sperm entry. The LH surge then causes the egg to resume "meiosis," or "reduction division," of the number of chromosomes from forty-six to twenty-three, an absolute genetic necessity before the sperm's twenty-three chromosomes can unite with the egg. So a lot more is happening under the stimulation of FSH and LH than just "ovulation."

The most effective and powerful method for stimulating your ovary is the drug Pergonal. The reason that Pergonal is so effective is that it is a purified preparation of FSH (with some LH also) which directly stimulates the ovary in the early part of the cycle to make better and more follicles. Pergonal does not just act indirectly by stimulating the pituitary gland to make more FSH (as Clomid does); Pergonal is the FSH itself. Thus it is more direct and potent than any other treatment utilized for stimulating ovulation. But Pergonal only sets the stage for proper ovulation by inducing the formation of good follicles in the first half of the cycle. For ovulation to occur, you then need an injection of HCG (the equivalent of LH) when the follicles are mature and ready. Since LH is not available as an injectable drug, we must use an equivalent, called HCG (human chorionic gonadotropin).

LUPRON TO PREVENT PREMATURE LH SURGE

It is important in the follicular phase of egg maturation that not very much LH be present. Naturally there is going to be some LH in Pergonal, but this is an insignificant amount as long as the pituitary does not respond with a "premature" LH increase. In a normal cycle, as the estrogen level goes up toward mid-cycle and surges to a high level around day twelve or thirteen, this estrogen surge stimulates the pituitary to suddenly release a huge amount of LH, the so-called "LH surge." This LH surge causes the mature egg to resume "reduction division" (meiosis), and the follicle to ovulate within twenty-four to forty-eight hours later. If the LH goes up too early before the egg is ready, it is much less likely to fertilize, and the pregnancy rate is much lower. Premature LH rise seems to "poison" the egg in some way, so LH must only be allowed to go up when the egg is mature and ready for the ovulatory surge. Also, in IVF or GIFT cycles, care is taken not to lose the eggs by premature ovulation prior to follicle aspiration, and this is another reason to prevent LH surge. For this reason it has become very popular to give a drug called Lupron beginning on day one of the cycle because it prevents a premature LH release.

The only reason the pituitary can secrete FSH and LH is that the primitive region of the brain, the "hypothalamus," releases a short brief pulse of GNRH hormone every ninety minutes. A drug like Lupron (or in Europe, Buserelin) is a GNRH "agonist," which means it first stimulates, and then completely prevents the pituitary from releasing GNRH.

Therefore, when you start on Lupron, for the first three days there is a tremendous increase in the pituitary's release of FSH and LH. But after five days the pituitary has become "down regulated" and then it is completely incapable of releasing any more LH or FSH on its own until the drug is stopped. (Once the drug is stopped the pituitary begins to function normally again very quickly.) Thus, if a woman is started on a Pergonal regimen, placing her on Lupron first will completely control the pituitary and prevent an early slow-rise of LH, which could poison the egg, or a premature LH surge which would cause you to ovulate unpredictably too early, before the egg is ready.

Lupron can be administered in either of two fashions. It can be started in the luteal phase of the preceding cycle or on day one of the stimulated cycle. If Lupron is given during the luteal phase of the previous cycle, then after about five days the pituitary is "down regulated." By the time you start your first injection of Pergonal (usually on day one, two, or three of the next cycle) your pituitary will not be able to release its own FSH or LH and thereby interfere with the Pergonal regimen. Many doctors prefer this "luteal phase Lupron" approach because they don't want LH levels to be elevated in the early part of the cycle.

On the other hand, if you want to reduce the overall amount of Pergonal that has to be given, or if you want to get greater stimulation in a woman who has resistant ovaries, you could give Lupron beginning day one of the cycle, and take advantage of the early stimulatory effect of Lupron on your pituitary. By day five of the cycle, the pituitary will no longer be stimulated, and the benefit of LH suppression will have begun in plenty of time for there to be no risk of a mid-cycle LH rise.

There is a great deal of debate about which is the best way to administer Lupron, beginning in the luteal phase or in the follicular phase. Needless to say, the results with both approaches are quite good. Both approaches accomplish the remarkable objective of preventing early LH rise and dramatically improving the pregnancy rates with Pergonal stimulation, whether using just intrauterine insemination, intercourse, or GIFT and IVF.

HOW IS PERGONAL MADE? WHAT IS IT?

Pergonal and HCG are "natural," not synthetic, hormones. The way in which this drug was prepared is at once humorous and probably would want to make any infertile woman who has benefited from it cry.

As you get older and go through menopause, your ovaries eventually run out of eggs and shrivel up into very small, pea-sized, atrophied organs that no longer make estrogen. In women who have passed the age of menopause their pituitary makes enormous amounts of FSH in response to the lack of "negative" feedback from the ovaries. When the ovary is no longer present, your FSH level goes sky high. Since FSH is excreted largely in the urine, the urine of a postmenopausal woman has enormous amounts of FSH (as well as LH) in it.

Serono, a drug company in Italy that produces Pergonal, simply needed to find a way of harvesting huge amounts of this FSH-rich urine in an efficient manner so that it could be processed for extraction of FSH. So they arranged for nunneries to have central processing vats in which all of the postmenopausal nuns would urinate. Instead of just having volunteers bring in daily bottles of urine (which is a cumbersome way to commercially collect enough urine to prepare Pergonal), they simply collected the urine from huge vats in institutes like nunneries. Obviously, these postmenopausal nuns were more than excited to donate their services for this enterprise because they knew that it would lead to hundreds of thousands of infertile women being able to get pregnant.

Naturally there is some LH in human menopausal gonadotropin. This can't be avoided because postmenopausal women will have increased LH as well as FSH. The amount of this LH, however, is physiologically not very significant. Nonetheless, Serono does have another menopausal gonadotropin called "Metrodin," which is purified FSH with all of the LH removed. Interestingly, this Metrodin that the company went to great lengths to manufacture is not very potent compared to Pergonal, which has led us all to conclude that some LH, though only a small amount, is required along with FSH to stimulate proper follicular development even in the early phase of the cycle. Nonetheless, many clinics will stimulate you with a combination of Pergonal and Metrodin out of the fear that giving Pergonal alone with its LH contaminant might raise the LH level a little too high. We have not found that to be a problem however.

We have already said the Pergonal merely sets the stage for

maturation of the egg, but ovulation does not take place unless HCG (human chorionic gonadotropin) is administered. Why not just give an injection of LH? Why give HCG? For that matter, what is HCG? We don't have any preparations of LH that are potent enough to mimic the normal mid-cycle LH surge. So HCG is used in its place because it is so readily available and has the same exact physiological effect.

HCG (human chorionic gonadotropin) is the hormone produced by the placenta of pregnant women to stimulate the ovary to make the progesterone and estrogen necessary to maintain the pregnancy. Therefore, this drug is easily obtainable by purifying the urine from pregnant women. It may not be LH, but it does the same thing LH does, and it is readily available.

Pergonal is extremely expensive. A single vial costs $40 and a monthly cycle can vary from $800 to $1,500, not including the cost of ultrasound ($400–$600) and daily estrogen tests ($300–$500). It is so potent that its dosage must be monitored daily by blood estrogen levels and ultrasound of the ovaries. Therefore, the decision to use Pergonal should not be taken lightly. Yet it is so much more effective than less expensive alternatives that it is the major "workhorse" of most infertility centers. The only problem is that the company has a worldwide monopoly which allows it to charge whatever exorbitant amount of money it desires. If it had competition, the costs might be more affordable.

Hyperstimulation Syndrome

When Pergonal was first available, doctors did not know about the importance of monitoring daily estrogen levels, and ultrasound wasn't available. There was a high incidence of multiple births and serious "hyperstimulation syndrome," and even a few deaths. With modern monitoring (daily) of blood estrogen levels, ultrasound evaluation of the follicles, and appropriate modification of dosage, these dangerous complications should not be a problem. One to 3 percent of women undergoing Pergonal therapy will get a mild degree of hyperstimulation despite the most careful monitoring. The rare patient today who develops severe hyperstimulation must go into the hospital, have intravenous fluids for several days, and wait for her ovaries to reduce in size and for her body to readjust. This unlikely complication should not scare you away from Pergonal because nowadays we are quite well equipped to handle it.

The cause of "hyperstimulation syndrome" is that ovaries with all of these budding follicles are loaded with estrogen. When you ovulate from a large number of follicles a huge amount of estrogen-rich fluid is poured directly out of the enlarged and fragile ovaries into the abdominal cavity. This estrogen then coats the "peritoneal" surface of the abdominal cavity and causes it to become very permeable to fluid leakage. Fluid (serum) literally pours out of your bloodstream into the peritoneal cavity because of the "leakiness" of the abdominal cavity's lining caused by this large amount of estrogen-rich fluid. Your abdomen swells, you get lightheaded with relatively low blood pressure, and you may get dizzy because of decreased blood volume. At one time this was a very dangerous condition only because it was not fully understood.

Doctors would treat this condition in the past by withholding fluids under the mistaken impression that this would somehow or other prevent the abdominal cavity from filling with so much fluid. The problem is that the blood volume that is lost has to be replaced with intravenous fluid. Secondly, something has to be done to eliminate the continued irritation of the lining of the abdomen with this estrogen-rich fluid. We now know that by putting a small "paracentesis" catheter into the abdomen and draining all of this fluid, the patient is made much more comfortable, she can breathe more easily, and by getting rid of this estrogen irritation, fluid leakage into the abdomen slows down dramatically. Thus, even in the very rare cases of severe hyperstimulation syndrome, knowledgeable treatment makes the likelihood of any dangerous outcome very remote.

Many women will have mild degrees of hyperstimulation syndrome with a little bit of lower abdominal swelling, discomfort, and dizziness. This does not require hospitalization, just a little bed rest at home. It is only the rare, severe cases that require hospitalization.

Interestingly, a woman going through GIFT or IVF is much less likely to develop hyperstimulation syndrome of any kind than if she is receiving Pergonal and IUI treatment alone. The reason is that the ovarian follicles are emptied by a needle, and very little estrogen-rich fluid leaks into the abdominal cavity. Thus, despite overproduction of large numbers of eggs (greater than twenty), it is very unlikely that hyperstimulation syndrome will develop. Thus not only is GIFT and IVF more likely to result in a pregnancy than a standard Pergonal cycle, but is also less likely to result in the complication of hyperstimulation syndrome.

The worst cases of hyperstimulation syndrome occur when a woman becomes pregnant. This is because her placenta is making HCG and stimulating the ovaries to continue to pour out large amounts of estrogen-rich fluid. So although it is a very unpleasant side effect to endure, hyperstimulation syndrome often means good news.

RESULTS AND MULTIPLE BIRTHS

More than 90 percent of patients can be induced to ovulate with Pergonal. About 10 percent per month will get pregnant, but some will not unless they go to higher percentage procedures like GIFT. These are dramatic figures, since the group of patients who receive Pergonal would not be likely to have conceived without it. Anywhere from 10 to 25 percent of the pregnancies are multiple births, which are usually twins, but can sometimes be triplets, and very rarely quadruplets. These women require a great deal of FSH activity to stimulate proper follicle development. This obviously results in many follicles and more than one ripe ovulation.

With any infertility treatment designed to stimulate ovulation, there is a risk of multiple births. Twins and triplets create obstetrical problems, but the couple is usually happy with such an outcome. Quadruplets or quintuplets are generally an extremely dangerous complication. The likelihood of multiple births is extremely low, but if it occurs, it can be a disaster. The odds are that most such children will die or be severely retarded, and the mother runs a much greater risk of danger to her life and health as well. Any couple entering treatment for infertility must be aware of this risk, however small it may be.

The risk of multiple births can be kept down by the doctor not administering HCG if the woman has a huge number of follicles. Actually, it should be understood that going to a GIFT or in vitro fertilization (IVF) procedure reduces the risk of multiple pregnancies even further because the doctor is able to obtain every one of the eggs and put back only the number that he thinks would safely give the best chance of pregnancy.

Another option which every couple must think about carefully and decide ahead of time is "selective reduction." With modern ultrasound techniques the embryonic sac can be detected as early as four weeks after fertilization, and before the sac gets very big, the ultrasonographer can very easily insert a needle and remove some of them. To some, such a procedure might carry a moral or ethical problem, and each couple will have to decide whether they will take advantage of this modern option that could convert the potential tragedy of quintuplets into the joy of healthy twins. Most religious leaders who have pondered this problem have decided that since this procedure, "selective reduction," salvages the lives of at least two or three of the fetuses, and reduces dramatically the obstetric risks to the mother, it is ethically quite justifiable.

MONITORING PERGONAL
AND TIMING WHEN TO GIVE HCG

Pergonal will only mature the eggs and prepare the follicles for ovulation. Resumption of genetic preparation of the egg for fertilization, and then ovulation, must be induced at the appropriate time by the injection of HCG. If the follicles develop too rapidly and the estrogen level climbs out of control, it is a warning that it would be dangerous for this woman to ovulate. As long as she is not given her HCG injection at mid-cycle, the woman will not develop hyperstimulation syndrome. She can then be given a month or so to rest, and her ovaries will shrink back to a more normal size. But if she is given HCG when her ovaries are too enlarged, the follicles may have reached enormous proportions, producing inordinate amounts of estrogen, and the ovulation induced by HCG could be the intra-abdominal catastrophe already discussed. Despite severe ovarian enlargement, with ten to thirty follicles and a sky-high estrogen level, she will be in no danger as long as HCG is not administered. Furthermore, if she decides to do GIFT or IVF, even a huge number of follicles and a very high estrogen level is not really dangerous, because the follicles will be aspirated.

How does the physician decide on which day to give HCG? How do we know that the egg has matured enough that it is ready for the LH stimulus to resume meiosis, and that the follicle is mature enough and ready to proceed with ovulation? With modern ultrasound imaging, the function of the estrogen level has become much less important than the actual visualization of the follicle. The estrogen level is just a confirmation that the follicle is mature, but most of our decision making is based upon the actual size and appearance of the follicles.

When the leading (or biggest) follicles have reached greater than 2.0 cm (four-fifths of an inch) in diameter, they have reached the stage of maturity where they are ready for HCG. At this stage each mature follicle should be releasing about 200 picograms per ml of estrogen. Thus if one has ten mature follicles in the ovary, the estrogen level at this point should be about 2,000 picograms per ml. If one has five mature follicles in the ovaries, the estrogen level should be around 1,000 picograms per ml. So the time to give HCG is judged by the follicular size, and it is verified that the eggs are mature by seeing whether the estrogen is at a high-enough level for that number of follicles. For IVF or GIFT the more follicles the better. We're happy to have more than ten or twenty. With just Pergonal and IUI, it is better to have a smaller number (three to six would be ideal). Sometimes it is very hard to adequately control the number of follicles achieved in an ovarian stimulation, and for that reason once again GIFT and IVF are procedures which in many respects are simpler than just plain Pergonal stimulation with IUI.

INDICATIONS FOR USING PERGONAL

Typical cases of successful pregnancy achieved with Pergonal teach us a great deal about what does and doesn't cause infertility. In the late 1970s, when it was generally postulated that Pergonal must only be given in the most recalcitrant cases of nonovulation and never without a clear-cut diagnosis, I was approached by a woman who had been trying unsuccessfully for ten years to get pregnant. Her husband had been told by a local urologist that his sperm count was "too low" (40 million per cc with 90 percent motility). They had gone through as detailed an ovulatory workup as was available in the late 1970s. As far as one could tell, her ovulation was normal, her cycles were regular, her laparoscopy was normal, and there was no tubal disease. No one was willing to treat her because they did not have any diagnosis other than the so-called low sperm count in the husband, which was not really a valid diagnosis anyway.

I knew her biological clock was ticking, and I also knew there were complex genetic processes taking place during the monthly cycle of ovarian stimulation that went beyond the simple issue of whether or not the woman was ovulating. I knew it would be considered quite radical at that time to administer Pergonal to such a patient, but with ten years of infertility behind her, and approaching her late thirties, I went ahead and gave it a try. She got pregnant during the first cycle.

The first scientific paper openly advocating the use of Pergonal therapy in patients with idiopathic infertility (infertility of unknown cause) came from Dr. Alan De Cherney of Yale University. He openly attempted "empirical Pergonal therapy" for patients in whom he had no idea why they were infertile. Most previous studies for Pergonal always tried to come up with some kind of diagnosis no matter how shaky it might have been. Dr. De Cherney noted a 12.7 percent pregnancy rate per cycle using Pergonal in couples with long-term infertility of unknown origin, and his control group of patients undergoing no treatment had only a 1 percent pregnancy rate per cycle. De Cherney was the first to openly suggest what was for some reason embarrassing to most of us to discuss so frankly: the administration of Pergonal to couples with documented long-term infertility of unknown origin despite the lack of a clear-cut diagnosis of poor ovulation.

No longer do we have to struggle to try to manufacture a diagnosis of some kind of ovulatory defect in these patients. Now it is known that there is a tremendous amount of preparation the egg must go through during the first half of the cycle in order to be fertilized, and these preparations are aided by an increased level of FSH. Ovarian stimulation is useful in most cases of infertility not caused by tubal blockage because it enhances whatever subtle defect might exist in the whole process of egg maturation and preparation for fertilization.

Directions Which My Patients Follow for Pergonal Treatment

Pergonal, Lupron, and HCG must all be given by injection. They cannot be given as a pill. The following is the protocol I usually recommend for my patients (see "Pergonal Regimen Summary Chart," page 262). Begin by giving yourself daily Lupron injections. Day one of your cycle, the first day of menstruation, is the day you start Lupron. Day three of your cycle will be the first day you receive Pergonal. The Lupron injections will continue until the day of your HCG injection.

You will need to have a preliminary ultrasound to be sure there are no ovarian cysts. If there are large cysts, they will be aspirated before beginning Pergonal. On the third day of Lupron injections you will begin Pergonal, referred to as "day one of Pergonal." On days one through three of Pergonal you would usually receive three ampules of Pergonal each day. On day four of Pergonal you will start daily monitoring, which includes rapid estrogens and ultrasound. You find out in the afternoon, based on these results, how much Pergonal you are to receive that afternoon or that evening.

When your estrogen levels are in the appropriate range (usually between 600 and 2,000 pg/ml, but more specifically about 200 pg/ml per mature follicle on ultrasound), and you have at least one follicle greater than 2.0 cm in size on ultrasound, that means that your follicles are ripe enough for ovulation to be triggered. On that day you no longer take Pergonal but rather an injection of 10,000 units of HCG. Normally nine to ten days of Pergonal are necessary before the follicles are ripe enough for HCG. The HCG triggers ovulation between thirty-six and forty-eight hours after injection. Timing of intercourse is critical. You should start having daily sex beginning the day after HCG and continue until the ultrasound shows disappearance of at least

PERSONAL REGIMEN SUMMARY CHART

month/year _____ Cycle of Pergonal

Patient Name: _____
Day 1 of menses _____/_____ Norlutate/Lupron began _____
_____/_____ Patient told no sex after Lupron begins

Day of Week	Date	Day of Pergonal	Follicle Sizes Right	Left	Estrogen Level	Rapid LH	Medication/SS Lupron/Pergonal/HCG (How Much)	Patient Received Prescription Date	Initial
Monday	1/1/90						Norlutate 10 mgs. daily begins		
Wednesday	1/10/90						Last day of Norlutate 10 mgs. daily		
Saturday	1/13/90						Lupron 0.2 mL. daily injections begin		
Monday	1/15/90	1					Pergonal 3 amps		
Tuesday	1/16/90	2					Pergonal 3 amps		
Wednesday	1/17/90	3					Pergonal 3 amps		
Thursday	1/18/90	4					Pergonal 3 amps		
Friday	1/19/90	5					Pergonal 3 amps		
Saturday	1/20/90	6					Pergonal 3 amps		
Sunday	1/21/90	7					Pergonal 3 amps		
Monday	1/22/90	8					Pergonal 3 amps		
Tuesday	1/23/90	9					Pergonal 3 amps		
Wednesday	1/24/90	10					Last day of Lupron medication 10,000 units of HCG		
Thursday	1/25/90								
Friday	1/26/90								
Saturday	1/27/90								
Sunday	1/28/90								
Monday	1/29/90						Progesterone ½ cc daily injections begin and continue x 6 weeks		
Friday	2/9/90						Beta HCG blood test		

_____/_____ This is the date menses began

PLAN PER DR. SILBER IF NO PREGNANCY THIS CYCLE:
_____ Skip 1 cycle, then Pergonal
_____ Other:

Receipt #:

H-81/08-23-89

one follicle, indicating ovulation. If you are having IUI, it should be performed on the day the follicle disappears.

PROGESTERONE INJECTIONS

Because Pergonal cycles sometimes exhibit early cessation of progesterone production and subsequent loss of pregnancy, you may require progesterone injections beginning two to five days after HCG. The package insert from the FDA on progesterone may scare you quite unnecessarily because it alleges in big, bold letters a risk of fetal damage from progesterone injections. However, no physicians I know of who specialize in infertility or in vitro fertilization anywhere in the world feel that this warning is valid. Progesterone is just the natural hormone you normally make during pregnancy to allow the embryo to implant and grow. You would not be taking any synthetic progesteronelike substances, but rather just the same, exact progesterone your body should normally be making. Nonetheless, any pregnancy carries the risk of fetal abnormality, however low, and it would be foolish not to acknowledge such a risk. I sincerely do not believe that progesterone (or any of our treatments for that matter) in any way increases that risk. Progesterone is just a natural hormone that your placenta needs to keep the pregnancy alive.

The absurdity of government involvement in this field is exemplified by such a stupid FDA warning packet on progesterone. In fact, Lupron, which prevents the premature LH surge and has been responsible for almost doubling the pregnancy rate with GIFT and IVF, is approved by the government *only for use in cancer of the prostate*. Virtually no one uses it for cancer of the prostate since better treatments are available for that, but every infertility specialist in the world uses it for ovulation induction, despite no FDA approval. The FDA is so burdened by congressionally mandated bureaucracy that no intelligent review by the government of any aspect of this field seems possible. So don't let the package insert on progesterone worry you.

NORLUTATE FOR TIMING THE CYCLE

Sometimes your cycle will come at an inconvenient time for you, your husband, or even your doctor. If that is the case, the first day of Lupron and Pergonal treatment can be delayed by taking a simple progesteronelike pill called Norlutate during the follicular phase of the cycle before. The dosage is 10 mg per day (two tablets). This pill will "put you on hold" quite safely until it is time to start day one of Lupron and Pergonal treatment. In fact, this approach, called "programming" your treatment cycle, allows us to schedule the days your husband has to be available months ahead of time. You're usually likely to require eight to ten days of Pergonal. So we can plan rather precisely when you will have either your GIFT or IVF procedure, or sex. You just discontinue Norlutate three days before we wish to begin Lupron plus Pergonal. We plan ahead what day (plus or minus one, or at most two) that you want your GIFT on, and just count back to figure out when to stop Norlutate, and start Lupron and Pergonal.

If it is just a matter of delaying the cycle for a few days, another scheduling approach is simply to "keep you on hold" with Lupron alone, and not begin Pergonal injections until the timing is appropriate. But Lupron is much more expensive than Norlutate. However, Norlutate has an additional benefit over and above the convenience of scheduling. If there has been any excessive endometrial buildup from poor ovulation and subsequent unopposed estrogen effect, the progesteronelike action of Norlutate will guarantee a clean menstrual slough before starting the Pergonal cycle.

PREGNANCY TESTING

With modern blood tests we can tell if you are pregnant quite reliably even *before* you realize your period is late. The fetus begins to make its own HCG around day seven after fertilization. By day fourteen after fertilization your blood level of HCG is high enough to determine pregnancy unequivocally. The "pregnancy test" is simply a measure of HCG in your blood or urine. If you have it, then you have to be pregnant. By getting several more HCG levels on your blood at intervals of a few days, it can be assessed to some degree if the pregnancy is likely or not to miscarry. The progesterone injections you may be taking will not in any way interfere with this determination.

If your HCG (actually it is called "Beta-HCG") is positive at fourteen days after ovulation or GIFT, you should continue taking progesterone (if you are taking it) for six more weeks. If your Beta-HCG is negative, it should be repeated again. If still negative, then discontinue progesterone, and wait for your period. If your period starts before HCG testing, just discontinue progesterone, don't bother with the HCG testing, and again contact your doctor on the next cycle. You should usually skip a cycle before trying again.

SUBSEQUENT PREGNANCIES WITHOUT TREATMENT

Whatever it is that is wrong with the hormonal cycle of infertile women and is corrected with Pergonal, it sometimes remains corrected for subsequent cycles. It's as though once the ovary gets stimulated properly, in some cases it then responds normally to the body's own FSH in a proper fashion in subsequent cycles. The most remarkable example of this in our practice was a woman in her early thirties who had been trying to get pregnant for eight years unsuccessfully. When we put her through a Pergonal cycle for GIFT, we found all of her follicles were completely empty and devoid of eggs. We tried again in a second cycle, this time using huge doses of Pergonal.

We were finally able to get five good eggs from her ovaries after the fourth cycle of treatment. Three of those five eggs fertilized in vitro with her husband's sperm, but unfortunately, she did not get pregnant during that cycle. We were all very sad about it because so much effort had gone into these four cycles of massive Pergonal therapy. Yet, the very next month she became pregnant on her own without any further treatment whatsoever. I have never seen a more dramatic case of Pergonal correcting some kind of ovarian problem of which we have a very poor understanding, so that in subsequent months the woman was able to get pregnant on her own. Of course this does not happen in the majority of cases. Most couples need to come back and go through ovarian stimulation, IVF, or GIFT again to get pregnant. But the fact that some couples have a permanent correction of their problem indicates that there are some mysteries about ovarian function we don't understand.

WHEN DO WE GO TO GIFT OR IVF?

If your husband's sperm count is good and you stimulate well, you should have an 8 percent chance of pregnancy per cycle with Pergonal or Pergonal and IUI. If your husband's sperm count is low, the monthly chance for pregnancy with Pergonal will naturally be lower. (Accurate figures as to what that monthly chance of pregnancy is when the husband's sperm count is low cannot be given). If you do not get pregnant after several cycles of Pergonal, or if your husband's sperm count is very low, I suggest proceeding to in vitro procedures, like GIFT or IVF, that offer much higher pregnancy rates per cycle.

CHAPTER 11

IVF (In Vitro Fertilization) and GIFT (Gamete Intra Fallopian Transfer)

INTRODUCTION

On a Tuesday evening, July 25, 1978, at 11:47 P.M., the world's first human test-tube baby was born. Louise Brown was a beautiful, normal, five-pound, twelve-ounce girl with blonde hair and blue eyes. Dr. Robert Edwards and Dr. Patrick Steptoe, in a little clinic near Manchester, England, were responsible for this giant step forward into the "brave new world." Dr. Edwards's first statement upon seeing the child was, "The last time I saw the baby it was just eight cells in a test tube. It was beautiful then and it is still beautiful now." The child's mother, Leslie Brown, and father, John Brown, had been married for nine years and were unable to have children. The problem was that the wife's tubes were so badly destroyed by scars and inflammation that surgery could not help her. Her ovaries and her uterus were normal, however, and all that was required was to take an egg from her ovary, mix it with her husband's sperm in a test tube, and then transfer the two-day-old embryo into her womb to grow for the next nine months into a full-term baby.

This achievement was the culmination of twelve years of painstaking research by the two doctors. Their experiments had begun many years before and involved an incredibly complicated variety of techniques which had to be tested over and over again in animals before being tried in humans. Determining the composition of the fluid in which the sperm and egg are to be bathed, the best time to remove and reimplant the egg, and monitoring the hormone levels of the mother prior to the retrieval of the egg; all required years of patient effort. Their work was not funded by the medical hierarchy, and even after their first successful result, they were ridiculed because it was so difficult at first to make it happen again. Drs. Steptoe and Edwards courageously ushered in a new era that makes it possible today for virtually any couple to have a baby.

As with all other advances relating to reproduction, no matter what politicians, theologians, and medical critics may think, test-tube fertilization has been widely accepted by the public. Since 1985, modifications of the original IVF technique (including "GIFT" and "ZIFT") are producing pregnancy rates of 20 to 55 percent per cycle, and have revolutionized the treatment of infertility. IVF and GIFT today are the dominant form of therapy for childless couples.

The elegance and simplicity of the techniques for test-tube fertilization and GIFT do not require the bureaucracy of an enormous medical center. Research in this area was severely retarded in the United States because in 1975 federal support for research into in vitro fertilization was halted because of a fear that such research was not "ethical." Most of our early knowledge in this field in the United States had to be "imported" from Europe and Australia. Not only did our government refuse to recognize it, but even the first IVF clinic in America (Norfolk, Virginia) which was completely privately funded had to go through tremendous obstacles to get permission to get started. Political activists protested this tampering with nature. But infertile couples continued to support this developing field with *no government* research funding whatsoever. Now, because of privately funded improvements, this is the single-most successful treatment available for infertility today.

As I wrote in a series of predictions in *How to Get Pregnant*, *all* of which have now come true: "Now that we have already stepped over into that brave new world, think of the other possibilities. What if a woman has had a hysterectomy? She has no uterus at all, but does have normal ovaries and a fertile husband. It would now be possible to remove one of her eggs through the laparoscope, fertilize it in a culture dish with her husband's sperm, and then implant this new embryo into another woman, who could act as a 'surrogate' mother. Then when the baby is delivered nine months later, it could be turned over to the mother who originally provided the egg. From the opposite point of view, what if a woman had a perfectly normal uterus and a fertile husband, but her ovaries were incapable of producing eggs? An egg could be extracted from a donor through the laparoscope, fertilized with her husband's sperm, and then implanted into her own uterus." Now such treatment is commonplace. More importantly, for all types of infertility, not just the dramatic ones described above, the success rate is so good with the new technology that couples have less of an agonizing wait and are more likely than ever to achieve their dream.

WHAT IS GIFT? ZIFT? AND IVF? HOW DO THEY DIFFER?

At first it might be confusing to hear all the different acronyms like IVF, GIFT, and ZIFT, but in truth these are all just minor variations of the same technology. When Steptoe and Edwards first reported on IVF, the pregnancy rate per cycle was no more than 2 percent. This made it simply an exotic procedure, too expensive for most, and not likely to result in very many happy couples. Even though the pregnancy rate with in vitro fertilization improved in the mid-1980s, the true pregnancy rate per cycle (taking home a baby) was still about 8 percent.

In fact, shortly before his death in 1989, Dr. Steptoe presented a review of almost a thousand babies born at his clinic in England since 1978, with the pregnancy rate for embryo transfer a very respectable 19 percent. However, after subtracting the number of women who did not stimulate to make eggs, the number of pregnancies which resulted in miscarriage, and the number in which there was no fertilization of the eggs, the true pregnancy rate per cycle was still only 8 percent, even in their experienced hands.

So although in vitro fertilization was an exciting, new horizon for infertility treatment, it remained just a curiosity for most patients and, indeed, in the eyes of most fertility specialists it took a back seat to the plodding, conventional treatments.

What led to the sensational popularity of the new technology, with IVF clinics springing up everywhere, was the improvement in pregnancy rates caused by a few very minor technical modifications, and that's what GIFT and ZIFT represent. (GIFT is an in vitro–type technique developed in 1985 by Dr. Ricardo Asch which has helped to revolutionize and popularize the new in vitro technology because it gives pregnancy rates two to three times higher per cycle than those achieved with standard IVF. However, GIFT can only be performed if the patient has normal fallopian tubes.)

With classic in vitro fertilization, sperm and eggs are mixed in a culture dish, put in an incubator, and the eggs are allowed to fertilize. Two days later the fertilized egg or embryo is replaced in the woman's uterus. The laboratory technology for this in vitro fertilization is so good that with the exception of men with extremely poor-quality sperm, there is very little difficulty for most infertile couples to obtain fertilization in a test tube. The only stumbling block to the wider success of in vitro fertilization is not any difficulty in getting fertilization to occur, but rather in getting the transferred embryo to *implant* in the uterus and result in a pregnancy. Hundreds and thousands of fertilizations were accomplished in IVF laboratories around the world bypassing all of the hurdles presented by infertile couples, but when those precious embryos were replaced in the uterus, only a small percentage of them were able to "implant" and become babies.

GIFT was introduced to solve that implantation problem. With GIFT everything proceeds the same way as with classic IVF except that sperm and eggs are placed directly into the fallopian tube (rather than in a laboratory culture dish) and allowed to fertilize there, so that by natural processes the fallopian tube would then move the embryo down into the uterus at the appropriate time (see Figure 27). This procedure was originally looked upon condescendingly by the early in vitro fertilization (IVF) centers, because they were very skeptical about the results. However, leading centers worldwide soon made it quite

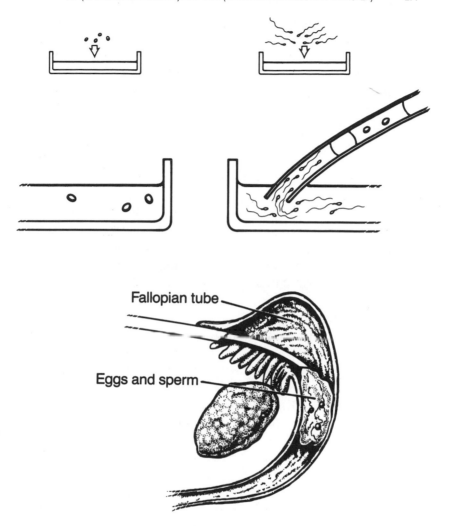

Figure 27. In the GIFT procedure, sperm and eggs are injected directly into the fallopian tube without their needing to be fertilized in a laboratory.

clear that although success rates may vary for IVF and GIFT, in almost all centers performing both procedures the implantation and therefore pregnancy rate for GIFT is about two and a half to three times greater than that with in vitro fertilization.

There is a popular misconception that the reason for that improved pregnancy rate with GIFT over IVF is that if fertilization is allowed to occur naturally in the fallopian tube, a greater pregnancy rate will be obtained than with fertilization occurring in a culture dish in a laboratory incubator. This is not the case, and this is not the rationale behind the GIFT procedure. If in vitro fertilization is performed and the embryos are placed back into the fallopian tube instead of into the uterus, the pregnancy rate is just as high as with GIFT. The issue isn't whether fertilization can occur more readily and properly inside the body than in a petri dish. The issue is where that embryo is positioned. If the embryo is put in the fallopian tube, the *implantation rate* is almost three times higher than when the embryo is placed in the uterus. There is something about direct transfer of the embryo into the uterus which in some way irritates it and makes implantation much less likely. That is the reason for the high success rate of GIFT compared to classic in vitro fertilization.

For several reasons there will always be some controversy about whether to have in vitro fertilization or GIFT. With in vitro fertilization it can actually be determined whether the husband's sperm can fertilize his wife's eggs, so there is tremendous diagnostic value out of IVF which you don't get from GIFT. With GIFT you never find out whether the eggs were fertilized.

That's why the "ZIFT" procedure was developed. ZIFT is a modification of GIFT and IVF, in which the embryo, called a "zygote," is placed in the fallopian tube, rather than the uterus, after fertilization. Normally with IVF, the "test-tube" embryo is placed in the uterus. Normally with GIFT, the sperm and eggs (no fertilization has taken place yet) are placed in the fallopian tube. With "ZIFT," sperm and eggs are allowed to fertilize in the laboratory, but resultant embryos are placed into the fallopian tubes rather than the uterus.

GIFT and ZIFT are virtually identical in results. The only difference is that with GIFT only one short forty-five-minute operation is required. With ZIFT you first have to go through egg aspiration and in vitro fertilization, and then two days later you have to go through another procedure for the embryo transfer into the fallopian tube.

A second reason why classic in vitro fertilization may be favored over GIFT is that results with IVF have improved so much that most good centers now are getting reliable 15 percent take-home baby pregnancy rates. These improved results have been due to better hyperstimulation of the ovary, and particularly the use of GNRH agonists, to improve the quality and number of the eggs obtained from the wife. Nonetheless, every improvement in IVF pregnancy rate the different centers have enjoyed has resulted in a corresponding improvement in GIFT pregnancy rates so that GIFT still remains two and a half to three times more successful per cycle attempt than IVF.

A third reason that IVF may be preferred in many centers is that with ultrasound-guided aspiration of the eggs, the IVF can be done completely as an outpatient procedure under mild sedation or very light anesthesia. GIFT, however, whether through the laparoscope or "minilap" incision (one to one and a half inches), does require a minor operation and general anesthesia. If one sets up a large office-based in vitro fertilization program, one does not have the flexibility of being able to offer GIFT to the patient. GIFT requires an operating room. Therefore, one's investment is much less with IVF, and one can run a privately operated clinic. It is for this reason that many people will only perform in vitro fertilization and not offer GIFT to their patients despite GIFT having almost three times the pregnancy rate per cycle.

There is of course a fourth reason why IVF is needed: if the fallopian tubes are damaged, GIFT and ZIFT are not possible. In these cases the fallopian tubes must be completely bypassed. Indeed that was the original reason for which Steptoe and Edwards developed the whole in vitro fertilization procedure, for uncorrectable tubal blockage. This still remains an absolute indication for in vitro fertilization as opposed to GIFT or ZIFT.

GIFT involves all of the methodology used for standard IVF. It's just that instead of putting sperm in the culture dish with the egg to make an embryo in the incubator, the sperm and the egg, after appropriate preparation, are taken out of the incubator and placed directly into the fallopian tube and allowed to fertilize there. Then the rest is "natural," and if fertilization takes place, the embryo is passed into the uterus several days later.

Sperm and egg cannot just be placed this way into the uterus since fertilization will not take place there. If there are no healthy fallopian tubes, trying this procedure by placing sperm and eggs into the uterus before in vitro fertilization just won't work. That is why if the fallopian tubes are damaged, fertilization must first be obtained in the laboratory and the resulting embryos (not just sperm and eggs) placed into the uterus.

One of GIFT's major advantages is that the technique relies to a far greater degree on the body's natural processes and time-table to produce pregnancy. It is not as though fertilization in the test tube is any worse than in the body. The issue is *how* the fertilized egg gets into the uterus, because that is what influences whether it will implant. It does not appear that fertilization in the fallopian tube is any better than in an incubator. The difference is *where* the end product is placed. Placement in the fallopian tube gives a higher pregnancy rate.

To prepare her body for the GIFT procedure, the woman receives hormones (as described in the previous chapter) to stimulate development of the ovarian follicles, saclike structures that contain the eggs, just like with IVF. Administering Pergonal increases the chances of retrieving many ripened eggs, each one capable of being fertilized. During the administration of the Pergonal regimen, the patient is carefully monitored with daily estrogen levels and ultrasound scans. When the eggs are ripe, HCG is given, and thirty-six hours later the patient undergoes the GIFT or IVF procedure.

Approximately three hours before the surgery, a semen sample from the husband is obtained and washed (see Chapter 10).

The eggs are then obtained by transvaginal needle aspiration (without a surgical incision) via an ultrasound guide. The fluid containing the egg is placed in a laboratory dish and observed under a microscope. The egg is located and its stage of maturity noted. It is then carefully placed in culture media and put in the incubator. (The details of egg and embryo culture will be explained in the next chapter.)

Up to four or more eggs may then be returned to the patient; this is performed surgically either though laparoscopy or a small "minilap" incision (1 to 1½ inches) in the lower abdomen, under general anesthesia. Sperm and eggs are then sequentially loaded into the catheter which is introduced into the patient's fallopian tubes. Usually two or more eggs are placed in each tube. The patient generally stays overnight in the hospital and goes home the next day.

Again, it must be explained that, done properly, GIFT uses *all* of the same techniques as IVF. The egg must be cultured, and sperm washed the same way as for IVF. GIFT must not be viewed as a "shortcut" approach to IVF, or the eggs and sperm will not do well. GIFT simply offers a greater pregnancy rate by allowing the fallopian tubes to transfer the embryo to the uterus at the right time and atraumatically, as in nature.

GIFT offers several other social advantages over classical IVF. There are no religious objections to GIFT. The Catholic Church and Orthodox Judaism fully approve of it. More importantly, the pregnancy rate is much higher because the embryo is transported naturally from the fallopian tube into the uterus several days after fertilization, rather than being injected into the uterus after growing for two days in a laboratory incubator.

RATIONALE FOR DOING GIFT PROCEDURE IN ALL CASES OF INFERTILITY WHERE NO TUBAL DISEASE EXISTS

There are a significant and disturbingly large number of patients who are not able to get pregnant despite perfectly normal ovulatory cycles, lack of any physical tubal damage or obstruction, absence of endometriosis, and normal healthy male sperm. In short, they have "nothing" wrong with them. There are also a number of patients who have problems such as ovulatory dysfunction who are successfully treated with Pergonal but still don't get pregnant.

In these cases as well as virtually any other so-called "diagnosis" for infertility (other than tubal disease) including endometriosis, cervical factor, autoimmunity, and luteal phase defect, the GIFT procedure has a higher success rate than conventional treatment. Therefore, after conventional treatment has failed, GIFT is the best next step.

If the male has a lower sperm count, GIFT may help solve that problem also by placing the smaller number of sperm that are actually necessary to fertilize the egg directly into the fallopian tube. Even though a fertile man may ejaculate as many as 200 million sperm into the vagina, only about 100,000 sperm get into the uterus, and only several thousand get into the fallopian tube. Thus, if sperm are placed directly into the fallopian tube via the GIFT procedure, the man does not need to produce a large amount of sperm.

Many cases of infertility are "idiopathic." This means that doctors really don't know why the couple is not getting pregnant and don't even pretend to know why. For these cases also, by bypassing all of the normal reproductive processes, it is possible to achieve high pregnancy rates despite not knowing what the problem is. No matter what the cause of infertility, if the fallopian tubes are normal, GIFT is an appropriate treatment.

Go to GIFT Sooner

The monthly pregnancy rate with GIFT is so good it always saddens me to see a couple that has been through years and years of costly and often painful conventional treatment just give up when they are confronted with the amount of effort they will have to put into a single GIFT cycle. It is really not that difficult for the patient and represents only the most minor surgical procedure, but the trouble of daily tests and shots can be overwhelming after they have already gone through years and years of failed treatment. It makes me wish that instead of thinking of GIFT, ZIFT, or indeed IVF as last-resort procedures, if we suggested it to the patient earlier, they wouldn't be so emotionally down already. GIFT should be an enthusiastic, exciting adventure rather than an ordeal with effort at the end of a long dark tunnel.

A patient from a few years ago was a nurse who counseled couples on the scientific use of rhythm methods of birth control. She obviously knew her cycle inside and out and was extremely knowledgeable. Her menstrual cycle was that perfect model chart that you see in a lot of the textbooks, with a temperature rise on day fourteen, a drop on day twenty-eight with menstruation, and perfect, regular cycles like clockwork where you can predict almost to the hour when she expects to start her next period. In fact, all of her studies and her husband's tests were completely normal, and yet with properly timing their intercourse to make sure never to miss the day or two before she ovulated, for many, many years they still had not gotten pregnant.

When she came in she did not want to go through any of the preliminary treatments like intrauterine insemination, Parlodel, Clomid, or even Pergonal plus intrauterine insemination. She asked point-blank to be put in our GIFT program. I explained to her that this is not our usual pattern and that we would rather put off doing GIFT or IVF-type procedures until she had gone through many cycles of Pergonal and intrauterine insemination and had had at least several years of confident, conventional therapy for their infertility. She told me that this was baloney, she understood everything that was involved, she looked at the statistics, she did not want to "mess around" with less effective remedies just to appease the doctor's sense of guilt. She was a strong feminist and told me exactly what she wanted to have done. I agreed, and after the first cycle with GIFT she became pregnant with twins and is quite delighted.

This woman avoided years and years of Clomid plus intrauterine insemination, Parlodel, laparoscopic surgery for minimal lesion endometriosis, months and months of Pergonal plus intrauterine insemination. She explained to me that if she had to go through all of these cycles without a pregnancy, she would lose her zeal for pursuing treatment any further. That's why she wanted to go right for the procedure that carried the highest yield immediately. As it turns out, she was right.

On the other hand, this same woman had a friend she referred to us who had been through three years of Clomid, hystersalpingograms, and laparoscopic surgery, and nine cycles of Pergonal and intrauterine insemination, and she and her husband were "fed up." It is only reasonable that she had been placed on so many cycles of Pergonal plus intrauterine insemination, because of an initial diagnosis of irregular menstrual cycles and poor ovulation. Her husband's sperm count was normal and everything else about her was normal. Yet despite the "reasonableness" of putting her on all of these cycles of ovulatory stimulation, they so exhausted her that when she saw us and the option of GIFT was presented she had heard all she really wanted to and wasn't going to go through anymore.

One of the leaders of our GIFT/IVF support group in St. Louis had a similar story and almost decided not to go through GIFT. Fortunately, she decided to give it one last try. She got pregnant and delivered a normal baby with her first cycle. She had gone through eight years of infertility with the diagnosis of poor ovulation and irregular cycles all of her life. She had already had three D & Cs (dilation and curretage) for irregular bleeding and had been on Clomid for years. She then gave up treatment for several years, and when we saw her hysterosalpingogram, it showed tremendously heaped-up, cobblestone-type lesions inside the uterus, which looked like multiple fibroids. In truth, when we did hysteroscopy we realized that this was just "endometrial hyperplasia," i.e., the potentially precancerous heavy buildup of a constant estrogen-dominated follicular-phase endometrium with no progesterone effect.

She went on an entire month of Norlutate (a high-dosed synthetic progesterone), and then had an enormous period correcting years of endometrial buildup, without the need for another D & C. She then went through the GIFT procedure and got pregnant. We solved her problem of her endometrial precancerous endometrium and got her pregnant all in the same treatment cycle.

It could be argued that this woman should have gone through ovulatory stimulation with Pergonal before resorting to GIFT. That would only have given her an 8 to 10 percent chance of pregnancy per cycle, whereas GIFT was able to give her a 45 percent chance of pregnancy per cycle. She was emotionally at the end of her rope, and had had enough procedure and many medications over the last eight years to no avail. The right approach was to dispense with preliminaries and go right for the highest-yield procedure even if it did involve a minor surgical operation.

Most of the aggravation and expense the patient goes through in a GIFT or IVF cycle is the stimulation and monitoring of the ovaries. By the time she has been through her Lupron, Pergonal, Metrodin, and HCG, along with daily ultrasound and blood estrogen tests, she has already done all of the work. The major effort for patients going through GIFT or IVF is the stimulation, not the actual IVF or GIFT procedure itself.

Another reason for going to GIFT sooner is that in so many infertile couples now in their thirties who want to have a child, both the husband and the wife have very responsible positions, and it is often very hard to find the time to devote going through an entire cycle without interruption for business trips, meetings, and so forth. Why not give them, therefore, the best possibility for pregnancy resulting from the Pergonal stimulation? It may seem radical to suggest this, but with this kind of couple, why not go to GIFT right away and dispense with the prerequisite of many cycles of unsuccessful Pergonal and IUI?

What about the couples who go through several cycles of GIFT right off the bat and still don't get pregnant? How are they going to feel after putting their time and effort into a high-tech procedure and coming out of it still without a baby? They understand ahead of time that despite the high pregnancy with GIFT there is a chance that they still would not be pregnant after going for the highest-yield procedure. At least there will be no lingering doubt in their minds that perhaps they hadn't yet given it their best shot. The benefit of having gone through GIFT unsuccessfully is that couples know that they have given it their all.

WHAT IS "ZYGOTE INTRA FALLOPIAN TRANSFER" (ZIFT)?

If there is a question of the sperm's ability to fertilize the egg, due to either a low sperm count or the quality of the sperm, it may be suggested that ZIFT be performed instead of GIFT. With ZIFT, the eggs are retrieved, the same as for GIFT; however, the eggs and the sperm are then fertilized in the laboratory, and usually two days later the resulting embryos are placed into the fallopian tubes. The only reason for doing ZIFT in preference to GIFT is if there is any question about the ability of the husband's sperm to fertilize the wife's eggs. This is just like classic IVF. The only difference between classic IVF and ZIFT is where the embryos are placed after fertilization. With classic IVF they are placed into the uterus nonsurgically, and with ZIFT they are placed into the fallopian tubes surgically.

There is another advantage to ZIFT over GIFT in cases of severe "male factor" infertility aside from seeing whether fertilization is possible. If there is very poor sperm but huge numbers of eggs (ten to forty), it is possible that only a few of those many eggs will fertilize. Those are the ones to put back in. With GIFT, if there are forty eggs, doctors don't know which ones to replace.

As with GIFT, the eggs are retrieved by ultrasound-guided needle aspiration under light sedation in the operating room. This involves no surgical incision, there is virtually no pain afterward, and a woman would be able to go home only two hours following the procedure. Then, two days later, she would be admitted to the hospital in order to undergo transfer of the embryos into her fallopian tubes. This minor surgical procedure, identical to GIFT, is performed under general anesthesia and does involve some moderate postoperative pain. Therefore, it may be necessary with this second procedure to stay in the hospital overnight. All of the ovulatory stimulation treatments —egg aspiration, treatment of the husband's sperm, HCG determinations—are the same for ZIFT as for GIFT and IVF.

GIFT, ZIFT, and IVF are, for the most part, the same procedure, involving the same ovarian stimulation, daily estrogen monitoring, daily ultrasound visualization of the follicles, the same method for needle aspiration of eggs, the same preparation of the sperm, same method of culturing eggs, as well as replacement of either sperm and eggs, or embryos, back into the woman after retrieval. The differences between these three procedures are only slight, but can vastly affect the pregnancy rate and are each appropriate for certain specific patients. In the majority of patients with idiopathic infertility, or for that matter any infertility other than tubal disease in which the husband's sperm quality is adequate, GIFT has the highest percentage of success and is the simplest of the three procedures. However, if there is any question about the fertility of the husband's sperm or if the couple has gone through several GIFT cycles already unsuccessfully, it is necessary to know for sure whether or not his sperm can fertilize in a test tube.

WHAT IS THE RATIONALE FOR
THE ZIFT PROCEDURE?

With ZIFT, there is the advantage of the greater implantation rate by placing the embryos in the fallopian tube rather than the uterus (see Figure 28). Unlike GIFT, the transfer is delayed for several days in order to find out whether or not the eggs have actually fertilized in vitro. There have been many speculations that perhaps fertilization in vitro is not as good as fertilization in the fallopian tube, and ZIFT would, therefore, yield lower pregnancy rates than GIFT. On the other hand, it has also been speculated that fertilization in the test tube with poor-quality sperm would be better than fertilization in the fallopian tube, and, therefore, ZIFT would yield higher pregnancy rates than GIFT with "male factor" infertility. Both of these specu-

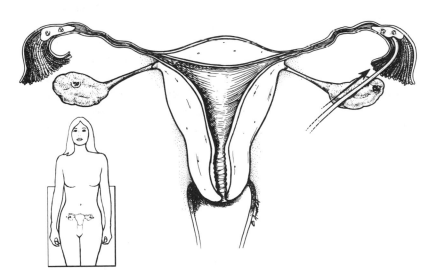

Figure 28. In the ZIFT procedure, eggs would have already been fertilized and growing for the previous two days in the laboratory and placed in the fallopian tube in a fashion similar to that of the GIFT procedure.

lations have been proven to be incorrect. Fertilization in the culture dish is just as good as fertilization in the fallopian tube, and, furthermore, it's not any better.

There is one advantage to ZIFT. In very special patients with severe "male factor" infertility, it would give a higher pregnancy rate than GIFT. A study verifying this situation was first worked out by Dr. Paul Devroey from Brussels, Belgium, one of the pioneers of the ZIFT procedure. If you have extremely poor-quality sperm from the husband, but a very fertile wife who yields large numbers of eggs, by performing fertilization in the laboratory culture dishes it is not infrequent to find that although the sperm are quite terrible and unlikely to fertilize any eggs, if you have twenty-five eggs, and only two of those fertilize, then you know which two eggs to place in the fallopian tube. If you were to perform GIFT on such a patient, you would not transfer twenty-five eggs because of the serious risk of severe multiple pregnancy that would involve. But with ZIFT, you can select the few that do fertilize and put those in two days later.

In our work with epididymal sperm aspiration for congenital blockage of the male sperm ducts, we often get incredibly poor sperm samples that have been stored up in the area near the outlet of the testicle for many years and have very poor motility and poor fertilizing capability. However, these men's wives are usually quite fertile (remember, with azospermic husbands only 5 percent of the wives have an infertility problem themselves), and often yield very large numbers of eggs. We have found with such couples that when greater than ten eggs are obtainable from the wife in a cycle, the pregnancy rate is 50 percent. However, with such miserable sperm, when fewer than ten eggs are obtainable, we rarely get a pregnancy. This is because when we have so many eggs, even if we only get two or three fertilizations, that is enough with a ZIFT procedure to get a high pregnancy rate. If we were to do GIFT on such patients, we would never put all twenty-five eggs back, but only take the best four or five, and then the statistical chance of any one of those four or five eggs fertilizing would be very low, even though if there were twenty-five eggs replaced, the chance of one or two of them fertilizing would be very reasonable. Since we can't take the chance, however remote, that all twenty-five of those eggs would fertilize, we simply can't pick the simpler option of GIFT for these patients, but must put them through the trouble of ZIFT. Remember, the only disadvantage of ZIFT compared to GIFT is that it puts you through two procedures instead of one. Otherwise, if it weren't for the issue of which eggs to replace, GIFT and ZIFT would have identical pregnancy rates.

Why not perform in vitro fertilization (IVF) on cases of severe "male factor"? The reason is that after you have gone through all the effort of obtaining huge numbers of eggs and fertilizing just a couple of them in vitro, you want to give them the greatest possible chance of implanting and forming a pregnancy. If you put these fertilized eggs back into the uterus, your chance of pregnancy would be somewhere around 15 to 20 percent. However, when you put these fertilized eggs back into the fallopian tubes, your chance of pregnancy is 55 percent. I'll give the details of pregnancy rates and implantation rates in more detail after we have discussed in vitro fertilization.

WHAT IS "IN VITRO" FERTILIZATION (IVF)?

If the fallopian tubes are damaged too badly, sperm and eggs *cannot* be put into them. In such cases, in order to achieve a pregnancy, fertilized eggs are placed directly into the uterus (classic IVF) (see Figure 29). Many studies have shown that if sperm and eggs are placed directly into the uterus, pregnancy will not occur. Fertilization can only occur 1) in the fallopian tube or 2) in a laboratory culture dish, but *not* in the uterus. Thus, if the fallopian tubes are damaged, the eggs must first be fertilized in the laboratory, and the resulting embryos are then placed into the uterus, usually two days later. This procedure achieves remarkable pregnancies in women with hopelessly damaged fallopian tubes. But the pregnancy rate is considerably less than with GIFT.

There are many who recommend IVF rather than ZIFT for "male factor" infertility. There is really no difference between IVF and ZIFT except *where* the already fertilized eggs or embryos are placed. With IVF, they are put into the uterus, requiring a very minor surgical procedure. When they are put

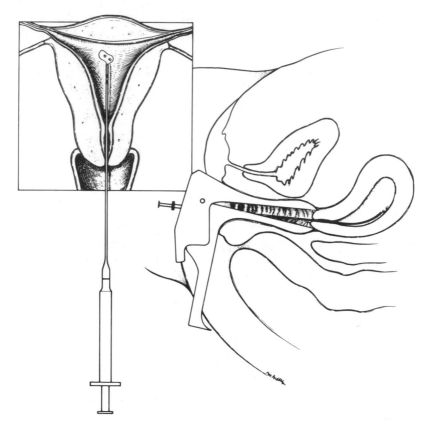

Figure 29. In classic IVF, fertilized eggs, or embryos, are placed without surgery directly into the uterus, and the fallopian tubes are not involved.

into the fallopian tubes, there is a much greater chance of pregnancy than when they are placed in the uterus.

The advantage of IVF, however, is that no surgical procedure is required. With GIFT or ZIFT there is. As with GIFT, the eggs are retrieved by ultrasound-guided needle aspiration under light sedation in the operating room. This involves no surgical incision and virtually no pain afterward. With IVF, a woman leaves the hospital directly from the operating room and comes back two days later to have the embryo (or embryos) placed into the uterus through the cervix with a tiny catheter (no incision and no anesthesia are necessary). Two hours later she is able to go home.

GIFT (or ZIFT) is preferable if there is no tubal disease because of the very high pregnancy rate per cycle. But IVF has the advantage of being an outpatient procedure, with less pain, and thus easier to undergo on repeated occasions than GIFT or ZIFT.

IMPLANTATION RATES WITH GIFT, ZIFT, AND IVF

The improved pregnancy rate with GIFT and ZIFT over IVF because of the greater likelihood of the embryo's implanting in the uterus requires some detailed explanation. We now have compiled data from Dr. John Yovich's center in Perth, Australia; Dr. Paul Devroey's center in Brussels, Belgium; our program in St. Louis; and Dr. Ricardo Asch's program in Irvine, California, on the relative pregnancy rates and embryo implantation rates for ZIFT, GIFT, and IVF.

First I'll explain what the "implantation rate" is. As you will recall, most of the embryos that one replaces in either IVF or ZIFT don't "implant" and therefore don't result in a pregnancy. For that reason, we always put in more than one embryo in order to increase our chances of a pregnancy occurring. When we do that, we take a chance, however slight, for a multiple pregnancy to occur. About 20 to 25 percent of GIFT or IVF cases are twins, and 2 to 5 percent are triplets. We take that risk of multiple birth because we know we are increasing the chance of pregnancy. Therefore, to simply compare pregnancy rates with IVF, GIFT, and ZIFT is not to pay attention to the fact that in some patients, two or three embryos may have been replaced, and in other patients, possibly five or six may have been replaced. In a few patients, maybe only one embryo was replaced. Therefore, in order to determine what is the chance that an embryo replaced by ZIFT or IVF will implant for a pregnancy, you compute what we call the "implantation rate." In a large group of patients, you add up the total number of fetuses ("fetal sacs") and divide that by the number of embryos (IVF or ZIFT) that were replaced, or by the number of eggs (GIFT) that were replaced, and you get the "implantation rate" per embryo (IVF and ZIFT) or per egg (GIFT).

With GIFT and with ZIFT, the pregnancy rate is 28 percent and 26 percent, respectively, in "male factor" infertility. When there is no discernible male factor problem, the pregnancy rate with GIFT or ZIFT per cycle is 50 to 55 percent. Note that there is really no significant difference in the pregnancy rates we've seen with patients undergoing ZIFT or GIFT. With in vitro fertilization (IVF), the pregnancy rate with male factor infertility is about 8 percent and with a normal male is about 22 percent. It is immediately obvious that the pregnancy rate with in vitro fertilization (IVF) is consistently about one-half to one-third that seen with GIFT or ZIFT.

We have consistently noted about a 30 percent overall fertilization rate per egg with "male factor" cases, and a 65 to 70 percent fertilization rate per egg in patients with "normal" sperm. Using this calculation, the implantation rate per egg transferred in normal men with GIFT was 12.5 percent. That means that 12.5 percent of the eggs transferred in a GIFT procedure resulted in a fetus when there were no sperm problems. You can see how transferring four or five eggs with a 12.5 percent implantation rate per egg would generate pregnancy rates in the range of 50 to 60 percent. When there was "male factor" infertility, however, the number of fetuses per egg transferred was only 5.7 percent, and again you can see how the transfer of four or five eggs in a male factor case yields a pregnancy rate in the 20 to 30 percent range.

Now if we calculate the implantation rate per "presumed embryo" with GIFT, figuring on a 30 percent fertilization rate for "male factor" patients and a 65 percent fertilization rate for "normal" males, in both cases we would come out with an implantation rate per "presumed embryo" of 18 percent in the normal male and 19 percent in cases with "male factor" infertility. Thus, whether fertilization occurs or not, or whether pregnancy occurs or not, with a GIFT transfer there is an 18 or 19 percent chance that an embryo formed in the fallopian tube will result in a fetus in the uterus. The implantation rate per embryo transferred for ZIFT is also 19 percent, and for classic IVF only 8 percent.

Pregnancy rates in many IVF programs are very high, and in others are very low. In any one period of time, some IVF centers may record pregnancy rates as high as 35 percent. During another cycle, however, their pregnancy rate may be considerably lower. There is a lot of statistical variation. What I have tried to give you in this summary is the distillation of a huge compilation of results from centers doing extremely careful work and involving patients with very long-standing infertility. Nonetheless, if you try to compare one center to another you will have a difficult time, because the centers which take on the most difficult patients, e.g., older women, or women with only a half an ovary left, or women with resistant ovaries from whom only a few eggs are obtainable, or a large number of "male factor" cases, you can see that the pregnancy rate from such an institution would be very low even though they might be extremely capable.

On the other hand, an IVF or GIFT program that took on many young patients from whom large numbers of eggs were obtainable, and tried to limit the number of "male factor" cases it tackled, would have a very high pregnancy rate. You cannot choose a center by comparing the overall pregnancy rates of one center to another. You must get the details, understanding that unfavorable factors for pregnancy rate per cycle include poor-quality sperm, wife over thirty-five years of age, and fewer than ten eggs obtainable with modern hyperstimulation protocols because of resistant ovaries.

To summarize, if your fallopian tubes are damaged, there is no choice and no thinking involved. Simply go to IVF (which means in vitro fertilization with transfer of the embryo to the uterus). However, if your fallopian tubes are normal and you suffer from any other type of infertility, GIFT and ZIFT have the benefit of higher pregnancy rates per cycle, but the disadvantage of involving a minor surgical procedure.

CHAPTER 12

Step-by-Step Details of How "Test-Tube" Babies Are Made

Now that you have a general overview of what GIFT, IVF, and ZIFT offer, and how they are performed, with a realistic view of results and a basis for comparing these three different modes of the same new technology, I'll try to go into the step-by-step detail, the fascinating, exciting adventure that each one of these procedures entails. I suggest that they not be viewed as a horrendous ordeal, but rather as an exciting adventure during which you can thrill to the view of your own eggs developing on the television screen on an ultrasound monitor, following every step of the procedure with the same excitement that I look forward to with each patient.

As an athletics coach of young children, I know how badly they want to win each game, and how seriously disturbing a loss or a "failure" can be. You may not get pregnant in any given cycle, but with this available technology and with the choices you have open to you notwithstanding donor insemination, egg donation, or even having someone else carry your genetic baby for you, with this new technology virtually everyone is able to have a baby. But it may take persistence and confidence.

In a recent CBS documentary titled *24 Hours*, a couple was filmed who had gone through eight previous in vitro fertilization (IVF) attempts without a pregnancy. But they were still trying, for their ninth time, when many would have given up and might have viewed an optimistic approach such as mine in this chapter with bitterness. But they did get pregnant on their ninth try. It is now clear that the chance of pregnancy per cycle stays relatively good even after as many as six or seven previous cycles in which no pregnancy occurred. The new technology raises your chance of pregnancy per cycle of treatment dramatically, and it stays good per each attempt even if you've failed in previous tries.

It is true that those who have previously gotten pregnant with in vitro fertilization have an increased pregnancy rate per cycle when they come back to try to have their second child. But for any given couple, their chance of pregnancy per cycle is still fairly constant, and if you stick with it, sooner or later you have a good chance of getting pregnant. Thus, I hope you will go through the rest of this chapter with the same sense of excitement that I have about witnessing the miracle of fertilization and conception.

HORMONAL STIMULATION NECESSARY TO OBTAIN MORE THAN ONE EGG AND HORMONAL TIMING OF THE PROCEDURE

The stimulation protocol for GIFT or IVF is the same as described in the chapter on Pergonal. Most centers use a combination of Lupron and Pergonal, often supplemented by Metrodin (like Pergonal but a pure preparation of FSH with no LH at all). First you are asked to have an ultrasound examination on day one or day two of your cycle to make sure there are no ovarian cysts. You begin self-injections of Lupron either in the luteal phase of the previous cycle or on day one or two of the GIFT or IVF cycle and continue these injections through the day you receive HCG. On the third day of your cycle, usually you will begin Pergonal. This will be called "day 1 of Pergonal." On day one through day three of Pergonal you would usually be administered two to three ampules of Pergonal each afternoon. On day four of Pergonal you would start having your blood drawn every morning for a rapid estrogen level and have an ultrasound examination. In the afternoon you are told how much Pergonal to receive that day. Under most circumstances you would be getting two or three ampules of Pergonal per day for a total of nine or ten days. The Pergonal dosage and timing will depend upon what the estrogen and ultrasound demonstrated that day.

When your eggs are ripe and ready, which is usually between day eight and day ten of Pergonal (but depends entirely on what your particular ultrasound and estrogen levels show), you will be told to have an HCG injection instead of Pergonal. This would normally stimulate ovulation to occur sometime between thirty-six and forty-eight hours later. The reason for giving you the HCG during a GIFT or IVF regimen is not to make you ovulate, but rather to make the eggs resume "meiosis," i.e., "reduction division" to half the normal number of chromosomes. Without this cellular event, fertilization cannot occur. The GIFT procedure is therefore performed thirty-six hours after the HCG injection. This will give HCG the maximum amount of time to prepare the eggs for fertilization, but will still allow us to aspirate them before they are ovulated and therefore lost.

You will get your HCG injection exactly thirty-six hours prior to the scheduled GIFT or IVF procedure. This means that if the procedure is planned for 11:00 A.M., your injection of HCG should be given at 11:00 P.M. two days before. If the procedure were planned for 10:00 A.M. the HCG injection would be given at 10:00 P.M. two days before. If the procedure is planned for the afternoon (for example, 2:00 P.M.), that would mean your HCG injection would have to be given at the rather inconvenient hour of 2:00 A.M. No matter what time of day the procedure is scheduled for (always two days from the day when the follicles are mature and ready), the HCG is injected *exactly* thirty-six hours ahead of that time. The husband would provide a sperm specimen for washing and preparation approximately three hours before the GIFT or IVF procedure.

Although your ovaries are likely to produce a normal amount of progesterone after the GIFT or IVF procedure, we can't take that for granted. Sometimes the ovaries stop making progesterone too early after the egg aspiration procedure and the pregnancy could be lost without assuring that there is progesterone support. Thus although it may not be 100 percent necessary, it is safer to go on an injection of one-half cc of progesterone per day beginning either the day of the IVF transfer, the day after the IVF transfer, or two or three days after the GIFT procedure. These injections are much easier to give to yourself than Pergonal because they are only a small volume of fluid (one-half cc). You would normally take the progesterone for about six weeks after the procedure because most likely by that time the placenta is beginning to make its own progesterone anyway.

You'll remember in the chapter on Pergonal, we were concerned about too much stimulation to the ovaries resulting in "hyperstimulation syndrome" or multiple births. For IVF and GIFT we don't have that concern. For IVF and GIFT, we want to get as many eggs as we possibly can to maximize the chance of having good eggs for fertilization. Furthermore, we don't have the same fear of hyperstimulation syndrome because all of the follicles will be aspirated and there won't be this huge leakage of estrogen-rich fluid into the abdomen.

Generally you can roughly estimate the fertility potential of the wife by how well she responds to the Pergonal stimulation regimen. If she generates large numbers of eggs, then each one of those eggs is more likely to be mature and fertilizable, resulting in a pregnancy. If it takes a tremendously increased dose of Pergonal to squeeze out whatever eggs we can get, the pregnancy rate is lower even with the same number of eggs. Although there is tremendous variation, the older the woman, the fewer eggs we are likely to be able to get from ovarian stimulation. Sometimes young women will have resistant ovaries that require huge doses of Pergonal, and sometimes women in their late thirties will yield large numbers of eggs with just normal doses of Pergonal. There is a lot of individual variation. But by and large, the older the woman, the fewer eggs we are likely to get and the more Pergonal she is likely to need to stimulate follicle development. Over forty years of age, we almost always have to give large doses of Pergonal (anywhere from four to ten ampules per day) in order to get a reasonable number of eggs for IVF or GIFT.

Four years ago, we performed Pergonal and intrauterine insemination (IUI) on a thirty-six-year-old lady who got pregnant with the first cycle, had her baby, and was just delighted. Now, just four years later, she is forty years old, and she did not respond at all to the usual dose of Pergonal. We were not able to get any follicular response and so we pushed her all the way up to ten ampules of Pergonal per day. The chance of her getting pregnant with just Pergonal and IUI again at age forty now is very low, and this lady should not hesitate to go with GIFT cycles every time because she is reaching the end of the line. Of course, with the new technology, there is never an "end of the line" because if she is willing, we can always get her pregnant with donor eggs. But we will discuss that in more detail in a later chapter.

OBTAINING THE EGGS

In the early days of in vitro fertilization (IVF), the eggs were always obtained via laparoscopy. This meant that IVF required a surgical procedure to obtain the eggs, and then the embryos were replaced nonsurgically in the uterus. With the advent of transvaginal ultrasound and transvaginal-guided needle aspiration of the eggs, all that has changed (see Figures 30, 31, and 32).

Ultrasound is performed just as described in the earlier chapters on diagnostic techniques. You can actually see on the ultrasound machine the echoes created by the tip of the needle. Thus, just by pushing the ultrasound probe directly against the ovaries through the vaginal wall, the needle can be inserted right into the follicle by visualization on the television screen. You can actually see the needle puncture the follicle, and as gentle suction is applied, you can see the follicle completely empty.

The egg is not contained in the fluid of the follicle. Rather, the egg sits on a stalk attached to the follicular wall. Thus, as this fluid is coming through the needle into the suction trap, the egg is almost never located in this first part of the fluid. As the follicle wall becomes completely collapsed, the egg gets drawn into the needle only at that point and literally gets pulled off the stalk attaching it to the follicle wall. The needle is then inserted into the next follicle closest to the first one that was punctured. The fluid from the next follicle then washes the egg through the needle and tubing into the suction trap test tube.

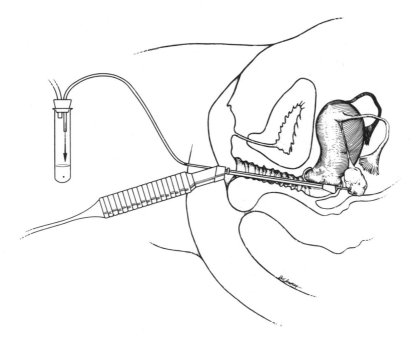

Figure 30. Diagram illustrating placement of the ultrasound probe for transvaginal needle aspiration of eggs.

Meanwhile, as this second follicle collapses completely around the needle, its egg also gets drawn up into the needle.

Some infertility centers flush and irrigate the follicle without going to the next follicle until the egg is obtained from the follicle that was just punctured. Other centers find this an unnecessary time-consuming procedure. When the procedure is finally completed and all the follicles have been emptied, the needle is removed from the ovary and culture media is suctioned through it to get any remaining eggs that might be caught in the tubing.

The fluid that is aspirated will either be clear yellow or somewhat bloody. If the fluid is very bloody, it means that the "follicle" was truly an endometrioma, a big cyst of the ovary containing endometriosis tissue.

Transvaginal aspiration is much more efficient than laparoscopic aspiration because with laparoscopy you can only see the follicles on the outside of the ovary. With the ultrasound you

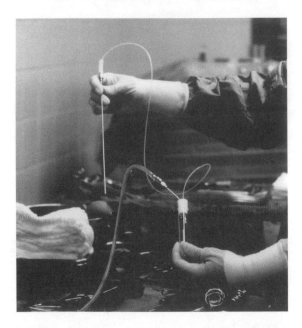

Figure 31. Picture of suction trap and tubing for collecting the eggs.

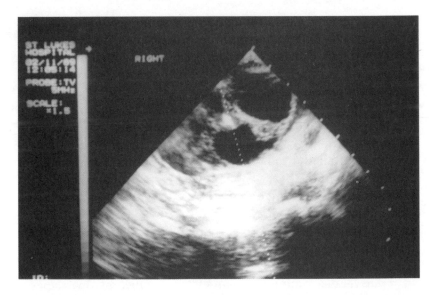

Figure 32. View on ultrasound screen of needle about to enter large follicle.

can see right through the ovary and can see every follicle. This allows you to guide your needle into every single follicle and completely empty the ovary of every possible mature egg, quite unlike laparoscopy where you are limited to what you can visualize on the surface.

The procedure, of course, is somewhat painful, and, therefore, is best tolerated with light sedation or light general anesthesia. Some women can handle this without any sedation at all, but the vast majority need the services of an anesthesiologist. However, you wake up very quickly and if that is all that is being done that day to you (as for IVF), you can go home in an hour or two. You will have no pain from the procedure but might have some low abdominal aching simply because of the large size of your hyperstimulated ovaries.

If you were scheduled for in vitro fertilization (IVF), you will come back in two days and have the embryos replaced in your uterus in a procedure no more complex than a simple pelvic examination. If you are having ZIFT, you will come back in two days and have the embryos replaced in the fallopian tube via laparoscopy or minilap, small surgical procedures that require one day or, at most, an overnight stay in the hospital.

If you are having a GIFT procedure, you stay in the operating room after egg aspiration and your abdomen is prepared for laparoscopy or minilap. Meanwhile, the eggs that have just been retrieved via transvaginal aspiration are sitting in culture media in the incubator waiting to be loaded with your husband's sperm into a catheter for transfer into your fallopian tube.

Because of the tremendous increase in the number of eggs obtainable when Lupron is combined with Pergonal in the stimulation cycle, we're retrieving literally five times the number of eggs we used to retrieve in the mid-1980s. In the mid-1980s about three to five eggs were all you could expect to obtain with hyperstimulation and egg retrieval. Nowadays, in younger women, anywhere from twenty to forty eggs are obtainable. Even from women in their thirties it's frequent to get over ten eggs. It used to be feared that when more eggs were obtained, each one of these eggs was in some way of less quality than when smaller numbers of eggs were obtained. We now know that the opposite is true, and in fact pregnancy rates are higher in women from whom we obtain larger numbers of eggs.

PREPARATION OF THE SPERM

Sperm preparation for IVF, GIFT, or ZIFT is no different from what was described in the previous chapter on sperm washing. The husband provides a specimen about three hours before the projected time of the procedure. That provides sufficient time for the sperm to be properly washed, separated, and capacitated.

An unsettled question is just exactly how many sperm should be placed in culture with the egg or how many sperm should be placed in the fallopian tube. As you know, a normal male will ejaculate anywhere from 100 to 300 million sperm into the vagina, but only about 10,000 ever make it to the fallopian tube. In an effort to enhance the chances for fertilization, anywhere from 100,000 to 1 million sperm are placed in the fallopian tube during a GIFT procedure. Similar numbers are placed in the culture dish with the eggs for in vitro fertilization. The idea is that by providing more sperm around the egg than is normally found, we can increase the chance of fertilization.

You might ask why we don't put in 5 million or 10 million sperm. There are two reasons for this. The first reason is that if the egg is completely overwhelmed by too many sperm, there is a very slight risk that when one of the sperm fertilizes the egg, another sperm will get in before the normal "block to polyspermy" has been triggered by the first sperm to penetrate. In fact we know that in any IVF procedure, about 5 percent of the eggs will exhibit polyspermy (i.e., were fertilized by more than one sperm), and if allowed to enter the fallopian tube or uterus, they would not develop and most certainly would result in miscarriage. It used to be thought that this "polyspermia" was caused by having too many sperm in the vicinity of the egg. It is more likely, however, that polyspermia is caused by an inherent defect in a certain percentage of the eggs in their ability to create this hardening of the zona after the first sperm penetrates. Nonetheless, the fear of "polyspermia" is one of the reasons for not completely overwhelming the egg with millions of sperm in the in vitro culture conditions, or in the fallopian tube.

The second reason for not using more than a million sperm is that as the sperm burn up energy, they release metabolic byproducts in the culture media and can cause the acidity of the media to increase, having potentially toxic effects on the fertilization process. Both of these concerns may simply be theoretical but it has prompted most labs in the world to limit the amount of sperm in contact with the egg.

Nonetheless, if sperm quality is extremely poor with very low percent and quality motility, it is common to put more than a million sperm in contact with the egg. We have used this approach in our epididymal sperm aspiration cases and have achieved fertilization with huge numbers of sperm, most of which were very poor, producing embryos that were perfectly normal and which have resulted in healthy live children.

CULTURE TECHNIQUES FOR EGG AND SPERM

Culture Media

"Culture media" to scientists simply means a fluid which has the necessary ingredients in it for proper cell growth outside of the body.

A pure, nontoxic culture media with constant acidity, temperature, and no evaporation is critical if the egg and eventually the embryo are to survive in the laboratory culture dish or test tube. The egg, sperm, and embryo must find that the fluid they are to reside in for the next two or three days is just like what they would find if they were in the fallopian tube. They must be made to feel "at home" or they will *not* fertilize.

Scientists have been "culturing" cells outside the body for over thirty years, and so this is not really a new technology. There are many different types of culture media, but most of the ones that work have basically the same ingredients with only a few you need to be aware of. Neither you nor the physician performing the in vitro fertilization (IVF) has to know about each one of the many ingredients in a typical cell culture media.

Please refer to the list of ingredients in the cell culture media that our laboratory uses which is called "HTF" (see Table 4). All of the different cell culture medias that are used in IVF, including Earle's, Hams F-10, Menezo's B-2, BW&W, Krebs-

TABLE 4

"HTF" IVF MEDIA

Component	Bicarbonate Buffered	Air Buffered
	(concentration in mEg/L)	(concentration in mEg/L)
Sodium chloride	101.6	Same
Potassium chloride	4.69	Same
Magnesium sulfate, anhydrous	0.20	Same
Potassium phosphate, monobasic	0.37	Same
Calcium chloride, anhydrous	2.04	Same
Sodium bicarbonate	25.0	4.0
Hepes	**	21.0
Sodium pyruvate	0.33	Same
Sodium lactate	21.4	Same
Penicillin-G	100 units/ml	Same
Streptomycin sulfate	50μg/ml	Same
Phenol red	0.001 grams/100 ml	Same
Osmolality	280 ± 5	Same
pH	7.3–7.5	Same

Ringer's Lactate, have basically the same ingredients. There may be minor variations but they don't result in any difference in the ability of the sperm to fertilize the egg. These look complex to you because I'm showing you all of the components, but they're very routine and have been standardized for decades.

There are a few critical factors, however, that must be paid close attention to because the purity of the culture media is truly the single most important factor affecting whether or not an IVF program will work successfully or not. First, the water that these ingredients are dissolved in must be ultra pure. The water must be distilled many times, and all glassware in which it is prepared has to be carefully washed many times with water that has been ultrapurified in this manner. A little egg, $\frac{1}{200}$ of an inch in diameter and trying to get a start in life, is extraordinarily fragile. It will die in an instant if put in the wrong environment, and that fact is not visible, as it is with sperm, that stops moving when it dies. When an egg dies it looks perfectly normal. The only problem is it doesn't fertilize and it doesn't become a baby.

The next thing you will notice is that there are basically two categories of media, "bicarbonate buffered," and "air buffered." A "buffer" is an ingredient that keeps the acidity of the media constant. Acidity is reflected by the "pH." The higher the pH, the more alkaline the fluid, and the lower the pH, the more acid the fluid. The pH of all of our bodily fluids and in our cells is 7.4. This is a biological constant. When the acidity or pH of the fluid gets above 7.5, most cells, and particularly eggs, will die. When the acidity or pH gets below 7.35, again the cell will die. The "buffer" in the media is what keeps this pH acidity at a constant level and prevents its fluctuation. The reason this is necessary is that as a cell metabolizes, it releases acids, and the buffer is the ingredient that absorbs these changes in acidity and keeps the "pH" constant.

Life would be much easier in the in vitro fertilization laboratory if all we had to use was "air buffered" media, which means the pH stays constant in ordinary room air. The problem with "air buffered" media is that, over many years of experience, everyone has found that cells can only function in such a media for limited periods of time. You cannot expect a cell or embryo to live for hours and days in "air buffered" media. They need bicarbonate (baking soda) to live. That is why we have to use "bicarbonate buffered" media for all of our culture work, and can only resort to the convenience of an "air buffered" media for short periods of time in which we are doing grading, manipulation, or some other handling of the eggs or embryos outside of the incubator.

Why all this concern about "bicarbonate" versus "air buffered" media? The problem bicarbonate creates is one of the number-one issues in maintaining good results with in vitro fertilization. As the media is exposed to air, the sodium bicarbonate forms carbon dioxide gas (CO_2). You don't see anything, but the CO_2 just quietly evaporates, and if you check the media two minutes after it's been out of the incubator, you realize that the pH has gone up dramatically and the cell has, therefore, probably died.

You only know it died because no fertilization takes place. That's the problem with the necessity of using bicarbonate as a buffer. Left in room air, the CO_2 leaves, the pH goes way up in just a few minutes, and the egg dies. Nonetheless, we're stuck with it because that happens to be what human cells require. So what's the solution?

CO_2 Incubator

You have to put the "bicarbonate buffered" culture media in an incubator designed to maintain a constant concentration of 5 percent carbon dioxide (CO_2) in the atmosphere. With this 5 percent concentration of carbon dioxide in the atmosphere, carbon dioxide which would otherwise evaporate from the culture media is prevented from doing so. If your incubator isn't functioning properly and has a concentration of 10 percent carbon dioxide, the culture media will be too acid (pH less than 7.35), and the egg will die. If the concentration of CO_2 is only 2 percent, the media will become too alkaline (the pH will go over 7.5), and again the egg will die. Therefore, you must have an incubator that maintains a constant atmosphere of 5 percent CO_2.

But what about when we open and close the door of the incubator to take culture dishes out in order to transfer embryos to them? The more the door is opened and closed the more CO_2 leaks out. Therefore, without your even being aware of it, the pH of the media can go up, and again the egg can quietly and unobstrusively die. Keeping the carbon dioxide in the atmosphere constant and the pH in the 7.4 range remains one of the major issues of quality control for IVF embryo culturing.

Culture Dishes and Test Tubes Designed to
Keep pH Constant When Out of Incubator

Now that we have the problem of maintaining constant pH in the incubator solved, what about when we do have to take the culture dishes out into room air for brief periods of time? How much time are we allowed before either having to transfer the egg or embryos to an "air buffered" media or to get them back into the carbon dioxide environment of the incubator? Unfortunately, with most culture dishes, that period of time is only a *couple of minutes* at most.

Typical culture dishes have a broad surface area which allows one to easily visualize the egg or embryo under the microscope. You simply put the tissue culture dish on the stage of the microscope and the embryo comes right into view and can be manipulated quite easily. That is the advantage of these common, broad-based tissue culture dishes. However, the CO^2 evaporation is so rapid that within several minutes the pH has gone way too high and the egg will be dead.

On the other hand, if the eggs or embryos are kept in a small test tube, which has a much narrower area for evaporation, the pH of the media can stay constant in air for fifteen minutes or longer because of the reduced surface area for carbon dioxide evaporation. The problem with these test tubes is that it is very difficult to visualize the egg or embryo under the microscope in a test tube, and it is technically very demanding to remove these embryos from the test tube without the possibility of losing them.

The other approach for minimizing CO^2 loss and pH changes while the culture fluid is out of the incubator is an "oil overlay." With this technique a very small micro-droplet of culture media with sperm and egg in it is placed on the bottom of a broad-based culture dish but purified mineral oil or paraffin oil is laid over this droplet. With this approach you can take the culture dish out of the incubator for periods as long as half an hour without a serious risk that the pH will go up. Of course, there is some CO^2 evaporation even through the oil, but it is slowed down tremendously. This way we keep the pH stable for a limited period of time while the embryo is out of the incubator, but guarantee the proper pH while it is in the incubator.

EFFECT OF pH ON SPERM

All the time we have been talking about the extreme sensitivity of the egg to changes in pH, and how easy it is to quietly kill the egg with just a short exposure to the wrong amount of acidity. What about the sperm? Sperm are remarkably resistant to the pH changes that would normally kill the egg. In fact sperm can be washed with CO^2 buffered media in air with impunity. The pH will climb to levels as high as 7.8, and yet sperm motility and function will not be seriously hurt at least over several hours. We found that changes in the pH occasioned by using "bicarbonate buffered" media in air did no harm to the sperm over several hours. The sperm seem to handle an increase in pH quite well for several hours. But prolonged exposure to a high pH can harm the sperm. Some laboratories wash the sperm in "air buffered" media to make sure they are never exposed to these pH changes, and others wash them in CO^2 buffered media, placing them in the CO^2 incubator only after the wash has been completed. No significant differences in fertilizing ability are noted with either of these approaches.

OSMOLALITY OF MEDIA

You'll remember from our discussion on sperm washing that the "osmolality" of a fluid is the number of dissolved molecules in a given volume. The "osmolality" is *not* the density. If the ingredients of the fluid are composed of very heavy molecules, like with percoll, the density may be very high. All body fluids and cells have an "osmolality" of about 280. If the "osmolality" of the fluid around the cell is too high, then water leaks out of the cell into the surrounding fluid by "osmosis" and the cell shrinks.

If the "osmolality" of the fluid is too low, fluid will enter the cell by "osmosis," cause it to swell and certainly kill it. When vigorously active, motile sperm are placed in fluid of low "osmolality," they die instantly. The effect is quite dramatic and visible. When embryos are placed in fluid with low "osmolality" they swell and also die.

One would fear that while the culture media is sitting in a warm incubator over a period of several days, the "osmolality" of the fluid might go up as evaporation of water occurs. Protection against this is afforded by creating a 98 percent humidity saturation in the incubator. So now we know that a good incubator must maintain a constant 5 percent carbon dioxide level, and also a 98 to 99 percent humidity to prevent evaporation. The other constant which the incubator must maintain is temperature.

TEMPERATURE

Our normal body temperature is 98.6°F, or 37°C. Without this constant temperature, our normal biological processes simply would not proceed. The incubator maintains a constant temperature of 37°C for this reason. How sensitive is the egg, or the sperm, to changes in temperature? Actually, when the temperature goes down, the sperm movement slows down, but there is no major effect on the sperm's viability. When the temperature goes back up again, the sperm once again become vigorous. Remarkably, the same effect, although less easy to observe, occurs in eggs. When the temperature goes down this does no real harm to the egg. It simply slows its metabolism down, and fertilization and growth of the embryo are not going to occur. The egg and embryo must be at 37°C in order to grow properly. But a temporarily lowered temperature does not kill them.

What if the temperature goes above 37°C? A slight elevation of the temperature above 37°C can be very damaging to the egg. You won't notice what happened. The egg simply will not fertilize because it died from overheating. If the temperature in the incubator goes up over 98.6°F, the eggs quite literally get poached.

PROTEIN

The ingredient in culture media not yet mentioned is "protein." We know that sperm are not likely to capacitate well in the absence of "protein," and we know that the egg derives some nourishment from "protein" in the media. Very few in vitro fertilization (IVF) centers would risk trying to culture eggs or embryos without some type of "protein" added. The amount and type of "protein," however, vary considerably and may not really make a significant difference. The simplest approach is to draw the mother's blood the day before the procedure, separate off the serum from the red blood cells and add some of her serum to the culture media, usually in a concentration of 10 percent.

FILTERING

Finally, after this media is prepared and the serum added, before using it, we must be absolutely certain there is no bacterial contamination. To guarantee against that, it is pushed through a "millipore" filter into sterile tubes or culture dishes. This "millipore" filter is a remarkable little device you might be well advised to bring with you on camping trips to prevent getting infections from impure, unboiled water. It is simply a little disk that you place on the end of a syringe that is filled with media, or any other fluid for that matter, and you push the fluid out of the syringe through the "millipore" filter. The openings in this "millipore" filter are only twenty-two microns in diameter, and that allows them to filter out all bacteria and other microbes that could cause infections, virtually everything except viruses. You don't have to boil or sterilize the fluid (which would completely destroy many of the ingredients), but just push it through a "millipore" filter and you have instant sterility.

I've covered these details not to bore you, but to give you the fullest picture of the kind of perfect environment that has to be created to mimic the atmosphere of your fallopian tubes, so that the husband's sperm and the wife's eggs can get to know each other and fertilize. If the environment isn't exactly right, i.e., constant pH (acidity), constant "osmolality," and proper temperature, not to mention all the other ingredients contained in routine culture media, a woman's eggs will not survive and the man's sperm will not be able to fertilize them.

THE REMARKABLE INTRAVAGINAL CULTURING (IVC) METHOD OF CLAUDE RANOUX

Now that you have heard about the tremendous complexity of maintaining proper laboratory conditions for culturing the sperm, egg, and embryos so that you can have a baby, let me tell you about an extraordinary simplification very few people are presently doing yet (and may not care to do), but which underscores how extremely simple this whole in vitro fertilization (IVF) process can ultimately become. With the method that Dr. Claude Ranoux from Paris has developed, in vitro fertilization could very easily be transferred to the poorest, most remote regions of the world without any need for an expensive laboratory setup. It's so astounding that you scratch your head and laugh until you realize that a tremendous amount of scientific thinking went into this almost ridiculous-sounding simplification of the whole procedure.

This maverick scientist (who presently is at Harvard University) simply takes the wife's eggs, only 60,000 of the husband's sperm, places *all the eggs* and this small number of sperm in one little test tube, seals it hermetically with paraffin paper and tape much like any wife who has prepared food for freezing is familiar with, and then sticks this test tube inside the patient's vagina. He then fits her for a diaphragm to make sure the test tube doesn't fall out. She does whatever she wants for the next two days, comes back, and lo and behold there are perfectly normal embryos in the test tube. He then takes these embryos out of the test tube, and places them in her uterus just as for a regular, normal, in vitro fertilization procedure.

How in the world could something this simple, so very French-sounding, work? I've just spent most of a chapter trying to explain to you all of the very careful, rigid conditions which must be met for the egg to stay alive, for the sperm to fertilize it, and for the embryo to cleave and grow. How does he get good embryos by sticking a test tube full of media, sperm, and eggs into the woman's vagina for two days?

This absurd-sounding technique was very carefully thought out and here's how it works: The "bicarbonate buffered" culture media is placed in a small test tube filled right *to the very top*. All of the woman's eggs are placed in this test tube. The idea of this procedure is that if the tube is filled to the top, carefully capped and sealed so that there is no air in it, then there will be no chance for CO_2 evaporation, and the pH will remain constant.

What about maintaining a constant temperature? Well that is the simple French solution. By putting the test tube in the vagina, you are keeping it as well controlled at 37°C as in the most expensive laboratory incubator. In fact, unlike with laboratory incubators, you don't have to worry about sudden loss of electrical power in the middle of the night during a thunderstorm. This is a simplification of a procedure that otherwise requires unbelievable attention to detail for maintaining the constant and proper conditions that the body would normally maintain for a fertilizing egg.

EGG HANDLING AFTER RETRIEVAL FROM OVARY

The test tube containing the follicular fluid is immediately brought to the laboratory work table, which preferably is either in the operating room or directly connected to the operating room. The contents of the test tube are immediately emptied into a large petri dish. This petri dish is then scanned under the microscope to find the egg. The egg is truly an incredibly serene, beautiful object in contrast to the millions of frantically moving

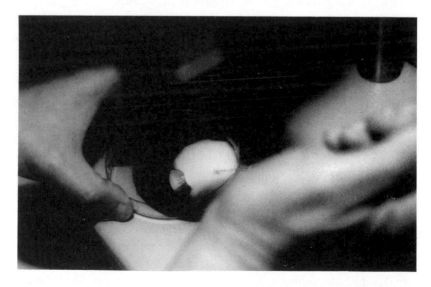

Figure 33. Picking up eggs from large petri dish using a small pipette.

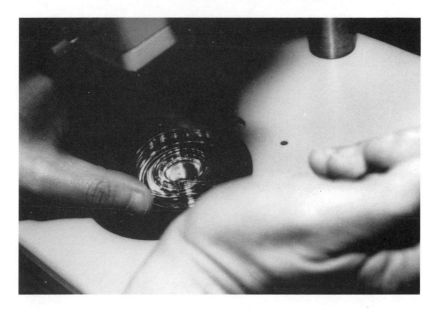

Figure 34. Transferring egg with small pipette into a grading dish.

sperm, only one of which will be able to fertilize the egg. When I'm looking at the egg I have a sinking feeling in my stomach that I'm looking at something that might someday grow up, and be able to write a poem. Sperm are very impersonal because any one of the millions of them might be the one to get into the egg. But the egg is something truly personal and exciting to look at.

The human egg is actually visible to the naked eye because of the sticky, gooey "cumulus mass" that surrounds it. A "bare" egg could never be picked up by the fallopian tube and so nature has provided this mass which cradles it and allows it to be grabbed on to by the cilia. On the other hand, in the laboratory dish, this substance clearly protects the egg and literally keeps it from contacting the glass, the tubing, or anything else it has to go through to make its way; and because of this, you can almost always find it in the petri dish even before looking through the microscrope.

The egg is picked up, of course, under microscopic control, with a small pipette (see Figure 33) and placed in what we call

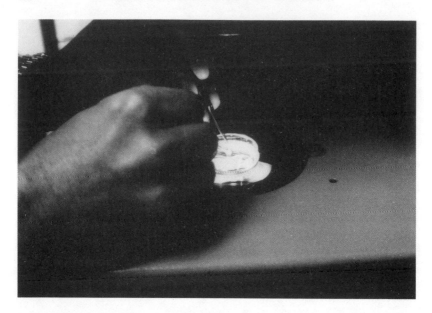

Figure 35. Dissecting cumulus mass off of a human egg with ultrafine microneedles.

a "grading dish." This "grading dish" is a smaller petri dish which has been filled with a small amount of culture media just prior to the grading procedure (see Figure 34). The reason for using such a small amount of culture media is to allow the egg to "flatten out" temporarily so that we can get a better two-dimensional view of it under the microscope and characterize its maturity and degree of fertilizability. However, the risk of using such a small amount of culture media over a broad-surface petri dish is that the evaporation is very quick.

We don't consider the cumulus mass a problem for sperm penetration under normal circumstances. But if there is any blood in it, if the sperm quality is extremely sluggish, or if there is any lint from the atmosphere attached to this sticky, gooey mass, then we dissect it off using ultrafine 30-gauge needles under the microscope (see Figure 35). We make sure to work extremely fast so that the egg is actually out of the incubator for no more than thirty seconds at most.

The egg is surrounded by "corona cells" which are closely

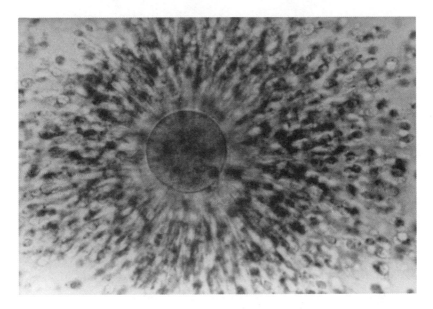

Figure 36. Picture of the sunburst appearance of a mature egg ready for fertilization.

attached to the zona pellucida shell. As the egg matures in the follicle under the stimulus of FSH and estrogen preparing to be ready for the LH trigger, not only does the egg grow from 20 microns to 140 microns in size, but the densely packed granulosa cells surrounding it begin to spread out circumferentially in a fan-shaped pattern like the spokes of a bicycle wheel. In fact, looking at a mature egg with a completely developed "corona" often reminds reproductive scientists of stylized drawings of the sun (see Figure 36). When you look at the sun, there is a center orb of brilliant light surrounded by flashes and streaks of hot gases extending and trailing off circumferentially outward from the sun's surface. In fact, that is the reason why these granulosa cells or the "corona" in a mature egg are classically referred to as the "corona radiata."

If the "corona" is widely dispersed and spread out in a beautiful fan-shaped pattern, that means that the cell is very mature and very likely to be fertilizable, particularly if the cytoplasm is clear and not clumpy or dark; such an egg would be graded as very high quality. Incidentally, if one were to look carefully, one would also almost always find in such eggs a first polar body indicating that the egg has received the LH trigger and is ready genetically for fertilization. However, in practice the first polar body is not often looked for because it may be difficult to find under an ordinary dissecting microscope.

If, however, the "corona" is tightly packed against the zona pellucida without very much spreading out, this type of cell is very immature, definitely not ready for fertilization, and most likely will not have a first polar body extrusion. Sometimes culturing such an egg for a period of twelve hours in the laboratory will allow it to mature sufficiently so that it may very well fertilize.

After the egg has been properly "graded" (and the "cumulus" dissected off if necessary), it is removed from this grading dish with "air buffered" media using a pipette and placed in the culture dish or test tube containing "bicarbonate buffered" media (see Figure 37). The culture dish or test tube is then immediately put back into the CO_2 incubator.

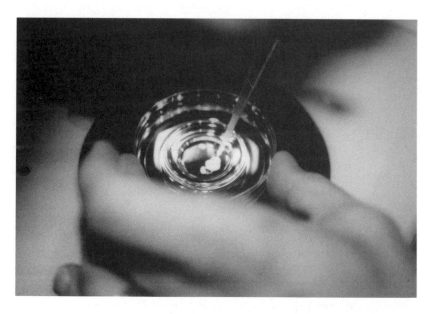

Figure 37. Transferring egg into culture dish with "bicarbonate buffered" media before placing in incubator.

PLACING SPERM AND EGGS INTO THE FALLOPIAN TUBE FOR GIFT

The eggs and sperm will remain quite safe in the incubator, while you are prepared for exposure of the fallopian tube either through a laparoscopy or through a tiny one inch incision in the lower abdomen called a "minilap." It usually takes a matter of ten or fifteen minutes, at most, to expose the fallopian tubes and get them in a position where the catheter can be easily inserted into the open fimbriated end. The surgery is extremely simple but, of course, must be performed delicately. Any rough handling of the fallopian tube that might stir up bleeding will hurt the chances for pregnancy. The most important thing, however, is to have the tube adequately exposed over a reasonably long length so that the catheter can be placed deeply within it. Very often GIFT programs have poor pregnancy rates because only the very tip of the fimbriated end of the fallopian tube is visualized and the catheter is placed only a short way inside. There is an excellent chance that the eggs will not remain in the fallopian tube for fertilization with such an inadequate placement.

Once the fallopian tubes are exposed, a small droplet usually containing anywhere from 100,000 to a million motile sperm is placed on a petri dish under the microscope. Then the culture dishes or test tubes holding the eggs are removed from the CO_2 incubator and placed on the microscope stage right next to the sperm droplet. Using a pipette, the most mature and fertile eggs are picked up and placed within the droplet of sperm. If four eggs are to be transferred, they are all four placed within this same droplet of sperm. If two eggs are to be transferred into each fallopian tube, then only two eggs are placed in this droplet of sperm. The entire sperm droplet containing the eggs is then aspirated into a small catheter using a tiny syringe on the end. The total volume of fluid containing this sperm and egg combination is usually no greater than fifty microliters at most ($\frac{1}{100}$ of a teaspoon).

This tiny volume of fluid containing sperm and eggs is then taken over to the patient. The catheter is inserted into the end of the fallopian tube to a depth of at least three or four centimeters (one and a half to two inches), and then injected. The catheter is then removed and carefully examined under the microscope to make sure that no egg has been accidentally left behind. If both fallopian tubes are going to be used, then two eggs (or more if it's indicated) are transferred to each side.

The question always comes up in GIFT as to how many eggs to transfer. The average number is four or five which gives quite good pregnancy rates and prevents too great a risk of triplets or greater. In older women in their late thirties and early forties, some would advocate transferring as many as eight eggs (and sometimes more), because the chances of developing a multiple pregnancy at that age are so incredibly rare. On the other hand, in a twenty-eight-year-old woman with donor sperm, the chance of a good fertilization and pregnancy is extremely high, and one would generally not transfer more than three eggs.

The entire GIFT operation from the beginning of egg aspiration to the placement of the eggs and the quick closure of the small incision, usually takes about forty-five minutes. The patient has minimal postoperative pain but may have enough discomfort to want to stay in the hospital overnight. The advantage of GIFT over ZIFT (in vitro fertilization with transfer of embryos into the fallopian tube two days later) is that it is done all in one procedure. The disadvantage of GIFT compared to ZIFT is that there is no proof of fertilization.

ADDING THE SPERM TO THE EGGS, CULTURING FOR IVF, AND TRANSFER OF IN VITRO FERTILIZED EMBRYOS

If in vitro fertilization or ZIFT is going to be performed (rather than GIFT), the patient leaves the operating room shortly after egg aspiration and goes home an hour or two later with very little pain at all. The sperm are then placed into culture dishes or test tubes containing the eggs (see Figures 38 and 39). If there are a lot of healthy, motile sperm and not too great a number of eggs, each egg is placed in its own tube or culture dish. Anywhere from 50,000 to 1 million motile sperm may be added

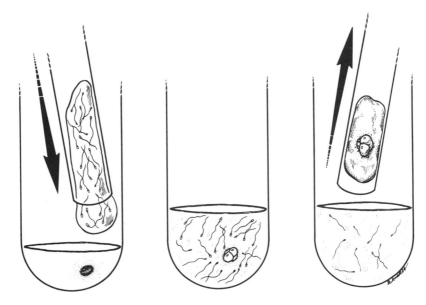

Figure 38. Diagram of sperm being placed in test tube with egg, resulting in four-cell embryo two days later and retrieval of four-cell embryo for transfer back to patient.

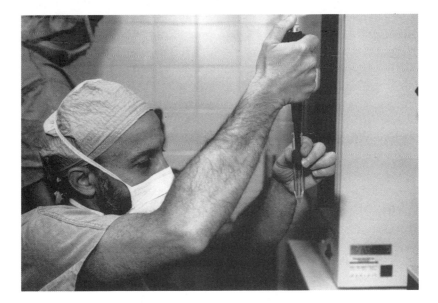

Figure 39. I'm preparing to transfer sperm from centrifuge tube into a culture dish.

to the culture tube or dish containing the egg. It used to be thought that a certain period of time was required for the egg to mature in culture and for the sperm to capacitate before this "insemination" procedure was performed. With modern stimulation protocols as discussed earlier in this section, one really doesn't have to go through this period of waiting. The sperm that has already been washed and therefore capacitated can be placed immediately in culture with the eggs.

Sometimes when the number of motile sperm available is extremely low, all of the eggs will be placed in one culture dish or test tube, and the total amount of the sperm that is available will be added to it.

Most laboratories check the eggs somewhere between thirteen and eighteen hours after "insemination" to see if "pronuclei" have formed and to see if the second polar body has been extruded. These would be clear indications that the egg has fertilized and that it will most likely undergo cleavage into an embryo. You should realize that at this point the egg may be fertilized but it is not yet really a new individual. The chromosomes have not truly met and united into a new cell. That is the process of "syngamy" where the two pronuclei seem to just miraculously move toward the center and become one. Usually this occurs sometime after eighteen hours. After syngamy and before cell division, you really can't tell whether or not the egg has been fertilized. Two days after the initial egg retrieval and insemination procedure, the embryos (if there are any) should be ready for transfer back to the patient.

Usually in two days, anywhere from two-cell to four-cell and occasionally six-cell embryos will be seen. Each one of these cells in a cleaving embryo is called a "blastomere." The quality of the embryo is judged by two factors: 1) how many blastomeres are present indicating the rapidity of embryo cleavage, and 2) perfect smooth roundness of each of those blastomeres (see Figures 40a–d). Often embryos will have uneven-shaped blastomeres or degenerating blastomeres, along with blastomeres that look quite healthy. Some of these relatively unhealthy-looking embryos turn into normal, happy, healthy, intelligent babies. On the other hand, an extremely poor quality embryo with mostly degenerating blastomeres and a very sluggish rate of cleavage will not develop into a pregnancy.

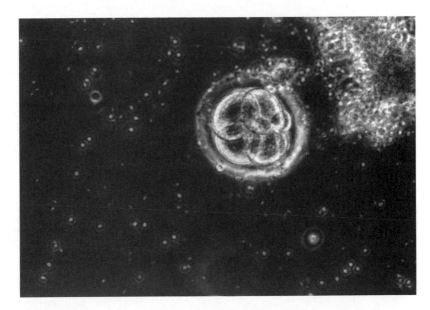

Figure 40a. Phase contract photograph of four-cell embryo with perfectly round blastomeres, indicating a high likelihood of viability. Notice tough outer zona pellucida with sperm still attached and loosely distributed corona cells in background.

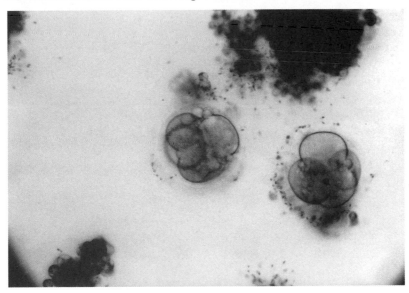

Figure 40b. Same embryos with bright field where sperm heads attached to outside of zona pellucida are more easily seen.

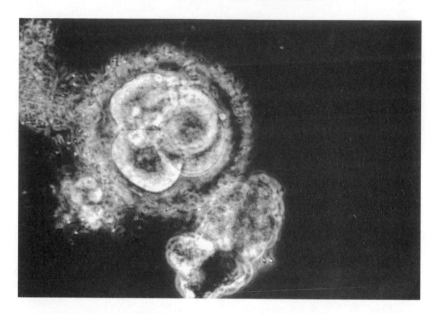

Figure 40c. Phase contrast micrograph of four-cell embryo with large numbers of sperm attached to outside of zona pellucida.

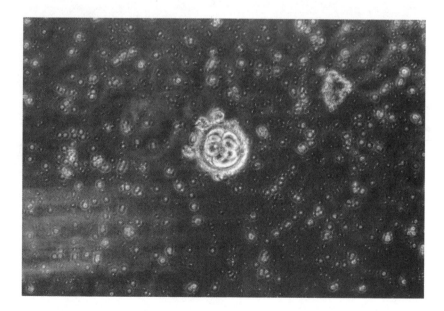

Figure 40d. Phase contrast micrograph of six-cell embryo with some of the round blastomeres.

Remember that eggs can undergo a cleavage-appearing process without any fertilization by sperm. This is called "parthenogenesis." Parthenogenesis is a regular method of reproduction
for honey bees and Amazon mollies that never works in humans.
So the physician must distinguish between a true fertilized egg
with healthy-looking, rapidly cleaving blastomeres, and the mere
appearance of fertilization by unhealthy-looking fragmentation.

The healthy-looking embryos are loaded into a catheter very
similar to the one used for the GIFT transfer. The same low
volume of fluid (about one hundredth of a teaspoon maximum)
is used for transferring two to five embryos.

The handling of embryos is truly thrilling and technically demanding (see Figure 41). You will notice that I refer to embryos
as rapidly or slowly cleaving, but I did not refer to them as
rapidly or slowly *growing*. In fact, the embryo does not grow at
all during the first six days of development. It divides into many

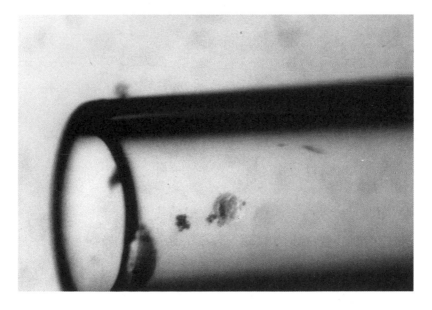

Figure 41. Tiny four-cell embryo near the tip of a tiny micropipette
blown up eighty times to demonstrate how delicate the egg is and
how easy it would be to lose.

cells so that by five days it is a "blastocyst." At this stage you can't tell one cell from another because there are so many of them compacted together. That large blastocyst at five or six days is no larger than the original egg it came from; the tough outer shell of the zona pellucida is an absolute limitation to the size of the cleaving embryo and it does not in any way "grow."

This ball of cells that is no larger than that original tiny egg (about 1/250 of an inch in diameter) and is no longer surrounded by a corona radiata, or a sticky, gooey cumulus mass, which otherwise made the egg so easy to handle. It is just a tiny, bare fragile little ball that even in a small culture dish looks like a mere speck in the universe. Although an egg was very impressive with all of its outer investments of corona radiata and sticky cumulus, it is hard to believe that this little speck of cleaving cells called an embryo can ever become a human being. Much more delicate than the egg, the embryo's membrane is more permeable (which ironically makes it easier to freeze an embryo than an egg because the cryoprotective agent can actually get in). Because it has no sticky mass around it, it poses a very big problem in doing a transfer procedure. It will not easily "lodge" in the area where it is injected. Care must be taken to be extremely delicate, and careful, so that the egg stays where it is supposed to stay and isn't accidentally yanked back as the catheter is pulled out.

When performing classic IVF (putting the embryos into the uterus through the cervix), one must place the transfer catheter deep into the uterus but not touch the back wall and thereby irritate it. After the embryos are inserted, the catheter should stay for a minute in that position and then be pulled back slowly and out. Dr. Alan De Cherney, head of the program at Yale University, had one of his graduate students calculate the force and the speed at which the embryo would leave the catheter if it were simply haphazardly injected without incredible care and attention to being delicate. They calculated that if injected too hard, the embryo could come flying out of that catheter at a speed of six hundred miles per hour as it hits the uterine wall. Not a very gentle way to start out life.

Sometimes the placement of the catheter through the cervix isn't all that easy and care and patience must be taken not to force it; only by careful slow exploration can the catheter negotiate the curvature of the cervical canal. When the catheter doesn't go in easily it would rarely be because the cervix is closed. The reason almost always is that the cervix pursues a curved course. The solution is to straighten out the cervix with a gentle sponge-type instrument so that the catheter can pursue a straight line without forcing or shoving it into the uterus. A traumatic transfer or a transfer that results in blood being seen at the opening of the cervix reduces dramatically the chances for pregnancy.

If a ZIFT procedure is going to be performed, the same technique is followed for loading the embryos into the catheter as for IVF or, for that matter, GIFT. The only difference from GIFT is that it is very easy to see the eggs and to load them with the sperm, but the embryos are much more delicate and are not automatically held in place by a sticky, gooey mass surrounding them. The catheter must be placed deeply within the fallopian tube (at least an inch or two) and there must be no tugging or bleeding or trauma. This can be performed (as with GIFT) either through a laparoscopy or a "minilap" procedure.

EMBRYO FREEZING

When many extra eggs or embryos are obtained for a GIFT or an IVF cycle, obviously they cannot all be placed back into the woman. It would create too big a risk of quadruplets or quintuplets or even greater. Some infertile couples will yield as many as ten to thirty eggs in a stimulation cycle. It would be a shame to waste these "extras" after the requisite three to five embryos (or eggs) have been replaced. It is for that reason that "embryo freezing" was developed.

Eggs cannot be frozen without killing them. However, embryos (and sperm also) can be frozen and preserved indefinitely and stored in liquid nitrogen tanks for future replacement into the uterus or fallopian tubes in a future cycle. In order for you to understand how we can actually hold this form of human life on call for future use without killing it, you need to understand how freezing normally does kill a cell or an organ.

Lowering the temperature to $-273°C$ does not poison any

metabolic processes. It just stops everything. One would, therefore, not logically expect freezing to harm the body at all. The
only reason that freezing kills comes from a peculiar property of
water (the cells in our body are over 70 percent water), is that
when the temperature reaches freezing, instead of just turning
solid, it crystalizes. We all know that ice cubes do not sink. The
reason is that when water freezes, unlike most other liquids, it
actually expands and forms a crystalline structure of much
greater volume. If you put an enclosed bottle of water in a
freezer, the water by virtue of freezing will burst the bottle.
Thus, when cells are frozen, they die only because the formation
of ice crystals *inside* them expand and damage the inside of the
cell.

The way this can be protected against is twofold: 1) get as
much water out of the cell as possible, and 2) get a "cryoprotectant" (literally an antifreeze solution) into the cell to prevent
formation of ice crystals. One reason that eggs cannot be frozen
without killing them, but embryos can be, is that the outer cell
membrane of the egg is not very permeable, and it is harder to
get water out of it and cryoprotectant into it. The reason that
embryos can be frozen and stay alive is that the moment the
egg is fertilized, the cell membrane begins to become more
permeable. The reason that a sperm is relatively easy to freeze
is that it is one of the few cells in the body that has hardly any
water in it. A sperm head is just solid DNA with virtually no
cytoplasm. There is hardly any ice crystal formation to worry
about.

The method for freezing extra embryos is relatively simple.
We place the embryos into a solution containing propanediol
(the antifreeze) and sucrose (a sugar that stays outside the cell
and thereby "pulls" water out osmotically). The embryos in this
solution are then aspirated into a tiny plastic freezing straw and
the ends are hermetically sealed. The straw is very carefully
labeled and placed into a programmed "freezing machine." The
temperature is then slowly reduced at a tightly controlled rate.
Once it is just below freezing, a crystal formation is induced,
and then the temperature continues to be slowly reduced to
about $-30°$ to $-40°C$. After that, the straw is immediately
plunged into the liquid nitrogen storage container.

The reason for the slow, carefully controlled freezing rate is that it allows ice crystals to first form on the outside of the cell. This increases the osmolality outside the cell and thereby draws more and more water out of it. Ideally, once the solution in the staw crystalizes, there is virtually no water left inside the embryo. All the ice crystals are left on the outside.

After thawing the embryos at a future date for putting them back into the wife, a similarly rigorous approach must be used, or they will die from what is called "osmotic shock." These dehydrated little embryos would swell and burst if just placed back into the body's normal osmotic environment. They must first be placed into successively less dilute solutions of sucrose to gradually get all the propanediol out and put small amounts of water back into the cell. Finally the embryos are fully restored, alive, and ready to start a new life.

Not all embryos survive this freezing and thawing process no matter how carefully it is performed. However, it is usually the least healthy embryos (that would have been least likely to result in a pregnancy anyway) that fail to survive the freezing process. That is why most programs freeze only the embryos that are completely normal looking. The others are left in culture to see if they can continue to develop. If they do, they are then frozen several days later. If they don't, then it means they never could have made it anyway.

The purpose of freezing embryos is not to tamper with life. These cells are not able to survive on their own if not replaced into the woman. If there are more embryos than can be safely put back into her, then freezing them is a way of maximizing their chance of eventually becoming a baby.

"NONSURGICAL" GIFT AND ZIFT PROCEDURES

Dr. Rob Janson and Dr. Jaco Anderson from Sydney, Australia, have been experimenting for many years with various catheters which they hoped could be threaded up through the cervix into the fallopian tube directly so as to perform GIFT or ZIFT without the necessity of an operation. If their efforts were successful, then ZIFT and GIFT, like classical IVF, would be completely nonsurgical. The results with this approach have been meager at best. The idea of this method is to thread a catheter that can be seen on ultrasound into the uterus and to place it near the "cornu" where the fallopian tube exists. Then with delicate manipulation (under ultrasound guidance) the catheter could in some way be negotiated through this very tight cornu into the ampulla of the fallopian tube. Then for GIFT, sperm and eggs could be injected; and for ZIFT, embryos could be injected.

The idea sounds great in theory, but there are a lot of problems with it, and it may never really work well. First, one of the major reasons that GIFT and ZIFT achieve a higher "implantation" rate than classic IVF may just be that the very process of entering the uterus in some way makes it less likely to accept the embryo for implantation. The best example one can think of is the IUD (intrauterine device) used for birth control. We've known for years that when any foreign object, no matter how small, is placed in the uterus, conception does not occur. The reason conception does not occur is that the uterus has been irritated by the IUD. So by placing a catheter up through the uterus into the fallopian tube to perform GIFT or ZIFT nonoperatively you may be defeating the very purpose of GIFT or ZIFT which is to leave the uterus completely unirritated. Unfortunately, pregnancies with GIFT using this nonsurgical transfer method are rare to nonexistent.

SEVERE "MALE FACTOR": THE BIGGEST PROBLEM IN REPRODUCTION

One issue that reproductive physicians agree on is that the major unsolved problem today is severe "male factor" infertility. We know that fertilization rates in vitro with men having low sperm counts average only 30 percent, compared to 60 to 80 percent with normal sperm. Forty percent of infertile couples have low sperm counts, but for the most part we are able to solve that problem simply by separating out the small number of good sperm they have and obtaining fertilization with the fewer sperm that are necessary for the fallopian tube or the culture dish. But there are some cases of male infertility in which the count is so extraordinarily low and the sperm so sluggish, or nonmotile at all, that we just don't get any fertilization despite optimum culture conditions.

There are two types of approaches being researched for this problem: one is to culture sperm and eggs in very concentrated sperm specimens in small microchambers or capillary tubes, or in small test tubes with low volumes of media. This way if there is just an occasional motile, fertile sperm capable of penetrating the egg, it will be more likely by random chance to strike the egg than if the mixture were placed in a standard culture dish or test tube. This approach works quite well.

"Micromanipulation" of Sperm

Another approach, however, as of yet unproven, is "micromanipulation." This technique was first used in the gene transfer technology for creating "transgenic" animals. Under a very high power "inverted" phase-contrast microscope, a very delicate micromanipulator geared machinery is attached to the stage of the microscope with extremely long, finely "pulled out" pipettes with microscopic tips and openings.

One of the pipettes, the "holding pipettes," has constant low-grade suction and an opening smaller than the egg (see Figure 42). It is used to "hold" the egg in place. The other pipette is used to direct a much sharper, even tinier-tipped micropipette directly into the egg. Originally this technology was used to inject foreign DNA (genes) into the pronucleus of an animal's fertilized egg to make a genetically engineered new animal.

There are hundreds of such "transgenic" animals now that have been injected with various genes for different biological and commercial purposes. For example, rats who were born after the growth hormone gene had been injected into their pronucleus at the "pronuclear" stage of fertilization make enormous amounts of growth hormone and in fact grow to be three times the size of a normal rat. Such "transgenic" animals can then be used for harvesting and purifying large quantities of growth hormone for medical usage for patients that need it. In the food-producing industry, transgenic cattle injected with growth hormone can yield tremendous volumes of milk, and for

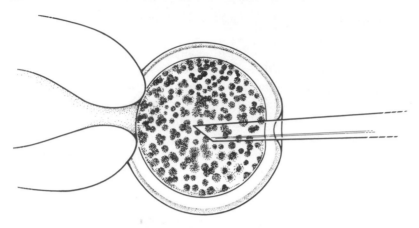

Figure 42. Egg being held in micromanipulator apparatus with holding pipette on left and puncturing micropipette on right.

the same amount of effort and expense on the ranch can result in the production of three times the quantity of meat.

For many years we have speculated about using this same technology to take a nonmotile sperm and directly inject it into the egg (see Figure 43a). I call this "fertilization by brute force," and as you can image the results with this are not much better than anything else that is done with brute force. The idea seemed extremely attractive but research on many animals has failed to demonstrate any more than what looks like pronuclear development. There have been other types of micromanipulation methods tried, including just making a hole in the zona of the egg to allow poor sperm an easier time getting in (see Figure 43b). With this approach there is no certainty that fertilization would not have occurred anyway in the successful cases, because success has only been reported with motile sperm.

Dr. Jacques Cohen in 1989 took eighteen couples with male factor infertility and performed this so-called micromanipulated "partial zona dissection (PZD)" on sixty-nine of their eggs. They reported a fertilization rate of 68 percent, but in their male factor patients without any micromanipulation they also had a fairly good fertilization rate of 47 percent (twenty-one out of forty-five). This would certainly not lead to any significant difference

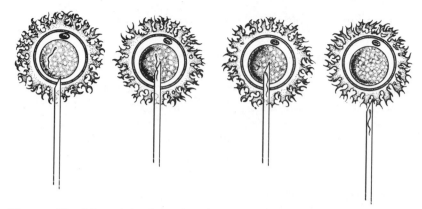

Figure 43a. Micro-injection of a single sperm into the egg itself.

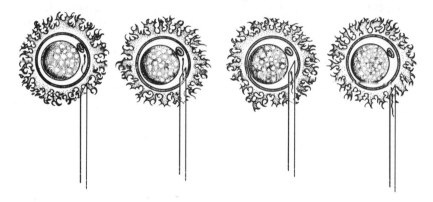

Figure 43b. Micro-injection of a single sperm through the zona pellucida into the egg itself.

in pregnancy rate; and indeed, when you analyze all of these numbers, the percent fertilization in those eggs that underwent partial zona dissection with micromanipulation is not significantly greater, as opposed to random variation, than those that did not undergo partial zona dissection.

There really has been no demonstration of fertilization and pregnancy caused by micromanipulation in types of patients where just normal laboratory in vitro fertilization techniques would not have just as easily allowed fertilization and pregnancy.

Remember, the biggest problem we deal with in interpreting any "male factor" infertility is that you must have controls. With very poor quality sperm we are able to obtain reasonable fertilization rates just by proper culturing techniques. The evidence is not clear yet that those fertilization rates can be improved by making a hole in the zona pellucida of the egg. In fact, doing so carries a tremendous risk that the embryo will not have the proper protection the zona affords it as it is growing up into a blastocyst in the uterus waiting for the time when it is ready for implantation.

Another approach to trying to micromanipulate sperm into the egg to fertilize by "brute force" that may have a future is "laser trapping" of the sperm pioneered by Dr. Yona Tadir from Israel while working at the Beckman Laser Institute at the University of California at Irvine. To watch video tapes of Dr. Tadir's experiments is truly a thrill beyond belief. He uses a very low-intensity beam laser directed under a high-power, phase-contrast microscope to actually "trap" the sperm optically. The laser is of low-enough power that it doesn't harm the sperm, and has a spot size as small as a sperm head. It works like a video arcade game.

You just aim this little laser spot at the rare or occasional sperm with good motility and good morphology. Once you "lock" the laser in on that sperm, it is totally under your control. You can see the tail wiggling frantically to try to get away but the head is held in place just like a collar that zoo keepers would use on the neck of a snake. Using the "joystick" attached to the laser, under microscopic visualization you can move that sperm anywhere you want to move it. You can take it off of its carefree, meaningless, joyless wanderings and bring it right next to the surface of the zona pellucida of the egg. Now it is true that you can lead a horse to water but you can't make it drink. Nonetheless, this laser trapping of the sperm, when it is more refined, will allow the sperm to be placed right next to the egg and will eliminate the difficulty that occurs when there are only tiny numbers of motile sperm that just by chance would never be likely to collide with the egg. This laser optical trapping of sperm won't be available other than for research for many years, and it may not turn out to improve fertilization rates in couples with poor sperm. But it holds promise for the future.

CONCLUSIONS

How Do We Pay for It?

Over $1 billion are spent on health care to try to help infertile couples get pregnant. A lot of this enormous cost is paid for by insurance companies only because of meaningless diagnoses that are used by health providers to avoid the word "infertility." While insurance companies will not pay for a diagnosis of infertility, they will pay for "disease"-sounding diagnoses such as "endometriosis" or "varicocele." Despite recommendations of the Congressional Advisory Panel in 1988 (which I was on) to call infertility an illness and to make payment for its treatment mandatory under health insurance policies, the U.S. Congress has done nothing except create some rumbling about the possibility of regulating in vitro fertilization. This very procedure, IVF, has made enormous technological leaps and continues to provide extraordinarily high pregnancy rates for hundreds of thousands of couples every year without any government research support whatsoever but purely through private funding. In vitro fertilization is not getting enough attention from the U.S. Congress to mandate that infertile couples have their medical care paid for by any insurance company that quickly pays for hemorrhoids or hysterectomy. There is so much payment by health insurance companies for ridiculous medical treatments adding into the billions and billions of dollars. Yet when a scientific advance comes along which would help couples with the tragedy of infertility have a baby, the only thing Congress can say is, "Well, maybe we ought to regulate it." Regulate what? The money isn't coming from the government, and it is not deriving from insurance companies out of any government mandate.

Insurance companies are paying only when a specific "pathologic diagnosis" is concocted. Heavy pressure has been placed upon insurance companies by consumer groups who recognize that this is at least as important a public health issue as coronary bypass, hemorrhoids, or unpleasant periods leading to hysterectomy.

Unfortunately, insurance companies do not realize (partly because of misinformation by Congress) that the new technology is much more cost-effective in the long run than the many tens of thousands of dollars that most couples wind up paying for conventional treatment that gets them nowhere. Several states, including Massachusetts, Maryland, and California, have mandated that health insurance companies pay for infertility treatment. But the federal government has done *nothing*, except to suggest regulating licensing of IVF clinics.

Among the examples of the silliness of government "regulation" to aid in the in vitro fertilization situation is that the very catheter that is most popularly used with the highest pregnancy rate for GIFT, ZIFT, and in vitro fertilization is the "Tom Cat," which was originally designed by Sherwood Pharmaceuticals for removing bladder stones from tom cats. Yet it is not legally sanctioned by the government or approved for use in humans. Therefore, IVF and ZIFT are "illegal" uses of the catheter. The catheters my Australian friends sent me in the early 1980s were made in St. Louis, purchased by Australians, and then sent back to me since I couldn't "legally" buy them because of government "regulation."

And consider government regulation of Lupron, the single most important drug coming out in the late 1980s to dramatically increase the pregnancy rates with in vitro fertilization and GIFT by preventing an early LH surge and ensuring the retrieval of large numbers of mature, fertilizable eggs. Yet the government will only "officially" allow us to use Lupron for cancer of the prostate, a condition for which very few physicians use it at all.

Finally, what about the "culture media." None of the culture media we use is legally sanctioned for human use. To get it sanctioned for human use would cost such incredible amounts of money and probably never pass any kind of bureacratic FDA evaluation. In fact, if an anti-fertility secretary of health (as there was during the Carter administration) didn't like in vitro fertilization on moral or ethical grounds, he or she could block the use of any culture media.

The fact is that it is the concerted intention to constantly improve this technology and help infertile couples in a laisse faire system combined with honest motivation on the part of leaders in this field to keep it clean and protect patients that has led to this dramatic improvement for all infertile couples. The government has been nothing but a hindrance, and, we have no doubt, it will continue to be a hindrance.

How does this technology get paid for? Infertile couples have lobbied legislators in many states and have gotten the legislators to pass laws mandating that the insurance companies doing business in that state include infertility as an illness and pay for its treatment. Maryland was the first such state to pass this law, pushed on by a consumer group in Baltimore.

Additionally the consumer needs to be knowledgeable about filling out insurance forms in such a way as *not to lie* but to emphasize the pathologic nature of their condition. Infertile women have a greater chance of developing cancer of the ovary and cancer of the uterus than fertile women later in life if their fertility problem is not treated. And while doctors cannot truly make a diagnosis of the cause of infertility in the majority of cases, they can at least call it "menstrual dysfunction" or "ovarian menstrual dysfunction" even though it is not known what is preventing pregnancy. With this kind of savvy and perhaps with a little help from your lawyer (as well as lobbying your legislature), the majority of the costs of this technology, which are less than the costs incurred by conventional treatment that no insurance company objects to, are being covered by insurance companies, whether they are aware of it or not.

What Are My Chances?

The original report of the Congressional Office of Technology Assistance in 1989 stated that out of 150 in vitro fertilization or GIFT programs, 50 percent had never had a pregnancy, and the overall pregnancy rate was only 7 percent. But since that time there has been an explosive improvement in our results which changes those figures drastically in most well-known programs.

• First, GIFT and ZIFT have been developed, which almost triples the live birth rate obtainable with classic IVF. Simply placing the embryos, or easier yet the sperm and the eggs, into the fallopian tube solves the number-one problem that used to haunt IVF clinics: low "embryo implantation rate." The implantation problem has been in a large measure solved by the introduction of GIFT and ZIFT.

• Second, ovarian stimulation protocols are far superior to anything that was available before 1989. In the U.S. government survey from 1989, 20 to 24 percent of IVF cycles had to be canceled because of an inadequate ovarian response with very few follicles due to stimulation protocols. This is an incredible failure rate when you can eliminate large numbers of women right from the starting gate from the possibility of having a success. Yet the same survey showed that when those couples were taken off of old-fashioned stimulation protocols and put on modern Pergonal, Metrodin, and Lupron protocols (most importantly Lupron), 90 percent of these "failures to respond" now responded with beautiful follicles and excellent mature fertilizable eggs. Not only are we able to get eggs out of women we couldn't get eggs from before, but we are getting more eggs. The greater the number of eggs we retrieve the greater the chance of pregnancy.

• The third reason for the tremendous improvement in pregnancy rate, just with IVF alone (leaving out GIFT and ZIFT), is that we have developed better, gentler methods for transferring the embryos into the uterus. This is simply a matter of physician awareness and experience. (It is not always the matter of having had a lot of experience. Some physicians with only a meager amount of experience got good results simply because they performed the transfer atraumatically and accomplished a deep placement into the uterus.)

• The fourth reason for the improvement in pregnancy rate is the much greater efficiency of egg retrieval. Before 1987, most egg retrievals for in vitro fertilization were being performed by laparoscopy, a clumsy process to go thorough, and a lot of eggs are left behind. With transvaginal egg retrieval, not only is surgery avoided, but more importantly, you can see the entire ovary—the outside and the inside—and collect every single egg that is available.

• A fifth reason for the dramatic improvement in pregnancy rates both with IVF and GIFT and ZIFT is the improvement of the sperm preparation. We are no longer using simple washes or swim-up techniques for male factor infertility. The sedimentation migration technique of Jondet's and the percoll density gradient method are allowing us to get better capacitated, more highly purified motile fractions of sperm.

In the United States alone there are more than 20,000 GIFT or IVF cycles performed per year, and this represents a fraction of the couples who need it. It used to be thought that only an elite core of centers performing huge numbers of cases of IVF and GIFT should be the only ones allowed to do this procedure because with their greater experience they would have a higher pregnancy rate. However, a detailed survey conducted by the American Fertility Society showed that small in vitro fertilization and GIFT programs in community hospitals were capable of obtaining extremely superb results even though it is true that some small programs also had extremely poor results. But if this information is available to the consumer, she can decide intelligently where she wants to go. By this process of natural selection, the better physicians directing the finer programs with the better results will flourish and the others will close down and die.

How Do I Decide Where to Go?

It usually won't do just to look at a single figure raw stating the pregnancy rate of a particular clinic. Pregnancy rates can be high or low depending upon whether the clinic sees easier or more difficult patients. In addition, clinics can give misleadingly inflated figures if they are not meticulously honest or include patients that miscarried in their pregnancy figures. Pregnancy rate is affected severely by the age of the patient, number of the eggs that were retrievable from a poorly responding ovary, and the quality of the husband's sperm. These are factors that the particular clinic has no control over and could seriously lower its success rate.

Other factors affecting you chances for pregnancy are the number of eggs or embryos that are placed in a GIFT or IVF/ZIFT procedure, and indeed whether the embryos are placed in the fallopian tubes or the uterus. You will be able to make that decision. Finally, and most hopefully, you can decide how many times you want to repeat the attempt. It used to be feared that couples who did not get pregnant in the first few attempts of IVF or GIFT would be highly resistant and unlikely to get pregnant in subsequent cycles. However, it is uncontrovertibly clear now that each time you try IVF (or GIFT) the pregnancy rate is no different than the first time you tried it, and the pregnancy rate per cycle for couples who have gone through as many as seven attempts unsuccessfully is no different than that of couples who are going through their first cycle.

Because we are all getting older each year, let's first take a look at the effect of age on the results. While the pregnancy rate with GIFT is over twice as high as that with classic in vitro fertilization, there is a dramatic drop-off in the likelihood of pregnancy for both GIFT and IVF for women over forty years of age. So if you are in your thirties, the longer you wait to get started with this treatment, the greater risk you are taking that in the long run you will be disappointed. I don't want to end that paragraph on a negative or sour note. If you do run out of fertilizable eggs, no matter what age you reach, even in your fifties, you would have an extremely high chance of pregnancy with GIFT or IVF using donor eggs from younger women. In fact, the chance of pregnancy is not really related to the age of the woman you are trying to get pregnant, but is strictly related to the age of the eggs you are putting in her.

Very clearly increased pregnancy rates are obtainable by increasing the number of embryos replaced (see Table 5). In the earliest days of in vitro fertilization only one egg was obtained, in a "natural" cycle, and therefore only one embryo was replaced. By replacing three embryos instead of one, even in the early years of in vitro fertilization there was a dramatic improvement in pregnancy rate. But notice once again that in couples over forty, the pregnancy rate is about half of what it was for couples under forty.

We know how many eggs to place in a GIFT procedure in specific types of patients in order to increase the chance of pregnancy and yet not create too great a risk of multiple pregnancy. For example, when up to eight eggs are transferred in younger women in their twenties, the risk for multiple pregnancy is dangerously increased; and when husbands have excellent sperm, the risks are even more increased. However, in older

TABLE 5

REASING THE NUMBER OF EMBRYOS REPLACED
(STEPTOE AND EDWARDS, 1987)

	40 Years Old or Over	
	Embryos Replaced	Pregnancy Rate
	(percent)	(percent)
	1	9.4
	2	13.2
	3	18.6

ets
rcent)

7 (6)
4 (6)
—

32 (4)

r number of

worst cases.

most difficult
ely and where
e of pregnancy

data that I am
rs the question
ertilization: Will
VF give the same
le? Or are those
ycles just wasting
? In other words,
nade it quite clear
ssibly longer) your
le is no lower than
or the first time. In
F, Dr. Jairo Garcia,
reports a cumulative

or sperm, the risk for multiple

women, and the decreased
vomen, does not apply when
an Craft from London has
l patients over forty, who
sfer of young donor eggs
regnancy rate per cycle
So forget about the age
ncy rates and risks of
out the age of the egg

ralian experience in
ship to the number
a low incidence of
e, and in one case
ryos is roughly
have to assume
to fertilize in
e cases of la
xtreme
This
t

TABLE 6

RISK OF MULTIPLE PREGNANCY RELATED TO NUMBER OF EMBRYOS TRANSFERRED TO THE UTERUS (AUSTRALIAN NATIONAL RESULTS)

Embryos Transferred	Singleton	Twins	Tripl
	(no./percent)	(no./percent)	(no./pe
1	104	1	
2	204	27 (12)	
3	208	84 (27)	1
4	151	52 (24)	
5	20	3 (13)	
6	1	1	
Totals	700 (78)	169 (19)	

1. Risk of multiple pregnancy increases with transfer of great
   embryos up to three.
2. But after three, up to six, no significant increase.
3. Probably because greater numbers are only transferred i

only transfer these large numbers of embryos in the
infertility cases where multiple pregnancy isn't lik
you want to increase as much as possible the chanc
occurring at all.

Finally, the most hopeful aspect of all of this
presenting for you (see Tables 7 and 8) answe
that has been haunting all of us doing in vitro f
coming back for subsequent cycles of GIFT or I
"relatively" good chance of pregnancy per cy
couples who don't get pregnant in the early c
their time coming back for subsequent cycle
loes persistence pay off? Recent data have
t for at least up to seven cycles (and po
e of pregnancy in each subsequent cy
vere just beginning IVF or GIFT f
u persist up to seven cycles of IV
at Greater Baltimore Hospital.

TABLE 7

PREGNANCY RATE BY NUMBER OF IVF ATTEMPTS RESULTING IN EMBRYO TRANSFER

IVF Attempts	Patients	Pregnancies per Transfer	Cumulative Clinical Pregnancy Rate
(number)	(number)	(no./percent)	(percent)
1	486	119 (25)	25
2	229	66 (29)	47
3	114	32 (28)	62
4	60	20 (33)	75
5	26	9 (35)	83
6	10	3 (30)	88
7	5	2 (40)	93

Dr. J. Garcia, *Journal of Fertility and Sterility* (1989).

TABLE 8

INTERPRETING TRUE PREGNANCY RATES WITH IVF

Pregnancy Rate
19.5%

A. 7,017   Cycles started
1,177 (17%) Abandoned
because of poor
stimulation

B. 5,840   Cycles went to
egg retrieval
870 (15%) None of the
eggs fertilized

C. 4,970   Cycles left
where
embryo(s) were
replaced
970   Pregnancies
310 (32%) Miscarriages
660   Live births

D. Pregnancy   970/4,970 = 19.5%
rate per
embryo
replacement

Pregnancy   970/5,840 = 16.6%
rate per egg
retrieval

Pregnancy   970/7,017 = 13.8%
rate per
cycle started

Live birth   660/7,017 = 9.4%
rate per
cycle started

Steptoe and Edwards, November 1987, AAGL Meeting, San Francisco.

pregnancy rate of 93 percent. In other words, even if you don't get pregnant in the first few cycles and you keep on coming back, the chances are 93 percent that in one of those seven cycles you will get pregnant. This used to be a controversial issue, but hard data from several sources have now verified this very optimistic outlook. Yet, the sad truth is that the vast majority of couples who don't get pregnant after two or three attempts of in vitro fertilization quit. What our evidence is telling us now is that you shouldn't quit. Whether you choose GIFT or in vitro fertilization of ZIFT, you should keep coming back and trying (unless the sperm simply don't fertilize the eggs during several attempts), because ultimately the chances are that during one of those cycles an embryo will implant in your uterus and make you pregnant.

CHAPTER 13

Obstruction to Sperm Outflow— Something in the Male We Can Actually Treat

Microsurgery is extremely effective in restoring fertility to oth erwise sterile men when the cause of male infertility is obstruction to sperm outflow. There are three major types of obstruction to sperm outflow. The most common is vasectomy in a man who has changed his mind and now wants to have children. The second is blockage in the epididymis caused by infection, which is prevalent in one-third of men in some parts of the world, but somewhat less common in the United States and Europe. The third is congenital blockage either in the epididymis or in the ejaculatory duct which often involves complete absence of the vas deferens. All three of these problems can be treated with very high success rates using modern microsurgical techniques.

VASECTOMY REVERSAL AND MICROSURGERY

Why Have a Vasectomy Reversal?

Vasectomy is one of the most common operations performed today in the United States, and it is the most popular method of birth control in the world. About 15 million American men have been vasectomized, and almost one-quarter of a million more undergo this operation every year. Despite careful counseling and warning that this procedure should be considered a permanent step, many men change their minds at a later date. A marriage can break up and the man may remarry several years later. In this new marriage both husband and wife generally find themselves wanting to have more children. The death of a child, an improvement in financial stability, or simply a change of heart with a desire for a bigger family, may result in intense regret at having been sterilized.

One patient of mine was working abroad and was only able to visit the United States two weeks every year. He and his wife had two healthy children and decided that their family was complete. On one of their trips back to the United States, the husband had a vasectomy performed. The day after his vasectomy, his wife was killed in an automobile accident and one child was in critical condition for several weeks. He knew just one day after his vasectomy that it had been a terrible mistake.

Our lives and our families are held together by such thin threads that few of us can feel quite comfortable, at least while we are young, with the decision to be sterilized. Another patient of mine had two healthy children, a wonderful wife, a beautiful home, and just about everything anyone could want out of life. When his third child, a boy, was born, it was an absolute culmination of all his desires. The patient waited several months to make sure the child would be healthy before having his vasectomy performed by a local urologist. One month after the operation he and his wife noticed a lump on the little four-month-old child's arm—which turned out to be a rare and incurable malignant tumor of the muscle. The child died four months later.

The couple knew that having another child would not replace the one they lost, but they simply had to have another child.

A fascinating example of how the most permanent decision not to have children can change with the times is that of a thirty-year-old man who came to see me for reversal of a vasectomy performed ten years earlier. He was known to have a family history of "polycystic kidney disease," which is hereditary and leads to complete kidney failure and death by the mid-forties. Because he had been advised that his life span would be short, he'd decided quite rationally, along with his parents' consultation, to have a vasectomy performed when he was twenty years old. Ten years later, kidney transplants became so successful that his expected lifespan changed dramatically for the better. His wife and he then naturally decided to have a vasectomy reversal.

I remember reading with extreme sadness a newspaper story about how the first baby born in 1990 in St. Louis was found dead in his crib of Sudden Infant Death Syndrome (SIDS) a month after its birth. Death in childhood is extremely common. I have hundreds of cases in my files of couples who thought they had all the children they wanted, but then when a child died, they wanted the husband's vasectomy reversed in order to have more. A nine-year-old son of one man I recently operated on was hit by a car in his neighborhood while riding a bicycle. The father was actually a vasectomy counselor at a Planned Parenthood Center and had warned over 10,000 men about not having a vasectomy until they were certain they would never want more children no matter what tragedy or accident might befall their family. Now he immediately wanted his vasectomy reversed.

These tragedies happen when you least anticipate it. One man had a two-and-one-half-year-old son who had become the pride of his family. He and his wife had been trying to have this child for years but needed to overcome first a prior infertility problem. He then had a vasectomy because he and his wife thought they could not afford any more children. Yet one day while visiting relatives, the boy pushed the button on the garage door opener and then tried to run under it. As the garage door came down upon him, it did not stop and go back up as it is supposed to, but because of a defect that no one was aware of, it crushed him to death immediately.

One rancher was shoeing his horse while his two-year-old was just standing around admiring everything his father did. The horse suddenly and unpredictably kicked and not another sound was heard. The patient remembers telling me how strange it seemed that one second his child was alive and the next he was dead and he hadn't uttered a sound. He couldn't even believe it had happened even though he was right there. Two months later, he desperately sought reversal of his vasectomy.

There are many other reasons why vasectomy reversal is so commonly sought after. I am an outdoors lover, and I realized on a recent trip to the far Arctic, in one of the most remote regions of the world, just how intense is the human will to reverse a previous decision to be sterile. I was traveling in the barren region of the magnetic North Pole thousands of miles from any populated area on a three-man expedition consisting of myself and two Eskimos. Kalook, my guide, had no idea that I was an expert on vasectomy. He just knew I was a doctor of some sort. He looked sad on the third day of our trip as he stared at the floor of the igloo and said to me, "I made a very bad thing last year." I asked what happened. He said, "The government sends a doctor to our camp every year, and last year he gave me a vasectomy." Kalook already had five children, quite enough according to the view of the government and the social worker who advised him. But Kalook deeply regretted that he could not have any more. He said, "I am so sorry I did that, I would like to have more children." I started to laugh, patted Kalook on the back and said to him, "My friend, you have come to the right igloo." For reasons that will become apparent by the end of this portion of the chapter, I could assure Kalook almost a 99 percent chance of having his fertility restored.

Several years ago, I reversed the vasectomy of a sixty-two-year-old man whose first wife had died and who was now re-married to a woman in her late thirties who had not been married before and had never had children. He already had five grown children and the question arose: Why should this man in his sixties want to try to start a new family? The fact is when he arrived at my office he didn't look his stated age but barely looked over thirty-five. His father, who came with him, was in his eighties, and his grandfather, who they left home to manage the ranch, was ninety-nine and leading a life certainly more active than mine. There was no question that despite his age and this unusual request, this man would be a great father, and because of his genes possibly even outlive his younger wife. Yet he had already had two attempts at vasectomy reversal which had failed. As this section of the chapter unfolds, you'll understand why they failed and how we were able to perform a delicate operation repairing the more delicate ductwork closer to the testicle (the "epididymis") and thus restoring this man's fertility. He has now begun a second family at almost sixty-five years of age.

A similar story unfolds about a marathon runner who has become a very close friend of mine. Now at the age of seventy he has three little children under the age of three (two are twins). When this man was fifty-five years old, he was running marathons regularly and only wanted his vasectomy reversed for intangible reasons he couldn't explain. I performed a reconnection of the vas according to the microsurgical technique which I had first described at the American College of Surgeons in 1975. Unfortunately, his vasectomy had been so long ago, and our understanding of the epididymis at that time was so poor, that this simple, though elegant, microsurgical reconnection of the severed vas did him no good at all, and he remained azospermic (no sperm in the ejaculate).

Three years later when I had discovered that the problem with cases like his is that pressure buildup from the vasectomy causes damage in the ductwork closer to the testicle (and after I had developed a more delicate microsurgical operation for bypassing that damage, "vasoepididymostomy"), I called him up to suggest he come back to St. Louis and let us give this new approach a try. When we bypassed the epididymal damage on the second operation, his sperm count returned to normal levels within six months, and although he was one of my earliest such cases, we have now performed thousands of such operations on men whose first vasectomy reversal had failed despite what appeared to be an accurate reconnection of the vas.

This man, who really did not foresee having more children, at age sixty-five married a thirty-five-year-old woman. Now, fifteen years after I originally met him and operated on him, he has three little children and, incidentally, he still runs marathons.

Fortunately, we have developed not only delicate new microsurgical techniques for reconnecting the vas, but also a dramatically improved understanding of the damage vasectomy can do to the more delicate ductwork of the epididymis (and how to correct that damage). Therefore, most such people now can once again father children.

The "Simple" Microsurgical Operation to "Reconnect" the Vas Deferens

Though it is easy to perform a vasectomy (it takes only five minutes in the doctor's office), it is very difficult to reverse it because of the microscopic size of the inner canal which carries the sperm. The outer diameter of the vas deferens is fairly thick, about one-eighth of an inch, and the tough outer muscular wall makes it feel like a copper wire through the scrotum. It is therefore an easy structure for the surgeon to identify and cut. But the diameter of the inner canal which carries the sperm is about one-seventieth to one-hundredth of an inch, or roughly the size of a pinpoint. This inner canal has a lining which is about three cells thick, approximately $1/2,000$ of an inch. Vasectomy had always been considered a relatively permanent condition because of the obvious difficulty in surgically reconnecting such a delicate, tiny tube. With the microsurgical technique that I developed in the late 1960s and early 1970s, this problem of reconnecting the vas deferens has now essentially been solved, but the problem in getting high success rates goes far beyond this "simple" microsurgical reconnection. Just "reconnecting the vas" will give only a 25 percent success rate because pressure damage closer to the testicle, in the epididymis, prevents sperm from ever reaching the vasectomy site. Over 90 percent success rates can still be achieved with microsurgery to bypass epididymal damage, but this surgery is much more delicate than just "reconnecting the vas."

But for the moment let's get back to the "simple" microsurgery for reconnecting the severed vas, since in some cases this is all that is needed. In order to achieve a nonobstructed reconnection, it is necessary to stitch accurately the delicate inner lining in a leakproof fashion using a thread invisible to the naked eye (see Figure 44). This surgery is performed under a microscope

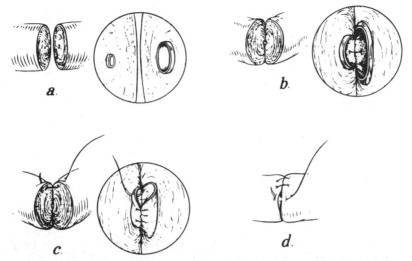

This rough overview illustration demonstrates the basic strategy of the two-layer microscopic technique. Because of the tiny inner lumen, compared to the thick outer muscularis, as well as because of the discrepancy in the size of the lumen (*a*), the mucosal lining is sutured first, picking up some inner muscularis (*b*) with it. The outer muscularis (*c*) is sutured separately. The sutures must be very tiny (*d*) so as not to create secondary inflammation or obstruction. By the time the last mucosal suture has been placed, a waterproof, sperm tight, leakproof reconnection of the inner lumen must have been achieved.

Figure 44.

with very high magnification, using delicate instruments especially designed for this purpose.

This microsurgical technique for reconnecting the vas is equally successful in cases where previous attempts at vasectomy reversal have failed. In these circumstances the scar tissue from the previous surgery may make the operation somewhat more difficult, but it should not interfere with obtaining an accurate reconnection. But if the failure of vasectomy reversal is instead due to blockage in the epididymis, just "reconnecting the vas" again won't work.

The use of a microscope alone does not ensure that an accurate reconnection will be achieved. The surgeon must spend a great deal of time practicing before he develops sufficient skill to do this sort of surgery with confidence. It is important to understand that even with very crude surgical techniques, some sperm can often be found afterward in the ejaculate. But the mere appearance of sperm in the ejaculate does not indicate any likelihood of fertility or subsequent pregnancy. If the amount and quality of sperm is poor, then pregnancy rates will still be very low.

Many patients are told that "too large a segment" of vas has been removed to allow a successful reconnection. They are told that their vasectomy cannot be reversed simply because the doctor who originally performed the vasectomy took out a huge piece of the vas rather than just severing it. Actually the majority of urologists take out an unnecessarily large piece of vas when they perform a vasectomy, but this in no way reduces the chance of a successful reconnection because we possess an enormous extra length of vas, far in excess of what is necessary for sperm to transit from the testicle into the ejaculate.

The vas is actually twelve inches long, although the portion in the scrotum is only an inch in length. Therefore, if a large segment of vas has been removed by vasectomy or even previous attempts at vasectomy reversal, there is always enough healthy vas left to free up and reconnect. Of course, this is a more difficult operation and will require a larger incision, but it is not really any more painful, and the success rate is absolutely unaffected by the necessity of making this larger incision.

One of my earliest patients was a very hardworking immigrant who was raising three beautiful children (two girls and a boy), holding several jobs, and saving up enough money to give them a home and the education he never had. Suddenly his boy came down with a rare and incurable illness, now called Reye's syndrome (caused by taking aspirin after the flu), which at the time baffled his doctors. The child finally went into deep coma and died. The man was beside himself with grief and decided shortly thereafter to go to one of the nation's leading medical centers in his region to try to reverse the vasectomy that had been performed only three years earlier when he thought his family was complete. The doctors at that medical center explored the patient's scrotum and found no vas deferens remaining to reattach. His previous doctors had removed all his scrotal vas. The doctor attempting the vasectomy reversal sadly closed the incision and explained to the patient that there was no hope.

One year later he chanced to read a newspaper article written by a former patient of mine, and he decided to come to St. Louis to see if anything could be done. As expected, we found there was no vas deferens left in the scrotum, but by extending the incision into the abdomen we were able to free his vas up enough to reconnect. The patient now has three more children, and he is working his head off trying to make enough money so they can all have an education.

I remember operating on one man in 1987 who had had simply the most incredible vasectomy I've ever seen in my life. The surgeon who performed his vasectomy must have been in just a terrible mood that day. Over four inches of vas had been removed on both sides. This meant that not only was the man's scrotal vas deferens completely gone, but much of his abdominal vas deferens had also been pulled out with it. It was really hard to believe. I've never seen another case quite that bad before or since. To reconnect that vas required a huge incision going all the way into the hernia region of the abdomen. We were able to free up the remaining portion of the abdominal vas sufficiently that it could come down into the scrotum and thereby reestablished his fertility. So previous surgery, no matter how messy, with enormous segments of scar and vas missing, should never be an impediment to obtaining a successful reversal of vasectomy in the proper surgical hands.

What Has Vasectomy Done to the Ducts of the Testicles?

After vasectomy, the testicle continues to produce fluid and sperm, which accumulates and dilates the entire sperm ductal system Fluid and sperm accumulate in the epididymis, the tiny, delicate twenty-foot-long canal (coiled up into a length of only one inch) that carries sperm out of the testicle into the vas deferens. In this area the sperm ductwork is only $\frac{1}{300}$ inch in diameter and the thickness of the wall of the epididymal duct is only $\frac{1}{1,000}$ inch. This buildup of pressure is usually not felt by the patient because the duct is so tiny that these events are usually not noticeable.

Eventually, the pressure builds up to a point where rupture or clogging occurs in the epididymis. This is the major culprit in the problem of restoring the man's fertility. It is what prevents patients from recovering normal fertility despite what might be a proper reconnection of the vas. The good news is that with extremely refined microsurgical techniques, the damage in this area can be repaired or bypassed, and the success rate for reversal of vasectomy can still be quite good. However, the technique requires so much practice and experience that not many surgeons are yet experienced with it.

Ironically, it is the sloppier vasectomies, the ones that result in sperm leakage at the vasectomy site, that have the best outlook for reversal. This is because these patients have a persistent low-grade leakage of sperm from the cut end of the vas deferens. A small lump, called a sperm granuloma, forms at the cut end of the vas deferens. This lump, which can be felt through the scrotum, is a dynamic structure, with sperm constantly leaking into it and being reabsorbed sufficiently to prevent the pressure increase that would normally occur. Patients with such a lump at the vasectomy site have the greatest chance of recovering normal fertility after a simple "reconnection" of the vas, and don't require bypass of the much more delicate epididymis.

Duration of Time Since Vasectomy

We originally demonstrated in 1977, that the longer the period of time since vasectomy, the worse the chance for success (despite an anatomically perfect reconnection of the vas) unless the surgeon knows how to perform epididymal bypass. At that time we knew nothing about the pressure-induced damage from vasectomy. All that was known was that the longer the period of time that the vas, epididymis, and testicle were subjected to the pressure increase caused by vasectomy, the less was the likelihood of restoration of fertility after simple reconnection of the vas.

In 1978, we discovered the cause of the problem. Hundreds of testicle biopsies on men with no sperm in the vas fluid showed completely normal sperm production. So why were we seeing no sperm in the vas fluid and having no success in patients who had been subjected to this pressure increase for prolonged periods of time? The answer of course was that the pressure buildup caused obstruction in the epididymal ductwork between the testicle and the vasectomy site. The longer the period of time since the vasectomy, the greater the likelihood of finding this epididymal damage.

We then developed a more intricate microsurgical operation in which we could locate the points of epididymal blockage where normal sperm were present, and bypass them. One of the first patients we tried this new operation on was a man on whom I had performed a beautiful vas reconnection in 1974, fifteen years after his original vasectomy. He had had no sperm in the vas fluid and he remained sterile despite a perfect vas reconnection. In 1979, after I moved to St. Louis, I let him know that we had discovered the cause of the problem, and invited him to come to St. Louis for an attempt at bypassing the epididymal blockage which we now expected to find. As it turned out, our concept was correct, and he now lives with three children and a very happy wife.

With "Modern" Vasectomies, the "Blowouts" Occur Much Sooner

It used to be that only a small percentage of the patients requesting vasectomy reversal within ten years had this epididymal problem. Unfortunately, the situation has gotten worse because of a change in the popular method for performing vasectomy. Whereas in the late 1970s, almost 90 percent of our patients had normal sperm in the vas fluid, today only about 20 percent of the patients have normal sperm in the vas fluid.

Blowouts and secondary blockages in the epididymis are now occurring very early after vasectomy. The majority of patients I see whose vasectomies were done even less than ten years ago have blowouts in the epididymis, almost half the patients whose vasectomies were done under five years ago have no sperm in the vas fluid, whereas in the 1970s almost all such patients would have had sperm in the vas fluid. If we are to maintain a high success rate for vasectomy reversal in the 1990s, it will require epididymal bypass operation rather than just the more simple microsurgical reconnection of the vas, and this applies to men whose vasectomies were recent as well as men whose vasectomies were a relatively long period of time ago.

The reason for the increased and earlier epididymal damage from vasectomy is the popularity of the cautery technique for vasectomy and the emphasis on getting a "leakproof" sealing of the cut ends of the vas. Because of a fear that leakage at the vasectomy site could lead to an occasional unwanted pregnancy after vasectomy (due to "recanalization" caused by the leaking sperm), urologists are using either cautery or very carefully applied clips to create an absolutely "watertight," "leakproof," completely solid seal at the cut ends of the vas. Thus, there is a faster and more severe pressure buildup, leading to earlier epididymal damage.

In fact, I recommend that if a vasectomy is being performed, the urologist should leave the cut end completely unsealed in order to avoid any pressure damage. I call this "open-ended" vasectomy (see Figure 45).

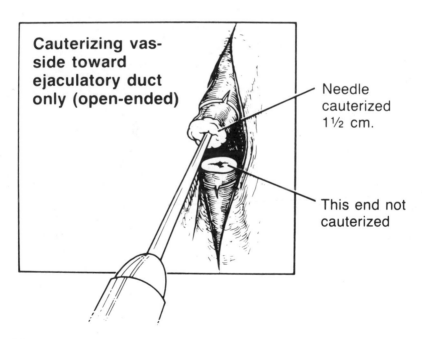

Figure 45. If the side of the vas draining fluid from the testicle is not cauterized and allowed to leak, the epididymis suffers no pressure damage and vasectomy reversal is much easier. This is the so-called "open-ended" vasectomy which I advocate.

How Is the Epididymal Blockage Bypassed?

I would like to roughly outline the operation required. Under the operating microscope, you can microsurgically cut the epididymis toward the testicle (see Figure 46) or cut into the epididymal tubule moving closer and closer to the testicle until there is suddenly a brisk outpouring of huge quantities of sperm under high pressure. We make small micro-incisions until we get past the area of blockage. Sometimes we find the blockage is "far" away from the testicle, and other times we find the blockage is extremely "close" to the testicle. In either event, we must bypass the blocked areas. The epididymal tubule is so fragile ($\frac{1}{1,000}$ of an inch in wall thickness) that it must be sewn to the inner lining of the vas with thread that is virtually invisible

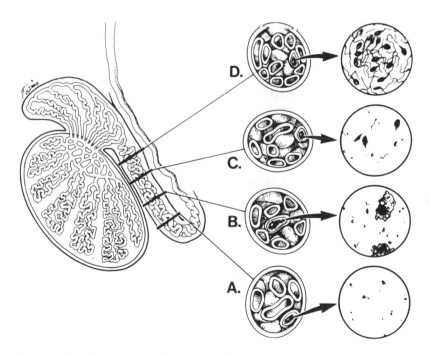

Figure 46. Microsurgically transecting the epididymis closer and closer to the testicle eventually gets beyond the areas of secondary blowouts and blockage where the reconnection to the epididymis has to be performed.

to the naked eye. An absolutely perfect connection of that inner lining of the vas to the opening in the epididymal tubule is essential (see Figures 47 and 48). As the drawings illustrate, there are two equally good ways to do this, "end-to-end" and "end-to-side." If a sloppily performed attempt at reconnection is made, sperm will just leak all over the place and result in scarring and either partial or total blockage.

Interpreting the Results of the Vasectomy Reversal Operation

If a man has *no sperm* in the ejaculate after surgery within a reasonable period of waiting, it is obvious that he has total blockage, and needs a reoperation. On the other hand, sometimes the man may just have *low* sperm counts with *poor* sperm quality and it must be determined whether this is due to partial blockage at the attempted site of reconnection. Most of the time low sperm count is caused by blockage rather than intrinsically poor sperm production. Couples may think they have had a successful reversal operation just because some sperm are present in the ejaculate in small numbers, but usually this is caused by severe blockage and an inadequate outflow channel for the sperm.

I remember seeing a fifty-year-old man, married to a twenty-seven-year-old woman. He was so dedicated to restoring his fertility that he had gone through three vasectomy reversals before I saw him. In every case, his vas had been reconnected by a competent microsurgeon who simply had no knowledge of epididymal physiology and never had any experience operating on the epididymis. His original vasectomy had been performed thirteen years earlier, and it was fairly obvious when we did his fourth vasectomy reversal that there was no sperm whatsoever in the vas. The answer to his problems was obvious. He had epididymal blockage very close to the testicle. We bypassed most of the epididymal tubule in order to get beyond his many areas of blowouts. After we did this, his sperm count went up fairly quickly and he and his wife now have two children. This man had had previous vasectomy reversal attempts that failed because the problem of epididymal blockage had not been addressed.

We now know that although remarkable maturational changes

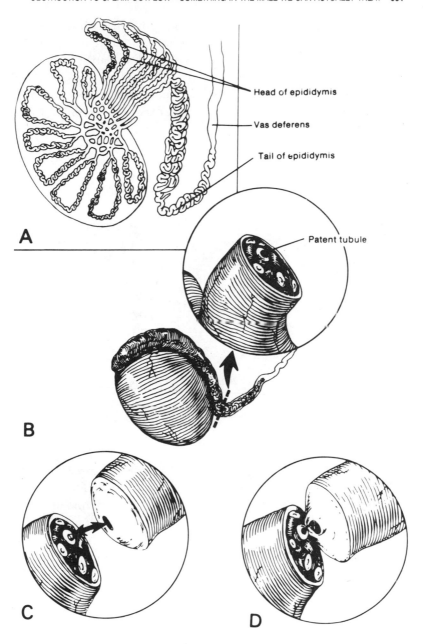

Figure 47. My original "end-to-end" technique for microscopic reconnection surgery of the tiny epididymal tubule to the vas.

occur in the sperm as they travel normally through the epididymis and acquire their ability to swim in a straight line and to fertilize, these changes do not require that journey, and can simply occur over a period of time. Therefore, bypassing epididymal blockage at almost any level, contrary to what we might have expected in the past, results in an excellent pregnancy rate.

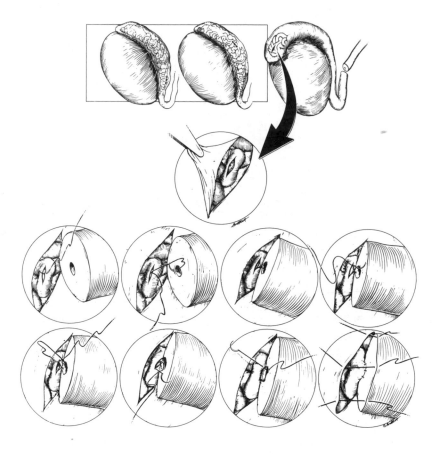

Figure 48. My refined, new "end-to-side" technique for bypassing epididymal blockage, requiring less surgical dissection than the original technique.

Recovery of Fertility After Vasectomy Reversal

Sperm counts do not return to normal immediately after vasectomy reversal. All of the old sperm which have been stored up over the years since the vasectomy have died of old age. This dead sperm material must be cleaned out after the vasectomy is reversed in order to make room for a fresh crop of sperm, which usually does not appear until about three months or more later. Also, the dilated epididymal duct may require many months to recover its microscopic muscular ability to transport the sperm by the slow pumping action which is called "peristalsis."

Usually if the microsurgery is performed well, most patients are fertile within a year and the wife gets pregnant within two years. However, occasionally a longer period of time is required for complete recovery of adequate sperm motility after vasectomy reversal. The best treatment for most men with *high sperm counts*—but poor motility—is time. On the other hand, if the sperm count is very low and the motility is poor, the problem is likely to be continuing obstruction, which requires reoperation.

When the patient has a normal sperm count after vasectomy reversal and the wife is not yet pregnant, it is important she be evaluated; the problem could be with her. Several years ago I operated on a history professor to reverse a vasectomy, and one year after the operation he had a perfectly normal sperm count with 55 million sperm per cc and 90 percent motility. His wife, however, had not gotten pregnant yet, and his local urologist decided without much thought to put him on hormone therapy. The wife had not been evaluated, but if she had been, they would have discovered (as I did on the telephone) that she had had irregular menstrual bleeding off and on for the last year and a half, and indeed had been placed on birth control pills temporarily by her obstetrician to regulate her periods. So how could she possibly get pregnant?

Some patients get pregnant remarkably quickly after the vasectomy reversal. I remember receiving a furious call from one patient six weeks after his surgery, extremely angry that his wife had just missed her period and her pregnancy test was positive. He was actually afraid that maybe this wasn't his child because he couldn't imagine that his sperm count could return to normal that quickly. Because most patients require more than three months to recover their fertility, this man was in a state of utter disbelief that his wife got pregnant so quickly. Yet his sperm count was excellent, and there was little doubt in my mind that it was his child. Genetic testing proved beyond a shadow of doubt that this indeed was his child. Most patients, however, don't get pregnant that quickly, and some require up to a year and a half and occasionally longer for the sperm count to rise to its maximal level, and for the motility to return to normal.

One patient from the Pacific Islands had no sperm at all in the ejaculate after bypassing epididymal damage until one year and four months after surgery, but the count was very low (6.5 million), and the motility was terrible. His count stayed in that range until three years and three months postoperatively when it finally went up to 23 million, the motility went from 1 to 20 percent, and his wife then got pregnant.

Another patient had sperm counts that were always high, in the range of 30 to 55 million per cc. Nonetheless, motility on some occasions would be absolutely zero, on other occasions 20 percent, then it would go back down to 2 percent, and then up to 60 percent, and then back down again to 0 percent. All this time the actual sperm count remained high, but the motility went from terrible to great to terrible. His wife became pregnant three and one-half years after the operation at a time when the motility jumped up to 60 percent. Since the sperm count remained normal and only the motility fluctuated, we have to assume that the epididymis had undergone some degree of damage in its ability to sustain and mature the sperm because of years of pressure buildup.

We had one case that broke our record in waiting for motility to return. This was a man who consistently demonstrated sperm counts of 100 to 150 million per cc after his operation. Yet the motility remained absolutely zero until five years and nine months after surgery. I had already given up on him and told the couple that the epididymis must have suffered permanent damage. Yet almost six years later, motility went up to 50 percent with good forward progression and his wife became pregnant.

The important point is in deciding whether a poor result after surgery simply calls for a period of waiting, or whether a new operation is required to bypass continuing obstruction. The answer to that question is as follows: If the patient has only undergone reconnection of the vas, the sperm count should return to normal by six months postoperatively. Otherwise you can be sure there is blockage. If the patient has required bypass of epididymal blockage, the sperm count may require up to a year and a half to come to normal levels. If after a year and a half there is no further improvement in sperm count, that means the patient has blockage. Remember: The most common cause of failure of vasectomy reversal is obstruction, either at the site of reconnection of the vas or somewhere in the epididymis. The solution to this problem is reoperation.

Sperm Antibodies

In Chapter 6 there is a detailed explanation of sperm antibodies and their effect on the ability of sperm to fertilize eggs. For over twenty years it has been speculated that the reason for the low success rate after vasectomy reversal is that the man develops antibodies to his own sperm and that these sperm antibodies prevent him from impregnating his wife even though a "successful" reversal operation has been performed. I have operated on hundreds of patients with very poor sperm quality and whose wife's failure to get pregnant was blamed on "sperm antibodies." After reoperating, the sperm count and the quality of motility improved almost ten-fold and then the wives did get pregnant. In fact, comparing the pregnancy rate of the wives of patients who had high sperm antibody levels versus those who had no sperm antibody formation after vasectomy, the pregnancy rate was no different. These studies were done at a time when the sperm antibody testing methodology we performed was state-of-the-art, and was supposed to be the explanation for low fertility after vasectomy reversal. Therefore, we think it is safe to conclude that most cases of persistent infertility after vasectomy reversal are not due to sperm antibodies.

This does not mean, however, that very sophisticated new methods of localizing sperm antibodies on specific areas of the sperm (explained in Chapter 6) might not provide useful information that could help us to decide whether in the occasional patient use of the new reproductive technologies like IVF or GIFT might be useful after a successful reversal operation. There may be a subtle reduction in the number of antibody-free sperm available for fertilization in a very small number of patients after vasectomy reversal, but this is a very tiny component of the much larger group who simply need to have a better operation performed on them.

The highest sperm antibody titers we've measured on a post-vasectomy-reversal patient is the man who got his wife pregnant earlier than any other patient we've seen (four weeks). Subsequently, he had another child with her and incidentally is now interested in having a vasectomy again. I remember a patient who underwent a vasectomy reversal in 1977 and who had a postoperative sperm count that was very high from the beginning (over 50 million per cc), but with poor motility. Several years went by and the wife did not get pregnant, and they told me that an "antibody specialist" had stated that her husband had a very high level of sperm antibodies and that he should have been tested for sperm antibodies before the reanastomosis. This doctor then recommended that the patient go on steroid medication, which, as has been explained before, can result in cataracts, infection, and destruction of the hip joint. I advised the patient and his wife's gynecologist that he should take no such medication. By two years and four months, the motility had come up to 70 percent and the wife got pregnant despite the fact that the sperm antibody titer remained quite high.

Recent sophisticated "immunobead" studies by Dr. Pasquale Patrizio from our group has demonstrated that even patients with antibodies attached to their epididymal sperm were able to fertilize in vitro and have pregnancies at the same rate as those with no antibodies at all. This study seems to close this issue quite definitively, but yet I'm sure this unnecessary controversy will rage on if only because many doctors are simply not that skilled in microsurgery, and get terrible results.

Does the Wife Always Get Pregnant After Successful Vasectomy Reversal?

Even when there is a perfectly normal sperm count and sperm motility after vasectomy reversal or vasoepididymostomy, the wife may not get pregnant. Among the patients who have had return of normal sperm counts and motility, 88 percent of the wives over a five-year follow-up period got pregnant. By all the parameters I could measure, the husband was fertile, but yet the wife did not get pregnant. Mysterious explanations like "sperm antibodies" used to be invoked to explain this discrepancy. But in truth no mysterious explanations are needed. Ten to 20 percent of any population of females are likely to have some degree of infertility and will not get pregnant without medical intervention.

I recently sent a couple with a clearly successful vasectomy reversal operation to a well-known fertility clinic in the local area where they live, because the wife was not pregnant yet after two years, with a sperm count of 5 million per cc, but excellent 90 percent motility. The doctor in charge sent them out in tears saying there was "no hope" because he had "never heard of a successful reversal." Yet at a different clinic six months later she became pregnant when *her* problem was treated.

There are countless cases of mine from around the country where the wife was told that because of sperm antibodies there was no chance for her getting pregnant despite the fact that the husband had a successful reversal operation. Sometimes she is told that the husband must undergo treatment of his sperm antibodies with dangerous steroid drugs. I always advise the gynecologist not to waste time with theories about sperm antibodies but rather to look more carefully at the female and to view them as any other infertile couple. The pregnancy rate with such "infertile" couples using the various treatments described in this book is no different than for any other infertile couple. The problem with couples that don't get pregnant on their own after successful vasectomy reversal (normal sperm after surgery) is simply an infertility problem of the couple independent of the fact that the husband has had a history of vasectomy and vasectomy reversal.

Results After Vasectomy Reversal

If there are no epididymal blowouts, we have a 98 percent success rate with simply reconnecting the vas. If there is epididymal obstruction requiring bypass, the success rate is 88 percent. Generally about 82 percent of successful cases get pregnant with no treatment of the wife. In those that don't get pregnant on their own, GIFT or treatment of the wife helps most of those get pregnant also.

OBSTRUCTION TO SPERM OUTFLOW IN PATIENTS WHO HAVE NOT HAD A VASECTOMY

When a man's sperm count is zero and a testicle biopsy shows normal sperm production, there has to be an obstruction somewhere along the duct that conveys sperm to the ejaculate. In some cases the man has actually been born with this obstruction and has never had sperm in his ejaculate. In other cases the obstruction results from an infection which leads to scarring. The obstruction is almost always in the epididymis (but there are occasional exceptions). With modern microsurgical innovations, identical to that described earlier in this chapter for vasectomy reversal, the outlook for correcting these obstructions is very good, but the surgery is delicate and intricate.

Prostatitis and other infections of the male genital tract are fairly common in young men. Occasionally an infection will spread down the vas deferens into the epididymis and cause a massive swelling of the scrotum. Often the infection is subtle and the patient does not know he has a problem until he tries to have children. Despite antibiotics and cure of the infection, the epididymis usually heals with scar tissue and becomes obstructed. Thus, an otherwise perfectly fertile man may have total obstruction to sperm outflow. The question is, when a man has azospermia (no sperm) how can doctors know the diagnosis is obstruction?

Testicle Biopsy

The diagnosis of obstruction in the male should really be quite easy. However, it is sometimes approached in a confusing way which can lead to an embarrassing situation for the urologist and a tragedy for the patient. Adherence to a few simple principles will avoid these difficulties and allow a proper decision to be made easily. *If a patient has a testicle biopsy which shows normal spermatogenesis (sperm production) and if he is azospermic (no sperm at all in the ejaculate), then he must have an obstruction.*

The only other piece of information which is necessary is whether or not the physician can palpate (feel) a vas deferens in the scrotum on physical examination. If the patient has congenital absence of the vas deferens, then a totally different surgical approach would be necessary, which will be described later in the chapter. But if there is a palpable vas deferens, and a normal testicle biopsy, in an azospermic patient, that is all the information you need to be certain that there is epididymal obstruction and that microsurgery is the appropriate treatment.

All other data are irrelevant, including a normal FSH level. The FSH level will be normal in a patient who is azospermic without obstruction if the early precursors of sperm production are present. A normal FSH does not in any way assure normal spermatogenesis. In fact, the majority of patients with azospermia and a normal FSH have "maturation arrest" (not obstruction) as the diagnosis.

It is true that if the FSH is elevated, there is inadequate sperm production, due to a small number of sperm precursors. Such a patient does not need a testicle biopsy. But most men with low sperm counts or zero sperm will have an FSH in the normal range. This does not mean that they have normal sperm production, and it does not mean that their diagnosis is obstruction. For that to be determined, a testicle biopsy must be performed.

The testicle biopsy will facilitate the husband's treatment only if performed and read by a physician who really understands how the testicle works. The biopsy involves taking a tissue sample through a small one-quarter-inch incision in the scrotum. The procedure should take no more than five minutes, but it must be done expertly. Testicular tissue is so delicate that if the surgeon handles it in the same way he would handle most specimens removed for biopsy from other areas of the body, the microscopic architecture of the specimen would be so shattered as to make it very difficult to interpret. Furthermore, if the tissue is not properly excised, or if it is placed in formaldehyde (the usual fixative for tissue specimens from almost anywhere else in the body), it would become distorted beyond recognition. The tissue must be placed in a solution which is gentler (either Bouin's or Zenker's). Though the biopsy is quite harmless, a man should not have to part with a portion of his testicle unless helpful information will be derived.

Contrary to expectation, the biopsy should not be very painful. The patient should have minimal temporary discomfort, which is relieved simply by Tylenol.

After the specimen is fixed and stained, it is examined a few days later under a microscope. If the specimen has been properly obtained, the doctor should be able to see a remarkable assembly line of sperm production. By looking at the various stages of sperm production he can tell whether there are an adequate number of precursors starting out at the beginning, whether there are weak spots, or whether there is a problem in the end stages of production when the sperm should be elongating and forming a tail.

If the testicle biopsy shows normal sperm production and the sperm count is zero, this indicates obstruction to the outflow of sperm. Such obstruction is virtually always in the epididymis.

The worst finding on testicle biopsy is a complete absence of any sperm or sperm-producing cells in the seminiferous tubules. The Leydig cells which make the male hormone testosterone are normal in these cases, but there are no sperm of any kind. There is no possible treatment for such a patient. He would have an elevated FSH and, therefore, never really needed the biopsy in the first place.

However, the most common pattern found on testicle biopsy in infertile men with no obstruction is "maturation arrest." In this case sperm production may be proceeding properly in the early phases, but further development into mature sperm is not occurring. This condition is untreatable, as explained earlier in the book.

Vasograms

When it is suspected that the vas deferens is obstructed, an X ray can be performed by injecting a radiopaque liquid into it. This test is called a vasogram. This X ray is not necessary (or advised) to diagnose obstruction. It should only be used as part of an operative procedure once the diagnosis of obstruction is made. The only two tests required to determine that there is obstruction to the outflow of sperm are a count that reveals no sperm in the semen and a normal testicle biopsy. In the presence of these two findings, obstruction will always be found somewhere, and a vasogram is not necessary to make that diagnosis. It is valuable only as part of the actual operation to correct known obstruction to sperm outflow just to assure the microsurgeon that the epididymis is the only site of blockage.

In fact, the X-ray dye should only be injected in the direction of the ejaculatory duct but *never* in the direction of the epididymis. Trying to visualize the epididymis could damage the epididymis further or cause "blowouts" and obstruction in an epididymis that is otherwise *not* blocked.

Microsurgical Vasoepididymostomy

If the cause of azospermia is obstruction, that is usually good news because the same microsurgical operations I have described earlier in the chapter will also correct the sterility of men who have blockage in the epididymis from "natural" causes. There is no difference in the return of fertility in sterile men whose epididymal blockage is caused by vasectomy, previous inflammation in the epididymis from infection, trauma, or in men who were born with congenital epididymal blockage. The surgical approach is identical to what was described earlier for vasectomy reversal patients, and the results are the same.

I had a patient from the Near East who suffered smallpox as a child and recovered from it. What many people may not realize is that anyone who survives smallpox is left permanently sterile because of the epididymal inflammation and subsequent scarring that smallpox inevitably causes. Smallpox was epidemic in the Middle East and India twenty to thirty years ago, and in fact it was one of the most common causes of sterility in India for many years. As soon as I see a patient from one of these areas with the typical scarred feature on his nose which unmistakably identifies him as having been a smallpox victim in childhood, I know that he is sterile from epididymal blockage, and I know that the blockage is in the head of the epididymis fairly close to the testicle.

When our first smallpox patient came to St. Louis years ago from Saudi Arabia, he was accompanied by his Egyptian physician and brother-in-law. They didn't really believe that his epididymal blockage could be corrected, because this patient had had an attempt at surgery eleven years earlier in London, which failed. Nonetheless, this gentleman wanted very badly to have a child and made sure his personal physician and brother-in-law were there to observe the entire operation. The patient's wife became pregnant six months later after the sperm count went up to over 50 million per cc with good motility. They were stunned because they knew that ten years earlier this kind of operation couldn't succeed. Since that time, all over the Middle East, it has become generally recognized now that epididymal obstruction, whether caused by an uncommon condition like smallpox, or more commonly a general infection, can be microsurgically corrected even if the majority of the epididymis has to be bypassed.

Similar realization hit the continent of Africa when a patient with a history of severe schistosomiasis of the bladder came to see me again because of azospermia. In America, most people have never heard of schistosomiasis, but it's probably the most common public health problem in the entire world. It infests almost all of Egypt and Africa and is caused by a parasite that invades the skin when one goes swimming or even wading in water that harbors the schistosomes. It can enter the liver, the bladder, and cause you to be extremely ill and die. Most Americans and Europeans have never even heard of this condition, but it is *the number-one public health problem in this area of the world*. When you survive a severe case of bladder schistosomiasis, you are left with epididymal obstruction. This patient left the little Midwestern town of St. Louis no longer sterile and it is now known in Africa that epididymal obstruction (the most common cause of infertility in Africa) is usually treatable with proper microsurgery.

Even in the Western world up to 30 percent of male sterility (complete azospermia) is caused by epididymal obstruction, but in the Western world, obstruction is more likely to be caused by gonorrhea, chlamydia, other sexually transmitted diseases, childhood trauma to the testicles, or congenital birth defects. Before ten years ago, with modern microsurgical technology, this condition was untreatable. It is now the most successfully treatable cause of male infertility.

Congenital Absence of the Vas Deferens

Congenital absence of the vas occurs in about 20 to 30 percent of men with obstruction to sperm outflow. Like all men with obstruction, the testicle is producing normal sperm. There is no testicular defect in these men and that's why over the last forty years this condition has been so incredibly frustrating. Experimental surgical pockets have been created to try to collect the sperm in a pool underneath the scrotal skin so that it could be aspirated by needle puncture in the office. Every kind of effort has been made to try to figure out a way of harvesting these trapped sperm and using them to inseminate and impregnate the wife, all unsuccessfully.

It was out of that frustration that Dr. Ricardo Asch from California and myself put our heads together and decided to embark upon a combination of in vitro fertilization and microsurgical aspiration of this epididymal sperm (see Figure 49). The idea was originally scorned because if the sperm were not able to traverse the epididymis, so the theory went, they would not be motile and would therefore be unable to fertilize. I knew, however, from our large series of vasoepididymostomies that sperm from absolutely anywhere, even the beginning-most regions of the epididymis, can indeed get women pregnant simply by maturing on their own.

An interesting observation that I had made in all the previous years of literally thousands of vasoepididymostomy operations is that in the obstructed system the sperm nearest the point of obstruction are usually dead because these sperm have been around for the longest period of time. They were the ones that reached the obstructed point first many years before and have already died of old age. But, sperm closer to the testicle have better motility. This is quite the opposite of what you might have predicted. Normally sperm farthest from the testicle are the most motile and the most fertile (see Figure 50) because

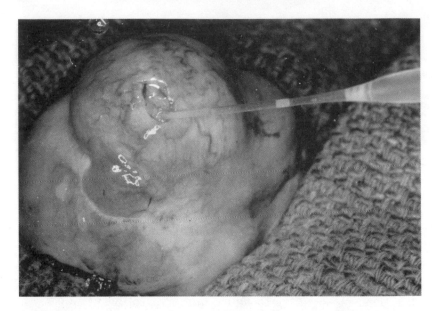

Figure 49. Photograph of microsurgical aspiration of sperm from the outlet of testicle in a man who was born with no vas and virtually no epididymis.

they have been "matured" by virtue of epididymal transit. What I found in obstructed men, where the sperm get out of the testicle but then can't go anywhere but stay in the epididymis, is the exact inversion of this situation. In the obstructed case sperm farthest from the testicle are the oldest and, therefore, have the worst motility or no motility. Sperm closest to the testicle are the most recently produced and, therefore, have the best motility. They have had enough time to mature on their own in the beginning regions of the epididymis, and therefore these sperm are able to fertilize, even though sperm farther from the testicle cannot.

Our postulate turned out to be correct. We have performed this procedure now on many men with congenital absence of the vas, always finding the most fertile sperm closest to the testicle. We have been able to obtain fertilization of at least one of the wife's eggs in 62 percent of the patients. Thirty-one per-

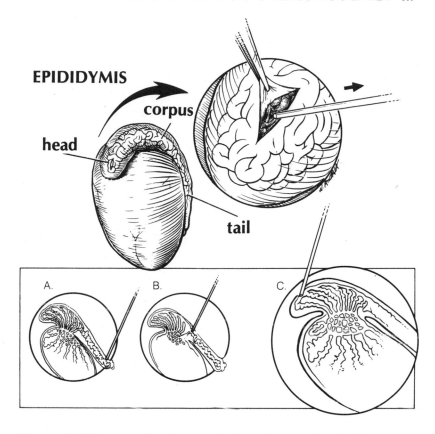

Figure 50. Diagram showing aspiration of sperm from different regions of the obstructed epididymis. The most motile, fertile sperm ironically are those which are found closest to the testicle.

cent of the patients achieved pregnancy and 25 percent delivered live, healthy babies (6 percent miscarried).

Several of these early patients keep in close communication. One of them has become a skiing partner of mine and is also a law professor who helps to figure out the legal and ethical aspects of the complex things we're doing with the new reproductive technology. Another is a religious fundamentalist who prays for me every day on the other side of the world. The third one is a policeman from another city who has made me an honorary member of the force, and whose wife became president of a support group for patients with congenital absence of the vas, recognizing that it is a much more common condition than is generally talked about. These are couples who several years before the writing of this book had no hope at all for having children. In fact, I maintained a list of over 1,000 such patients whom I had told to absolutely forget about ever having this problem solved because without enough epididymal length I thought there was no hope for any therapeutic approach to work. I guess, as Professor Donald Coffey from Johns Hopkins has pointed out, "Every pessimist in the history of the world has been proven to be wrong."

CHAPTER 14

Egg Donation
and Surrogate Uterus

SURROGATE UTERUS
(YOUR MOTHER CAN HAVE YOUR KIDS FOR YOU)

In 1980, I received a very sad letter from a twenty-five-year-old lady in the Bronx, New York, saying that when she had surgery for uterine fibroids, the doctor had to perform a hysterectomy, and now she desperately wanted to have children. Unfortunately, in 1980, I had to write to tell her there was no hope.

I did predict in my original book that with the new in vitro technology on the horizon, perhaps at some time in the future such a woman without a uterus could have someone else carry her genetic child for her. But by the time this futuristic medical prediction became a reality, this lady had already run out of eggs and was in menopause (of course, we can solve even that problem as you will see in the second part of this chapter).

In 1985, Dr. Wolf Utian and Dr. Leon Sheehan from Cleveland reported the first successful case whereby a woman with no uterus whatsoever was able to have her own genetic child. The story of this first case, reported in the *New England Journal of Medicine*, is absolutely spellbinding: A thirty-seven-year-old woman became pregnant, but the uterus spontaneously ruptured at twenty-eight weeks of gestation, necessitating a caesarean section and a hysterectomy. The baby girl subsequently died and the woman was left childless and *without a uterus*.

The couple, however, remained strongly committed to having their own genetic child and the wife asked that an embryo of hers be transfered to the uterus of a friend who was interested and willing to carry the child as a surrogate. The friend was a healthy, married young mother of two.

The reproductive cycles of the two women were synchronized (this will be explained later). Her eggs were incubated with sperm from the husband, and three days later an eight-cell embryo was transferred to the uterus of the surrogate. The surrogate became pregnant and nine months later delivered the healthy genetic baby of her ecstatic friend.

At the American Fertility Society meeting in 1986 a lady introduced herself and thanked me for the prediction that I made in my original book in 1980 about the solution to this very problem. She told me that the prediction in my book prompted her to go to the in vitro fertilization (IVF) program in her community, and she told them what she would like. Performing this kind of procedure is so simple that it turned out not to be a problem, and indeed, when I saw her at the Fertility Society meeting, her best friend was pregnant with her genetic baby and ready to deliver and give it to her in a couple of months' time.

A colleague of mine reports a very unusual "surrogate uterus" case of a patient that he had tried to get pregnant with either GIFT or IVF for five cycles unsuccessfully. The sixth time she was ready to undergo in vitro fertilization she came to the office with her sister, who was, by chance, at the exact same time in her cycle as she was. She was so convinced that there was something wrong with her uterus causing the embryos not to implant that both she and her sister talked the doctor into putting the embryos into her sister instead of her. They made all the appropriate legal arrangements and the next day placed the embryos into her sister's uterus. Her sister got pregnant and they were absolutely overjoyed because nine months later she would receive her own genetic baby, for which she had strived for years and years unsuccessfully.

We were approached by a twenty-nine-year-old woman who had had both her uterus and ovaries removed and desperately wanted to have a child. Her husband had perfectly normal sperm, and they both wanted a baby by her husband's sperm. For such a woman who does not have ovaries or a uterus, another option is possible.

The question for this patient is who would provide the eggs and who would provide the uterus? In her family, one of her sisters was willing to donate an egg, the husband of course would provide his sperm, and another sister would allow the eggs and the sperm to be transferred to her so that she could carry the baby. Thus, if your attitude is open enough, and you have loving friends and family who are willing to help, with the new technology virtually anybody can have a baby.

I want to emphasize that all of these cases are different from the famous "Baby M" surrogacy case that you've probably read about in the newspapers. *The "Baby M" case was not a surrogate uterus situation. It involved no medical technology whatsoever.* I believe it was probably an unethical and improper arrangement in which a paid, fertile woman was inseminated using the sperm of the infertile woman's husband. Then, after nine months, this "surrogate mother" was required to give her own baby up (and it was her genetic baby) to the couple from whom the sperm came. Despite the fact that all the adoption laws in every state in the country prohibit enforcing a prior arrangement for a woman to give her baby up for adoption—clarifying that any such prior contract has no legal validity and it is the woman's absolute right to decide after she has the baby, and that she must be given a period of one to six months to be able to retract her decision to give up the baby for adoption—despite all the legal and ethical protection that the mother of "Baby M" should have had, the police department hunted her down, took her baby away from her, gave the baby to the couple that had paid her to contract for these services, and then the judge presiding over this case (who was, in my opinion, mistaken, went against all prior legal precedent and did not allow the biological mother of this baby to keep her child).

The laws in every state in the union clearly assure that the husband who is living with the woman when she gets pregnant, no matter where the sperm came from, is the father of the child. The laws also assure that a woman carrying a baby for nine months does not have to give it up involuntarily. I feel Mrs.

Whitehead was forced to give her baby up to Mrs. Stern (who was not the biological mother) because the judge probably felt that these parents would do a better job of raising the child, even though the child wasn't theirs.

This kind of surrogacy is heinous and something reproductive physicians working in the field abhor. The new reproductive technology that we are advancing has nothing to do with such absurd violations of human rights. In fact, the new reproductive technology allows us to help women have a child in an ethical, moral manner without the temptation to resort to the scandalous-type "Baby M" behavior. "Baby M"–type pregnancies require no reproductive technology whatsoever. It can be arranged between any scheming lawyer and an unsuspecting client. Doctors have nothing to do with it. The problem is not that society needs to monitor physicians who are trying to help couples have babies, but rather it must monitor the lawyers and the judges who think that we need their protection to make sure we don't misuse the technology.

The most exciting and heartwarming case of surrogate uterus was reported in the *Journal of In Vitro Fertilization and Embryo Transfer* in 1988. In this situation, a twenty-five-year-old woman had lost her uterus from a hysterectomy necessitated by severe bleeding occurring in her previous pregnancy. The only way the doctors could save this young woman's life from this obstetric disaster was to remove her uterus. Yet she had normal ovaries and her husband had good sperm. What was the solution?

As it turned out, her forty-eight-year-old mother was quite willing to serve as a surrogate uterus to carry her daughter's baby. Their menstrual cycles were synchronized with birth control pills so that day one of the mother occurred simultaneously with day one of the daughter. The daughter was stimulated in the usual fashion for in vitro fertilization (IVF), her eggs were fertilized with her husband's sperm, and her embryos were transferred into her mother's uterus with a classic IVF approach. Astoundingly, the forty-eight-year-old mother became pregnant with her daughter's triplets. Nine months later, she gave birth to three healthy grandchildren which she then immediately turned over to her daughter and son-in-law.

In 1988, Dr. John Yovich from Perth, Australia, transferred embryos derived from the ovaries of a woman with no uterus to her sister who had voluntarily offered to carry the baby for her. Dr. Yovich did this "against the advice of local ethical committees." He decided to go ahead with this case because the patient did not have a functional uterus, the surrogate selected was a relative (indeed a sister), she was not expecting any financial reward, and there was a firm understanding that the infertile couple would become the legal parents. His decision to proceed was motivated by a wish to provoke the authorities into drawing up more reasonable guidelines on surrogacy so as to allow such couples to be helped. He felt that if the laws could specify unambiguously who should be regarded as the mother and that no advertising or payment was involved, it would serve the interests of the community.

Instead of receiving acclaim for his courageous decision and for the beautiful gift of triplets that this otherwise hopelessly sterile woman could never have had, he received rebuke from stodgy medical authorities who, at the instigation of the Australian government and partly as a result of their own jealousy, wanted to squash this young upstart before he would bring the wrath of the moralizing government down on their shoulders. If these medical authorities could offer him up as a sacrificial lamb, perhaps the government would leave them alone.

Surrogate uterus pregnancies are here to stay; they are morally and ethically completely proper, and they simply offer an opportunity for a relative or a loved one to voluntarily offer the greatest gift possible to a woman without a uterus. Although the procedure is simple now that you have read the rest of this book and understand how the new technology works, we should outline some of the methods for synchronizing the cycle.

What is critical about this technique is that both the cycle of the donor and that of the recipient be synchronized precisely. This work has been going on for decades in cows. Embryos from highly prized cattle would be placed in the uterus of very low milk-producing cows, who would then give birth to prize heifers. Since embryos could be obtained from the prize cows every month, it allowed a prize cow to deliver twelve heifers a year via the uterus of the surrogate cow rather than just one prize heifer a year. This vastly improved the efficiency of milk production in the world. Every time you go to the grocery store and realize how relatively inexpensive nature's most perfect food (milk) is, you realize that it is partly because of these reproductive advances that this product, milk, can be kept at such an otherwise unreasonably low price.

In humans, the synchronization is a little more difficult than in cows. There are two basic approaches: The first approach is what I'll call the "natural" approach, in which both women are placed upon either high-dose birth control pills or, my preference, which is Norlutate 10 mg a day, as described in Chapter 10. Norlutate started in the beginning of the follicular cycle puts them each on hold and can be discontinued at the same time for both of them.

The donor (who in this case is actually the patient) then undergoes normal ovulatory stimulation, usually starting several days after the recipient has stopped her Norlutate. This delay is because the donor undergoing stimulation is likely to be ready to release her eggs before the LH surge and progesterone rise of the recipient. The recipient under this "natural" approach receives no medication and is allowed to go through her normal cycle. The donor receives her HCG and two days later has her eggs retrieved. Her eggs are then cultured in vitro with her husband's sperm. The embryos are usually ready several days after the recipient's LH surge so that the timing comes out just right. If, however, the timing does not work out naturally, all that has to be done is to place the recipient on progesterone the day after the donor gets HCG. In this way the doctor can be sure that her endometrium has been properly prepared for progesterone so that when the time comes for the embryos to be transferred into the surrogate uterus, it will be ready.

It must be emphasized that there is a relatively narrow, three-day "window" for uterine receptivity to the embryo. This receptivity is maximum between the third day of progesterone secretion (or replacement) and the fifth day of progesterone replacement. In an idealized cycle in which ovulation occurs on day fourteen, this would mean that the ideal time of receptivity for the embryo to be transferred to the uterus would be days seventeen through nineteen. If the embryo is replaced during the time between the third day of progesterone to the fifth day of progesterone, there is the maximum chance of implantation occurring. If the embryo is transferred earlier or later than that, pregnancy is very unlikely. Thus synchronization is critical.

One key factor in synchronizing the cycles of donor and recipient is that the recipient must either start on progesterone (if she needs it), or be making her own progesterone one day after HCG is given to the donor. This would mean a GIFT procedure should be performed on the second day of progesterone administration to the recipient, and an IVF embryo transfer should occur on the fourth day of progesterone. So however you want to remember it, just realize progesterone must begin in the recipient, whether naturally or via injections, one day after the donor receives her HCG injection.

There is a more reliable, though perhaps not simpler, method of assuring synchronization. If you look at Table 9, you will see our protocol for synchronization, whether it involves a surrogate uterus or an egg donor to a postmenopausal woman. Whichever of these two situations is involved, this synchronization schedule works quite reliably. Both the donor and recipient are put on Norlutate to synchronize their cycles. The recipient goes on Lupron so as to completely suppress her pituitary.

Then on the first day the donor receives Pergonal, the recipient starts on Estrace (an oral, absorbable form of natural estrogen). The recipient's Estrace dose is gradually increased as in a natural cycle from 2 mg per day to 4 mg per day, finally to 6 mg per day. The length of the artificial follicular phase that she is on Estrace is not important; the only significant factor is when she goes on progesterone. Whenever the donor receives HCG, which is often (but not always) on the tenth day after Pergonal has begun, the recipient starts on progesterone one day after the donor has received her HCG. This always allows the synchronization to time out perfectly for either embryo replacement or GIFT, surrogate uterus cases, or egg donors.

One of the problems that could be anticipated with this is that after carrying a baby for nine months, a woman might decide to change her mind and keep it. This occurs very frequently with the kind of surrogate motherhood that the "Baby M" case exemplifies. Again I want to emphasize that we're not talking about that kind of surrogacy. When the baby does not genetically belong to the gestational mother who delivers it, in my experience the woman who carries the baby is usually very happy to give the child over to its genetic parents.

TABLE 9

PROTOCOL FOR SYNCHRONIZATION

	Egg Donor's Protocol	Recipient's Protocol
	Begin Norlutate on day 1 or by day 6 of menses.	Begin Norlutate on her day 1 or, if possible, near donor's day 1
		Take last day of Norlutate 10 mg (1 day before donor stops)
	Take last day of Norlutate 10 mg	Begin Lupron injections 0.2 ml daily (MUST BE ON LUPRON 6 DAYS BEFORE ESTRACE)
		Lupron
	Lupron 0.2 ml daily injections begin	Lupron
	Lupron	Lupron
1	Lupron and Pergonal (3 amps)	Lupron and Estrace 2 mg
2	Lupron and Pergonal (3 amps)	Lupron and Estrace 2 mg
3	Lupron and Pergonal (3 amps)	Lupron and Estrace 2 mg
4	Lupron, daily ultrasound and estrogen test, Pergonal	Lupron and Estrace 2 mg
5	Lupron, daily ultrasound and estrogen test, Pergonal	Lupron and Estrace 4 mg
6	Lupron, daily ultrasound and estrogen test, Pergonal	Lupron and Estrace 4 mg
7	Lupron, daily ultrasound and estrogen test, Peronal	Lupron and Estrace 4 mg
8	Lupron, daily ultrasound and estrogen test, Pergonal	Lupron and Estrace 6 mg
9	Lupron, daily ultrasound and estrogen test, Pergonal	Lupron and Estrace 6 mg
10	Lupron, daily ultrasound and estrogen test, HCG injection	Lupron and Estrace 6 mg
	Estrogen test	Estrace 6 mg and Progesterone 1 cc

Egg Donor's Protocol	Recipient's Protocol

Day of Pergonal

Follicle aspiration	GIFT procedure and Estrace 6 mg and Progesterone 1 cc
	Continue Estrace 6 mg daily and Progesterone 1 cc for 14 days
	On 14th day post GIFT, get a Beta HCG and, if positive for pregnancy, begin taking Estrace 8 mg daily and Progesterone 2 cc daily for 12 weeks.

EGG DONATION
(YOU CAN GET PREGNANT AFTER MENOPAUSE)

While I have written that it is easier to get pregnant when you're younger than when you're older and have urged women in their thirties not to delay high-tech treatment until it is too late, I'm going to turn around completely and point out that if you do delay too long and you have run out of eggs and entered menopause, it is really not too late to have a baby with the new technology. All that is needed is an egg donor, and you can still carry your own baby even in your late forties or fifties.

A typical case is a woman I recently saw who is presently in her forties, who first got pregnant seventeen years ago, and because she was not married had an abortion. She went on the birth control pill for ten years and finally fell in love and had a happy, stable marriage. She had been trying unsuccessfully to get pregnant in that marriage for six years. She had irregular, only occasional periods and was clearly about to go into menopause. We tried stimulating her with high doses of Pergonal but were unable to get any eggs. When I suggested the idea of getting a donated egg she jumped up with excitement and immediately had in mind two or three very good friends who were in their early thirties who she felt would be happy to donate. In fact, whenever we come across women like this, we find that usually they can find close friends or younger sisters who are more than happy to donate an egg.

You must understand that if you receive a donor egg, the genes of the baby will be a combination of your husband's genes and those of the woman who donates the egg. It will not be your genes even though you will carry the baby for nine months and deliver it. The question has to come up, whose baby is it? What are the psychological consequences of your carrying a baby that is genetically not your own? This has been going on since 1983, when the first case was reported in Australia, and I can say unequivocally that carrying that baby for nine months results in a solid, loving bond between the mother and the child, regardless of the genetic origin of the donated egg. This is really not greatly different from the artificial donor insemination discussed in Chapter 9. I would like to refer you back to that chapter where I talk about the issues of emotional bonding with the child, and where the child's personality, intelligence, value system, and even athletic ability come from—genes or environment? The fact that the child has been carried for nine months in the uterus results in a solid bonding between mother and baby.

The medical world was shocked to hear about the first pregnancy using an embryo from a donor egg in such a menopausal woman at Monash University in Melbourne, Australia, in 1983. Dr. Peter Lutjen and Dr. Alan Trounson and their colleagues were the innovators of this idea (which I had predicted in my first book three and one half years earlier). These brilliant reproductive scientists from Australia established what then seemed to be the impossible system of hormonal replacement for the menopausal woman that allowed her uterus to behave just like that of a woman in her twenties, allowing implantation of an embryo despite the fact that she had no ovaries to make the hormones which are normally necessary to sustain a pregnancy in the first three months.

This is a more complicated proposition than the surrogate

uterus, because the menopausal woman could not possibly carry the baby without three months of hormonal replacement. Dr. Zev Rosenwaks and Dr. Ricardo Asch then reported in 1986 and 1987 the first large series of pregnancies in menopausal women using donated eggs. Dr. Rosenwaks's patients all got pregnant with in vitro fertilization (IVF) and the transfer of embryos obtained from eggs of donors and sperm of the husband. Dr. Asch reported his pregnancies by the GIFT technique, transferring the egg of the donor along with the sperm of the husband into the menopausal woman's fallopian tubes.

Both Dr. Asch and Dr. Rosenwaks reported shockingly high pregnancy rates per cycle, much greater than anybody would normally anticipate. In fact, Dr. Ian Craft of London, England, later reported that much older women (late forties and early fifties) had no difficulty getting pregnant (greater than a 50 percent pregnancy rate per cycle) so long as the donor eggs came from young women. In fact, despite the age of the recipient, the real problem he was dealing with was too high an incidence of multiple pregnancies in women of such age that one would never dream such a risk could exist.

All of these pioneers in this field, Drs. Lutjen and Trouson, Dr. Rosenwaks, Dr. Asch, and Dr. Craft, concluded that the age of the uterus is not what is significant in the high pregnancy rate of these patients, but rather the fact that: 1) the eggs came from healthy younger women, and 2) the recipient's only infertility problem was that she had run out of eggs. With these two operative factors, pregnancy rate using GIFT and donor eggs in menopausal women is close to 60 percent, and using IVF is close to 30 percent. Those are simply astounding pregnancy rates, much higher than would be seen in a normal series of infertile couples.

There are basically three different ways of organizing an egg donor program: Dr. Asch's original study was with "anonymous" egg donors. That means that women undergoing GIFT or IVF who had extra eggs that could not be used agreed to give them to menopausal women who were on a waiting list and placed on the appropriate estrogen and progesterone regimen to synchronize their cycles artificially with the women who had the extra eggs to give. This source of eggs is beginning to dry up now that embryo freezing is more available.

The next approach is similar to that of running a sperm bank. The donor is paid just like a man giving sperm. A pool of available donors are stimulated with hormones, synchronizing their cycle and egg retrieval with the artificial cycle that the recipient has been placed on. There are some possible ethical problems associated with this approach in that women are paid to undergo drug therapy and invasive follicle aspiration to donate eggs to someone they don't know and don't care about. In other words, they are taking a medical risk (however slight) simply for pay. Regardless of some objections that might be raised ethically, this egg bank is doing rather well.

The third approach, which is becoming the most popular one, was pioneered by Dr. Mark Sauer from the University of Southern California Medical Center in Los Angeles. Dr. Sauer asks his patients to search among their younger friends or relatives for someone who is willing to donate an egg, to make all the legal arrangements privately with them, and then to go through a screening and counseling evaluation with him and his staff. Thus he has a "nonanonymous" program, and no one is being paid, but rather the gift is being made as an act of love. Anonymous, paid-for-hire egg donors bother most doctors ethically, and anonymous donors with extra eggs to give away simply are hardly available anymore. So out of necessity, Dr. Sauer's approach is becoming the approach that most are presently following.

Finally we need to talk about the technical aspect of: 1) synchronizing the cycles of the donor and the recipient, and 2) giving the proper hormone replacement (to these women who are not making any hormones on their own) so that their uterus is prepared for implantation of the embryo and to maintain the pregnancy until such time as the placenta starts making its own hormones by eight to twelve weeks of pregnancy. Once again, you should look at Table 9 because the protocol is virtually no different for surrogate uterus cases than it is for egg donation cases.

The only difference is that in the surrogate uterus case, the recipient is not the patient but rather the helper, and in the egg donation case, the recipient is the patient and the donor is the helper. The only other difference in the protocol is that if the recipient is truly menopausal, she does not need to be placed on Norlutate, and she does not need to be placed on Lupron, because she is simply not making hormones at all. She would begin Estrace, however, on the same day that you see on the cycle chart in this chapter. It is all timed out with the same goal in mind, that the recipient begin progesterone after proper estrogen priming, one day after the donor receives her HCG injection. That assures that either GIFT or IVF will be performed at that time in the progesterone part of the cycle where the window of receptivity for egg implantation is open. Between day three and day five of progesterone replacement is when the embryo must be placed in the uterus. By the same token, if the egg donation is being performed via a GIFT procedure, the egg transfer must take place between day one and day three of the progesterone replacement.

Even after it is clear that you are pregnant you will have to stay on estrogen and progesterone supplements for up to twelve weeks longer until the normal time in pregnancy when the placenta takes over the function of the ovary and produces all of its own self-sustaining estrogen and progesterone. This may require considerably less than twelve weeks, and the latest data from Dr. Rosenwaks indicates that by six weeks (contrary to our previous thinking) the placenta may be making enough estrogen and progesterone to sustain the pregnancy. The way to determine that is to get blood tests every week for estrogen and progesterone levels, and when the progesterone level begins to rise dramatically over what we know you're getting from replacement, then we know the placenta has taken over and you no longer need to take hormone replacements.

Before 1983, with Lutjen and Trounson's first successful case, this concept that a menopausal woman could carry a baby with the requisite hormone replacement to keep that pregnancy going until the placenta took over was quite revolutionary. Now it is taken for granted.

It seems like nothing can shock us anymore, that is until I came across a case which Dr. Asch and I discussed in great detail, only for its theoretical interest. I do many operations for young boys and adults with very high, undescended testicles that require opening up the abdomen, dividing the blood vessels supplying these abdominal testicles, and reconnecting them microsurgically to the blood vessels closer to the scrotum. This is a so-called "testicle autotransplant" for men born with testicles inside the abdomen (where the ovaries are normally found in a woman). When I operated on one such case several years ago, I was astounded to find an extraordinarily rare congenital abnormality. This man had a completely normal uterus, fallopian tubes, and upper vagina located within his abdomen. Nonetheless, he also had normal testicles, vas deferens, prostate gland, and penis typical of a normal genetic man. Of course, we brought the testicles down into the scrotum with this microsurgical operation so that they would be able to function and make sperm normally. But think of the possibilities.

His wife had no uterus. Therefore, with our technology we could have placed him on female hormones, taken his sperm and his wife's eggs, placed them into his fallopian tubes via a GIFT procedure, and gotten him pregnant. Obviously, this would be too much of an emotional burden for him or any other man to carry, so we never considered it seriously.

The only reason I bring up this fascinating case is to point out that as long as there is a uterus, a woman can become pregnant despite no ovary whatsoever; or as long as there is an ovary, even if she has no uterus, her eggs can be used to get a friend or relative pregnant with her baby. There are thus very few couples, no matter how severe their problem (if they have open minds), who can't have a baby through use of the new technology.

Index

Abdomen, examination of, 107–8
Acosta, Anibal, 142
Acrosome, 75–77, 78, 232
Acrosome reaction, 232, 233, 245
Adhesions, 210–11
Adoption laws, 269
African bushmen, 41–42
Age, likelihood of pregnancy with, 184–86
AID (Artificial insemination by donor), 183, 213–25
  AIDS testing, 217, 228, 229
  donor selection, 216–20
  legislation concerning, 216
  paternity issue, 213–16
  sperm banks, 218–20, 225–29
  technique of, 216–218, 222–24
AIDS, 42, 162, 165
  AID and, 217, 228, 229
Air-buffered culture media, 298–300
Amelar, Richard, 18–19
American Association for the Advancement of Science, 21
American College of Surgeons, 341
American Fertility Society, 368
American Urological Association, 132
Ampulla, 50, 70, 322
Anderson, Jaco, 321
Animal husbandry, 226

Animals
  infertility, 27–30
  mating habits, 37–38, 153
  seasonal timing of sex, 30–31
  sperm production, 32–34
  transgenic, 323–24
Anorexia nervosa, 90, 100
Anovulation, 93
Antibodies, sperm, 161–69, 355–56
Artificial insemination, 222–24
  in animal husbandry, 226
  See also AID
Artificial insemination by donor. *See* AID
Asch, Ricardo, 18–19, 23, 270, 285, 363, 377, 379
Autoimmunity, 162–69
Autotransplant, testicle, 379–80
Azospermia, 121, 220–21, 282, 359, 362

"Baby M," 16, 369–70, 373
Baker, Gordon, 133, 149, 150, 168, 183
Banks
  egg, 378
  sperm, 218–20, 225–29
Basal body temperature, 91–94, 191–94
BBT. *See* Basal body temperature

TABLE 5

EFFECT OF INCREASING THE NUMBER OF EMBRYOS REPLACED
(STEPTOE AND EDWARDS, 1987)

Less Than 40 Years Old			40 Years Old or Over	
Embryos Replaced	Pregnancy Rate		Embryos Replaced	Pregnancy Rate
(number)	(percent)		(percent)	(percent)
1	13.7		1	9.4
2	20.6		2	13.2
3	28.0		3	18.6

women whose husbands have poor sperm, the risk for multiple pregnancy hardly exists at all.

This decreased fertility of older women, and the decreased risk of multiple pregnancy in older women, does not apply when young donor eggs are used. Dr. Ian Craft from London has showed that in sixty-one menopausal patients over forty, who were no longer making eggs, the transfer of young donor eggs resulted in an excellent 46 percent pregnancy rate per cycle despite the older age of the recipient. So forget about the age of the patient in thinking about pregnancy rates and risks of multiple pregnancy; only be concerned about the age of the egg and the quality of the husband's sperm.

Table 6 demonstrates the combined Australian experience in one year with multiple pregnancy in relationship to the number of embryos that were transferred. They had a low incidence of triplets despite the replacement of four and five, and in one case six embryos. Remember, replacing five embryos is roughly equivalent to replacing eight eggs because you have to assume that only five out of those eight eggs are likely to fertilize in a GIFT procedure. Despite the replacement in some cases of large numbers of embryos the incidence of triplets was extremely low and quadruplets or greater was extremely rare. This lack of increase in multiple births with the transfer of greater number of embryos may simply be related to the fact that physicians

TABLE 6

RISK OF MULTIPLE PREGNANCY RELATED TO NUMBER OF EMBRYOS TRANSFERRED TO THE UTERUS (AUSTRALIAN NATIONAL RESULTS)

Embryos Transferred	Singleton	Twins	Triplets
	(no./percent)	(no./percent)	(no./percent)
1	104	1	—
2	204	27 (12)	—
3	208	84 (27)	17 (6)
4	151	52 (24)	14 (6)
5	20	3 (13)	—
6	1	1	—
Totals	700 (78)	169 (19)	32 (4)

1. Risk of multiple pregnancy increases with transfer of greater number of embryos up to three.
2. But after three, up to six, no significant increase.
3. Probably because greater numbers are only transferred in worst cases.

only transfer these large numbers of embryos in the most difficult infertility cases where multiple pregnancy isn't likely and where you want to increase as much as possible the chance of pregnancy occurring at all.

Finally, the most hopeful aspect of all of this data that I am presenting for you (see Tables 7 and 8) answers the question that has been haunting all of us doing in vitro fertilization: Will coming back for subsequent cycles of GIFT or IVF give the same "relatively" good chance of pregnancy per cycle? Or are those couples who don't get pregnant in the early cycles just wasting their time coming back for subsequent cycles? In other words, does persistence pay off? Recent data have made it quite clear that for at least up to seven cycles (and possibly longer) your chance of pregnancy in each subsequent cycle is no lower than if you were just beginning IVF or GIFT for the first time. In fact, if you persist up to seven cycles of IVF, Dr. Jairo Garcia, head of IVF at Greater Baltimore Hospital, reports a cumulative